Cure Models

Chapman & Hall/CRC Biostatistics Series

Series Editors
Shein-Chung Chow, Duke University School of Medicine, USA
Byron Jones, Novartis Pharma AG, Switzerland
Jen-pei Liu, National Taiwan University, Taiwan
Karl E. Peace, Georgia Southern University, USA
Bruce W. Turnbull, Cornell University, USA

Recently Published Titles

Bayesian Applications in Pharmaceutical Development
Mani Lakshminarayanan, Fanni Natanegara

Innovative Statistics in Regulatory Science
Shein-Chung Chow

Geospatial Health Data: Modeling and Visualization with R-INLA and Shiny
Paula Moraga

Artificial Intelligence for Drug Development, Precision Medicine, and Healthcare
Mark Chang

Bayesian Methods in Pharmaceutical Research
Emmanuel Lesaffre, Gianluca Baio, Bruno Boulanger

Biomarker Analysis in Clinical Trials with R
Nusrat Rabbee

Interface between Regulation and Statistics in Drug Development
Demissie Alemayehu, Birol Emir, Michael Gaffney

Innovative Methods for Rare Disease Drug Development
Shein-Chung Chow

Medical Risk Prediction Models: With Ties to Machine Learning
Thomas A Gerds, Michael W. Kattan

Real-World Evidence in Drug Development and Evaluation
Harry Yang, Binbing Yu

Cure Models: Methods, Applications, and Implementation
Yingwei Peng, Binbing Yu

For more information about this series, please visit: https://www.routledge.com/Chapman--Hall-CRC-Biostatistics-Series/book-series/CHBIOSTATIS

Cure Models

Methods, Applications, and Implementation

Yingwei Peng, Binbing Yu

CRC Press
Taylor & Francis Group
Boca Raton London New York

CRC Press is an imprint of the
Taylor & Francis Group, an **informa** business
A CHAPMAN & HALL BOOK

First edition published 2021
by CRC Press
6000 Broken Sound Parkway NW, Suite 300, Boca Raton, FL 33487-2742

and by CRC Press
2 Park Square, Milton Park, Abingdon, Oxon, OX14 4RN

CRC Press is an imprint of Taylor & Francis Group, LLC

Library of Congress Cataloging-in-Publication Data
Insert LoC Data here when available

ISBN: 9780367145576 (hbk)
ISBN: 9780429-032301 (ebk)

Typeset in CMR10
by KnowledgeWorks Global Ltd.

To our parents and our families.

Contents

Preface

Cure models refer to a class of survival models that deal with censored survival data or time-to-event data when some subjects in the study sample will not experience the event of interest, however long the follow-up is. In some cancer clinical trials where the event of interest is often the relapse or recurrence of cancer tumor after the treatment, it is possible that some patients will never relapse or their cancer tumor will never recur due to the effectiveness of treatment or other factors, and they are often deemed as cured. Analyzing the survival data from such trials using standard survival models that do not take the fraction of cured patients into account will lead to biased estimates and waste the information in the data, and cure models should be considered.

Cured subjects arise not only in cancer clinical trials but also in other disciplines. Examples are employees who never lose their jobs and marriages that never break in sociology studies, offenders who will not commit crimes again in criminal justice, companies and subjects who are never in default on loans in economics, and parts in a complex system that never fail, and so on. They are all can be viewed as cured subjects and cure models should be considered when analyzing time-to-event data arisen in the situations.

Cure models have sparked tremendous interest in academia, government, industries. Both the European Union (Francisci et al., 2009) and United States (Hudson and Collins, 2017) emphasize the importance of translating cancer discovery into cancer cure. Pharmaceutical industries are spending billions of dollars on immune-therapy of cancer to improve the survival and cure of cancer patients. A Google Scholar search shows wide applicability of cure models and active research activities around the world in this field. This field attracts many young statistical researchers and practitioners in many disciplines to seek applications of cure models in the disciplines. Thus, a book that focuses on cure models will be in high demand. The first book on cure models — *Survival Analysis with Long-Term Survivors* (Maller and Zhou) — was published in 1996, a time when the widely-used R program did not even exist and many interesting advances in cure models in the last two decades were not available yet. There are later books in survival models with chapters/sections devoted to some specific cure models. Some recent review articles provide reviews on more up-to-date cure models and are valuable for an overview of cure models. But they lack enough details for readers at different levels.

The authors of this book conducted extensive research and training in the field of cure models for years. The first author (Peng) offered several short courses in recent years on cure models, either by himself or with Jeremy

Taylor (University of Michigan), in various international venues including Joint Statistical Meetings, Boston, MA, USA, ENAR Spring Meeting, Baltimore, MD, USA, and the Institute of Statistics, Biostatistics and Actuarial Sciences (ISBA), Université catholique de Louvain, Belgium. In addition to seminars and presentations in international conferences, the second author (Yu) has extensive experience in the applications of cure models in public health, clinical trials and health economics and made notable contributions to the development and enhancement of cure modeling for the presentation and analysis of cancer survival data for the USA National Cancer Institute. Such experiences motivate us to write a new book on cure models that provides a comprehensive coverage of cure models with a focus on the developments in the last two decades and with enough and self-contained details for readers to better understand cure models in one book.

This book is appropriate for researchers and senior undergraduates or graduate students who have some basic knowledge of statistical modeling and survival models. The book is application oriented. We choose to skip details of relevant large sample properties and only provide brief technical results that are necessary to understand the methodology presented in the book. Instead, we try to provide some details on software packages that were developed for cure models and hope the details will enhance the applicability of cure models discussed in this book. The book may be used as a course spanning one or two semesters. We hope that this book will provide invaluable resources for statistical researchers in academia, policymakers in the public sector, and clinicians and biostatisticians in the biopharmaceutical industry.

We would like to thank the anonymous reviewers and many individuals, including Jeremy Taylor, Ingrid Van Keilegom, and Yi Li, for their valuable comments, and Eric Feuer and Angela Mariotto for their input and discussions during the preparation of this book. Our joint work with our collaborators and students in the past two decades had a great influence on this book, and we are grateful for many productive discussions with them. We are especially thankful to John Kimmel for his support, advice, and patience in the book publishing process.

Yingwei Peng
Binbing Yu

Glossary

i.i.d.: independently and identically distributed

AFT: accelerated failure time

AH: accelerated hazards

AIC: Akaike information criterion

ALL: acute lymphoblastic leukemia

AML: acute myelogenous leukemia

AO: Aranda-Ordaz

AR-1: first-order autoregressive

AUC: area under the curve

BCQ: Breast Cancer Questionnaire

BIC: Bayesian information criterion

BMT: bone marrow transplants

CAR: conditionally autoregressive

CEF: cyclophosphamide, epirubicin, and fluorouracil

CMF: cyclophosphamide, methotrexate, and fluorouracil

CML: chronic myelogenous leukemia

DIC: Deviance Information Criterion

ECOG: Eastern Cooperative Oncology Group

EM: Expectation-Maximization

GCV: generalized cross validation

GLMM: generalized linear mixed effect model

GMW: generalized modified Weibull

HLA: human leukocyte antigen

HN: half-normal

IO: Immuno-oncology

IPCW: inverse probability of censoring weights

IUT: intersection-union test

LR: log-rank test

LRT: likelihood ratio test

MCMC: Markov chain Monte Carlo

MVN: multivariate normal

MZ: test of Maller and Zhou (1995)

NB: negative binomial

NTM: nonlinear transformation model

OS: Overall survival

PFS: Progression-free survival

PH: proportional hazards

PHC: proportional hazards cure

PO: proportional odds

POC: proportional odds cure

PPHC: piecewise PHC

PSA: prostate-specific antigen

QEM: quasi-EM

RFS: recurrence-free survival

RMST: restricted mean survival time

RNPMLE: restricted nonparametric maximum likelihood estimation

ROC: receiver operating characteristic

SVM: support vector machine

SEER: Surveillance, Epidemiology, Endpoint Results

TS: two-stage

WLR: weighted log-rank test

YP: adaptive test of Yang and Prentice (2009)

1

Introduction

1.1 A Brief Review of Cure Models

1.1.1 Time-to-Event Data and Cured Subjects

In many scientific studies, researchers are interested in time to the occurrence of a specific event of interest. When analyzing time-to-event data, it often happens that a certain proportion of subjects may never experience the event of interest and are considered to be cured. Cured subjects are immune or non-susceptible to the event. Time-to-event data with cured subjects are abundant in population health and medical studies. In some diseases, there is strong biological evidence that, when considering endpoints other than a natural death, the event would never occur for some fraction of the subjects. The assumption that some individuals will never experience the event may also be based solely on empirical considerations, such as the presence of a large number of long-term survivors. Recent progress in the diagnosis and treatment of cancer has led to substantial improvement in cancer survival. If patients are diagnosed early and receive effective treatment, e.g., the targeted therapy or immunotherapy, a subpopulation of the cancer patients eventually become cured from the disease, which leads to some long-term survivors if the follow-up time is long enough. The presence of cured subjects is often suggested by a Kaplan-Meier estimate of the marginal survival function, which shows a long and stable plateau with heavy censoring at the right extreme.

In sociology studies, the rates of life-long marriage and permanent employment are important concepts of social stability. An employee who has been with the same company for a sufficiently long time may be considered as unlikely to join other companies (Yamaguchi, 1992) and can be considered as cured or immune to the event of joining other companies. In criminal justice, the recidivism rate is an important feature to determining the effect of rehabilitation to stop offenders from committing crimes again and those subjects who will not commit crimes again after a long time may be considered as cured (Schmidt and Witte, 1989). The concept of cured subjects has applications in economics. For example, when considering the probability of default and the timing of default on loans, a company or subject who is not in default for a long time may be considered as cured (Tong et al., 2012). In reliability studies, one complex system is often considered as being composed of some subsystems in series. Usually, the failure of any subsystem would lead to the failure of the entire system. However, some subsystems' lifetimes are long enough and even never fail during the life cycle of the entire system and they can be considered as cured. In political studies, the time to intervention over the course of a conflict and the conflicts that are never intervened for a long time may be considered as cured (Findley and Teo, 2006).

1.1.2 Survival Models and Cure Models

Standard statistical methods for time-to-event analysis, often called survival models, typically assume that every subject in the study population is susceptible to the event of interest and will eventually experience the event if the follow-up is sufficiently long. They do not account for cured subjects and can lead to biased estimates of the survival of susceptible subjects.

Survival models that take into account the possibility of cure are commonly referred to as cure models or cure rate models. A cure model allows a direct modeling of the cure proportion and the effect of covariates on the cure proportion. Additionally, the cure model also provides estimation and inference of the distribution of the survival time for uncured subjects or subjects who are not cured. Most of the existing cure models are modified survival models that include the probability of being cured. Based on how the cure proportion is introduced, the cure models can be roughly divided into two types: mixture cure models and non-mixture cure models.

Although the cure models have a shorter history compared to the standard survival models, they have been an area of active research in statistics since the early 1950s. The most widely used cure rate model is the mixture cure model which is also known as the standard cure rate model. This model was first introduced by Boag (1949). He introduced the traditional definition of a cured fraction for patients who have a specific illness, by a five-years survival rate. Although the definition of the cured fraction has changed and improved over the years, many authors developed and improved the original mixture model further. Berkson and Gage (1952) divided the population into two groups: susceptible individuals to the event of interest and insusceptible individuals. They suggested that a group of treated patients are considered to be cured if they have approximately the same survival distribution as the general population who have never had the disease of interest. Farewell (1982) used a mixture model as a combination of logistic model and Weibull distribution to model the toxicant and stress level for laboratory animals. Kuk and Chen (1992) proposed a semiparametric mixture cure model consisting of the logistic model for the probability of occurrence of the event of interest, and the proportional hazard model for the time to event of interest for uncured subjects. Maller and Zhou (1996) have collected a comprehensive account of mixture cure rate models with various survival functions. Goldman (1984), Taylor (1995), and Peng and Dear (2000), among others, have also investigated parametric, semiparametric, and nonparametric mixture cure rate models. Yu and Peng (2008) and Peng et al. (2007a) extended the mixture cure model to multivariate survival data. Both marginal survival models (Chen and Lu, 2012; Niu and Peng, 2014; Niu et al., 2018a) and random-effects frailty models (Peng and Taylor, 2011; Peng and Zhang, 2008a) have been proposed. More recently, Wu and Yin (2013) suggested quantile regression methods and martingale estimating equations for a better assessment of covariate effects on quantiles of a time-to-event of interest.

The non-mixture cure model is another type of cure models for modeling time-to-event data with a cure fraction. Non-mixture cure models were first introduced by Yakovlev et al. (1994a) and then discussed by Yakovlev et al. (1994b), Ibrahim et al. (2001), Chen et al. (1999), and Wang et al. (2012a). These models were motivated by an underlying biological mechanism for cancer cells, which assumes that the number of cancer cells after cancer treatment follows a Poisson distribution. Most of the current investigations on the non-mixture cure models are in the Bayesian context due to its special form. The non-mixture cure models can be expressed into the mixture cure models. However, the model interpretation, particularly the covariate effects on the distribution of the survival time of uncured subjects can have important differences between the two types of cure models.

Because of abundant time-to-event data with a cure fraction in many different disciplines, cure models have potentially wide applications in the disciplines. The novel applications of the cure models have help investigators understand the pattern and behavior of survival times after treatment or intervention. Particularly, in recent years there has been significant progress in the research and development of immune-oncology (I-O) therapy. Because the mechanisms of actions of immunotherapy are profoundly different from traditional chemotherapy and radiation therapy, the patient survival in the clinical trials of immunotherapy have demonstrated delayed clinical effects as well as long-term survival, and cure models can play an important role in revealing the complicated short-term and long-term effects of the therapy to cancer patients.

However, although there have been tremendous efforts and development in modeling of survival data with a cure fraction, there are very few books that provide a comprehensive coverage of the statistical concepts, methods, and applications of cure models. The applications of cure models, particularly those developed in recent years, in the disciplines are still limited, such as in the clinical literature (Othus et al., 2012; Yilmaz et al., 2013). The only published book that is devoted to cure models is Maller and Zhou (1996). However, it focused on large sample properties of estimation and tests for nonparametric and exponential-family based mixture cure models only and is not application-oriented. Moreover, the book was published more than 20 years ago and there has been no book since then that covers the rapid growth in research and applications of cure models in the last two decades. Ibrahim et al. (2001) devotes a chapter on specific Bayesian cure models. More recently there are a few review papers that cover more recent advances in cure models, such as Peng and Taylor (2014) and Amico and Van Keilegom (2018). Due to space limitations, the review papers do not include many details. Thus, a book that covers the rapid growth in research and applications of cure models in the last two decades and provides a comprehensive introduction of various cure models, their estimation methods and their applications using software programs that have been developed will provide a valuable resource for practitioners to apply cure models in various disciplines and for statistical researchers and students to further advance the investigation of analysis time-to-event data with a cure fraction.

1.2 Aim and Scope of the Book

The goal of this book is to give a comprehensive introduction to cure models. It includes many recent advances in cure model research. It covers both statistical methodology and applications of cure models in many disciplines with software packages. Particularly, this book provides extensive discussions about the applications of cure models in cancer research and oncology clinical trials. We hope this book may serve as a useful desk reference for scientists and researchers engaged in biological research and related areas, and biostatisticians who provide statistical support for clinical trials and public health decision-making. More importantly, we would like to provide graduate students with an advanced textbook with both statistical methods and real applications.

The scope of this book includes basics of the cure models as well as many recent developments related to the methodological issues and software implementations of cure models for right-censored time-to-event data subject to non-informative censoring. Due to the limited time, we are unable to include cure models that are developed for interval-censored data and truncated data. The software implementations are only limited to those developed in R (R Core Team, 2013), SAS™ (SAS Institute, Cary NC), WinBUGS (Lunn et al., 2000), and OpenBUGS (Lunn et al., 2009). Programs developed in other software environments, such as STATA, are not included.

The rest of the book is organized as follows. Chapter 2 introduces the basics of parametric mixture and non-mixture cure models and the EM-based estimation methods that have been pivotal in the cure model methodology. Model assessment methods and some existing R packages and SAS macros for parametric cure models are also presented with real-world data sets as examples. Chapter 3 focuses on the basics of the semiparametric and nonparametric mixture and non-mixture cure models, the estimation methods, and implementations in existing R packages and SAS macros illustrated with real-world data sets. These two chapters lay the foundation of cure models and are essential for understanding statistical estimation and inference of cure models. Chapters 4-6 cover more advanced topics in cure modeling. Chapter 4 covers various modeling approaches to multivariate, recurrent-event, and competing-risks survival data. Both marginal and random-effects (frailty) cure models are described. Chapter 5 describes joint models of longitudinal and survival data with a cure fraction and illustrates the advantage of joint models using a real case study. The joint models provide efficient and unbiased estimates of the trajectories of longitudinal data. Chapter 6 focuses on the statistical testing for the existence and difference of cure rates and also the identifiability and sufficient follow-up issues in cure model estimation. Bayesian methods have been widely used for survival modeling including cure models. Chapter 7 presents some new developments and models that emerged recently after the review of Bayesian cure models in Ibrahim et al. (2001). General implementations of Bayesian analysis using BUGS program are also presented. The last two chapters cover practical applications of cure models in public health research and clinical trials. Particularly, Chapter 8 presents the application of cure models in the population-based cancer survival analysis. Chapter 9 discusses statistical issues in the design and analysis of cancer clinical trials with a possible cure fraction. Comparisons regarding the relative merits and disadvantages of the adaptive design methods in clinical research and development are discussed whenever deemed appropriate. R programs that implement a suite of tools for applied researchers in clinical trials are provided.

In each chapter, whenever possible, real examples from clinical trials or public health research are used to demonstrate the use of cure models. If applicable, topics for future research are provided too.

2

The Parametric Cure Model

2.1 Introduction

This chapter focuses on cure models that are fully parametrically specified. The parameters in such models can be readily estimated using the maximum likelihood method, and thus the properties of the estimates can be established using the maximum likelihood theory. Parametric cure models also allow extrapolation in prediction, which can be attractive in practice. The chapter is organized as follows. Section 2.2 introduces parametric mixture cure models, followed by some common estimation methods for the models in Section 2.3. Section 2.4 presents some non-mixture cure models as well as parametric transformation cure models that unify mixture cure models and other types of cure models. Model assessment issues such as choosing appropriate parametric distributions, selection between mixture versus non-mixture cure models, and goodness of fit of cure models are discussed in Section 2.5. Finally, some software packages that can fit parametric cure models and an example data set for cure models are presented in Section 2.6. This chapter focuses on independent and right-censored data only. The censoring is assumed to be independent and non-informative throughout this book unless otherwise specified.

2.2 Parametric Mixture Cure Models

As discussed in Chapter 1, we consider a sample drawn from a population that consists of two groups of subjects: cured subjects who respond well to their treatments and never experience the event of interest regardless of how long the follow-up is, and uncured subjects who will experience the event given a sufficient follow-up. It is natural to consider a mixture model for such a population. Let T be the time to the event of interest and Y be the cure indicator with $Y = 1$ if the subject is not cured and $Y = 0$ otherwise. We assume $P(T < \tau | Y = 1) = 1$, where τ is an upper bound of survival time of uncured subjects. Usually, τ is set to ∞ for theoretical convenience, and in this case, $Y = 0$ is not observable and a cured subject with $Y = 0$ is always censored. Thus for a subject with a right-censored time, the value of Y is not observable and can be 1 or 0. However, it is possible to set τ to a finite value in practice, and in this case, $Y = 0$ is observable. For example, in a pregnancy study on time to abortion, $\tau = 20$ weeks is used because a pregnant woman is no longer considered susceptible to the event of abortion if the gestation age is 20 weeks or more.

Define $S_u(t)$ and $S_c(t)$ as the survival functions of the uncured and cured subpopulations respectively, i.e., $S_u(t) = P(T > t|Y = 1)$ and $S_c(t) = P(T > t|Y = 0)$ for any $t < \tau$. Following the definition of cured subjects, $S_c(t) = P(T > t|Y = 0) \equiv 1$ for any $t < \tau$, i.e., $S_c(t)$ is a degenerate survival function. The mixture cure model is defined by the following unconditional survival function of T for any $t < \tau$:

$$P(T > t) = S(t) = \pi S_u(t) + (1 - \pi)S_c(t) = \pi S_u(t) + 1 - \pi, \quad (2.1)$$

where $\pi = P(Y = 1)$ is the probability of being uncured. It is clear that the mixture cure model consists of two parts: one part is π, which is often referred to as the incidence part and describes the probability of being cured or uncured subjects, and the other part is $S_u(t)$, which is often referred to as the latency part and describes the distribution of the survival time of uncured subjects. This two-part structure facilitates the separate consideration of the effects of covariates on the cure probability and on the distribution of the survival time of uncured subjects, which renders appealing interpretation of covariate effects and easy generalization a mixture cure model to more complex situations. Because of the properties, the mixture cure model has been in use for near 70 years since it was first considered in the work of Boag (1949), and it is still attracting a great deal of attention.

The mixture cure model (2.1) is parametrically specified if both the latency submodel and incidence submodel are parametrically specified. In the following sections, we describe some parametric mixture cure models.

2.2.1 Parametric Incidence Submodel

Since Y is a binary variable, the only distribution for a binary variable is the Bernoulli distribution with the parameter π. Thus the specification of the incidence submodel of the mixture cure model is mainly focused on the specification of the functional form of the effect of $\boldsymbol{z}$, a vector of covariates (the first value of this vector is 1), and how it is linked to π. The most common parametric specification is the linear form of the effect $\boldsymbol{z}'\boldsymbol{\gamma}$ linked to π via a logit link:

$$\text{logit}[\pi(\boldsymbol{z})] = \boldsymbol{z}'\boldsymbol{\gamma}, \quad (2.2)$$

where $\text{logit}(\pi) = \log(\pi/(1 - \pi))$ and $\boldsymbol{\gamma}$ is a vector of the coefficients of the covariates in $\boldsymbol{z}$. For a particular covariate in $\boldsymbol{z}$, the corresponding coefficient in $e^{\boldsymbol{\gamma}}$ can be interpreted as the odds ratio of being uncured when the covariate is increased by 1 while other covariates are fixed.

Alternative link functions to link π and the linear predictor $\boldsymbol{z}'\boldsymbol{\gamma}$ can be considered. For example, one may consider the complementary log-log link function

$$\log[-\log(\pi(\boldsymbol{z}))] = -\boldsymbol{z}'\boldsymbol{\gamma}. \tag{2.3}$$

For a particular covariate in $\boldsymbol{z}$, the corresponding coefficient in $e^{\boldsymbol{\gamma}}$ can be interpreted as the relative log risk (not relative risk) of being uncured when the covariate is increased by 1 while other covariates are fixed. The probit link function $\Phi^{-1}[\pi(\boldsymbol{z})] = \boldsymbol{z}'\boldsymbol{\gamma}$, where $\Phi(\cdot)$ is the cumulative distribution function of the standard normal distribution, is another link function that can be considered. However, due to unavailability of the closed form in $\Phi(\cdot)$, there is no straightforward interpretation of $\boldsymbol{\gamma}$ under this link function.

The logit and probit links are symmetric in the sense that modeling $\pi(\boldsymbol{z})$ and $1 - \pi(\boldsymbol{z})$ are equivalent and the coefficients in $\boldsymbol{\gamma}$ only differ by a sign. The complementary log-log link, on the other hand, is asymmetric. That is, it approaches 0 slowly and 1 fast, and its models for $\pi(\boldsymbol{z})$ and $1 - \pi(\boldsymbol{z})$ are not equivalent. The differences between the links functions can be seen in Figure 2.1, where $\boldsymbol{z} = (1, z)'$ and a) logit link with $\pi(\boldsymbol{z}) = e^z/(1 + e^z)$; b) complementary log-log link with $\pi(\boldsymbol{z}) = \exp(-e^{-0.3665-z})$; c) probit link with $\pi(\boldsymbol{z}) = \Phi(0.6z)$ is plotted against z. All the functions leads to $\pi(\boldsymbol{z}) = 0.5$ when $z = 0$ and the parameters in the complementary log-log and probit links are chosen to produce curves close to the curve from the logit link. The figure shows the symmetry in the logit and probit links and minor differences between the two curves with extreme values of z. The complementary log-log link, on the other hand, is clearly not symmetric and displays noticeable differences when $z < 0$ while the curve fits the logit curve for $z > 0$.

It can be challenging to choose an appropriate link for a given data set in practice. When the sample size is large, one may consider to use

$$\pi(\boldsymbol{z}) = \left(1 + \lambda e^{-\boldsymbol{\gamma}'\boldsymbol{z}}\right)^{-1/\lambda}, \quad 0 \leq \lambda \leq 1 \tag{2.4}$$

based on the Box-Cox transformation (Box and Cox, 1964). It is easy to see that $\pi(\boldsymbol{z}) = e^{\boldsymbol{\gamma}'\boldsymbol{z}}/(1+e^{\boldsymbol{\gamma}'\boldsymbol{z}})$ when $\lambda = 1$ and $\pi(\boldsymbol{z}) = \exp(-e^{-\boldsymbol{\gamma}'\boldsymbol{z}})$ when $\lambda \to 0$. Therefore (2.4) includes both the logit link and the complementary log-log link as special cases. An estimate value of λ and its standard error may produce useful information to determine which of the two link functions is adequate for the data if it is not clear which link function should be used.

2.2.2 Parametric Latency Submodel

A parametric specification of the latency submodel of the mixture cure model involves a parametric specification of the distribution of $T|Y = 1$ and a parametric specification of the effect of $\boldsymbol{x}$, a vector of covariates, on the distribution. This is often achieved by writing $S_u(t)$ as a function of a parametrically

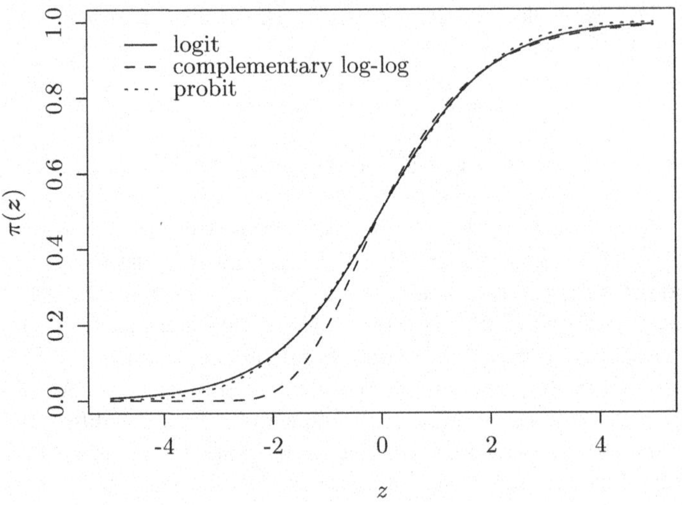

FIGURE 2.1
Comparison of three link functions for the incidence part of the mixture cure model.

specified baseline survival function $S_{u0}(t)$ and $\boldsymbol{\beta}'\boldsymbol{x}$, where $S_u(t) \equiv S_{u0}(t)$ when $\boldsymbol{x} = 0$, and $\boldsymbol{\beta}$ is a vector of the coefficients of the covariates in $\boldsymbol{x}$. The covariate vectors $\boldsymbol{x}$ and $\boldsymbol{z}$ may or may not include the same covariates.

2.2.2.1 Parametric PH Latency Submodel

One method to specify the latency part is to use the proportional hazards (PH) assumption:

$$S_u(t) = S_u(t|\boldsymbol{x}) = S_{u0}(t)^{\exp(\boldsymbol{x}'\boldsymbol{\beta})} \tag{2.5}$$

and $S_{u0}(t)$ is a survival function from a parametric distribution. For example, if $S_{u0}(t) = e^{-\lambda t}$, the survival function from an exponential distribution with rate λ, then $S_u(t|\boldsymbol{x}) = e^{-\lambda \exp(\boldsymbol{x}'\boldsymbol{\beta})t}$ is also a survival function from an exponential distribution with rate $\lambda \exp(\boldsymbol{x}'\boldsymbol{\beta})$. Similarly, if $S_{u0}(t) = e^{-\lambda t^p}$, the survival function from a Weibull distribution with shape parameter p and scale parameter λ, then $S_u(t|\boldsymbol{x}) = e^{-\lambda \exp(\boldsymbol{x}'\boldsymbol{\beta})t^p}$ is also the survival function from a Weibull distribution with shape parameter p and scale parameter $\lambda \exp(\boldsymbol{x}'\boldsymbol{\beta})$. Note that $\boldsymbol{\beta}$ in the above cases should not contain an intercept because it will not be identifiable from the scale parameter λ in the baseline distributions. The interpretation of $\boldsymbol{\beta}$ is similar to Cox's PH model. That is, for any covariate in $\boldsymbol{x}$, the corresponding coefficient in $\boldsymbol{\beta}$ is the log-hazard ratio if the covariate increases by 1 while other covariates are controlled.

The parametric latency submodel with the PH assumption is not widely used except for the cases discussed above because a semiparametric estimation method is available for the latency submodel under the PH assumption without specifying the baseline distribution parametrically, making a parametric PH model as the latency submodel less attractive.

2.2.2.2 Parametric AFT Latency Submodel

The parametric submodel for the latency part is more popular under the so-called accelerated failure time (AFT) assumption (Cox and Oakes, 1984), which can be written as follows:

$$S_u(t|\boldsymbol{x}) = S_{u0}(te^{-\boldsymbol{x}'\boldsymbol{\beta}}), \tag{2.6}$$

where $S_{u0}(t)$ is the survival function of a baseline distribution. If

$$\log(T|Y=1) = \boldsymbol{x}'\boldsymbol{\beta} + \sigma\epsilon \tag{2.7}$$

with σ as a scale parameter and ϵ as an error term satisfying $P(e^{\sigma\epsilon} > t) = S_{u0}(t)$, then $T|Y=1$ will follow the AFT model (2.6). Unlike the PH assumption, the AFT assumption allows direct interpretation of the effects of $\boldsymbol{x}$ on the $\log T|Y=1$ scale. Most of the parametric latency submodels based on the AFT assumption is via (2.7) by assuming a parametric distribution for $e^{\sigma\epsilon}$. For example, if e^{ϵ} follows the exponential distribution with mean 1 or if ϵ follows the extreme value distribution with survival function $P(\epsilon > s) = \exp(-e^s)$, then $S_u(t|\boldsymbol{x}) = \exp\left[-\left(te^{-\boldsymbol{x}'\boldsymbol{\beta}}\right)^{1/\sigma}\right]$. The corresponding mixture cure model is a Weibull AFT mixture cure model. It is well known such a latency submodel also satisfies the PH assumption and thus is also a Weibull PH mixture cure model (Farewell, 1982, 1986). If $\sigma = 1$, the model reduces to the exponential mixture cure model and is well studied in the early 1990s. See Maller and Zhou (1996) for the details.

There are many parametric distributions that can be considered for $e^{\sigma\epsilon}$ or ϵ when the Weibull baseline distribution is not appropriate. If the standard normal distribution is assumed for ϵ, then $S_u(t|\boldsymbol{x})$ is from the lognormal distribution (Gamel and McLean, 1994). Some multi-parameter distributions are proposed for ϵ as well, such as the extended generalized log-gamma distribution (Yamaguchi, 1992) with a density function

$$f_\epsilon(\epsilon) = \begin{cases} \frac{|q|}{\Gamma(q^{-2})}(q^{-2})^{q^{-2}} \exp\left[q^{-2}(q\epsilon - e^{q\epsilon})\right] & \text{if } q \neq 0 \\ \frac{1}{\sqrt{2\pi}} \exp(-\epsilon^2/2) & \text{if } q = 0, \end{cases} \tag{2.8}$$

or a generalized F distribution with density function

$$f_\epsilon(\epsilon; s_1, s_2) = \frac{(s_1 e^\epsilon/s_2)^{s_1}}{(1 + s_1 e^\epsilon/s_2)^{s_1+s_2} B(s_1, s_2)}, \tag{2.9}$$

where $s_1 > 0$ and $s_2 > 0$ and $\Gamma(\cdot)$ and $B(\cdot, \cdot)$ are gamma and beta functions (Peng et al., 1998). The complexity of the multi-parameter distributions makes the interpretation of the parameters in the latency submodel difficult. However, the fact that they include many simpler distributions, such as the Weibull, lognormal, and log-logistic distributions, as special cases makes them suitable to test the adequacy of the simpler distributions as the distribution for the latency part. See Section 2.5 for more details.

2.2.2.3 Other Parametric Latency Submodels

In addition to the PH and AFT assumptions above, there are other less known assumptions that can be considered for the latency submodel. The accelerated hazards (AH) assumption was first considered by Chen and Wang (2000) for survival data. It is in the following form when used as the latency submodel:

$$S_u(t|\boldsymbol{x}) = S_{u0}(te^{-\boldsymbol{x}'\boldsymbol{\beta}})^{\exp(\boldsymbol{x}'\boldsymbol{\beta})}, \tag{2.10}$$

where $S_{u0}(t)$ is a parametric baseline survival function. It may be easier to see how $\boldsymbol{x}$ affects the latency distribution under the AH assumption by the corresponding hazard function: $h_u(t|\boldsymbol{x}) = h_{u0}(te^{-\boldsymbol{x}'\boldsymbol{\beta}})$. Thus for a non-zero coefficient in $\boldsymbol{\beta}$, the corresponding covariate accelerates/decelerates the baseline hazard function. Due to the nature of the AH assumption, the baseline survival function can be from any distribution that is suitable for modeling time except for the exponential distribution. Unlike the PH and AFT assumptions above, the AH assumption allows a gradual effect of $\boldsymbol{x}$ on the distribution of T for uncured subjects. That is, if the baseline hazard function is monotone but not a constant, the hazard functions of two groups differ only when $t > 0$, and the larger the time t, the greater the differences in hazard.

The proportional odds (PO) assumption can also be considered in the latency submodel as follows:

$$S_u(t|\boldsymbol{x}) = \frac{1}{1 + [S_{u0}(t)^{-1} - 1]e^{-\boldsymbol{\beta}'\boldsymbol{x}}} \tag{2.11}$$

where $S_{u0}(t)^{-1} - 1$ is a parametric baseline odds function. Contrary to the AH assumption, the PO assumption implies that the hazard ratio of the uncured subjects approaches one as $t \to \infty$. That is, the differences in hazard will fade away under the PO assumption, making it suitable to model the effect of a covariate that diminishes as the survival time increases.

The four assumptions above are the examples of ways to specify the effects of $\boldsymbol{x}$ on $S_u(t)$ in the latency part. Determining an appropriate assumption among them for a given data set is important but not trivial. Hutton and Monaghan (2002) discussed issues of misspecification between PH and AFT assumptions for models without a cure fraction. Figure 2.2 displays two hazard functions from two groups under the four assumptions when one hazard function is a linear function of time. One may choose an assumption based on how the hazard ratio changes. For example, if the hazard ratio is a constant, the

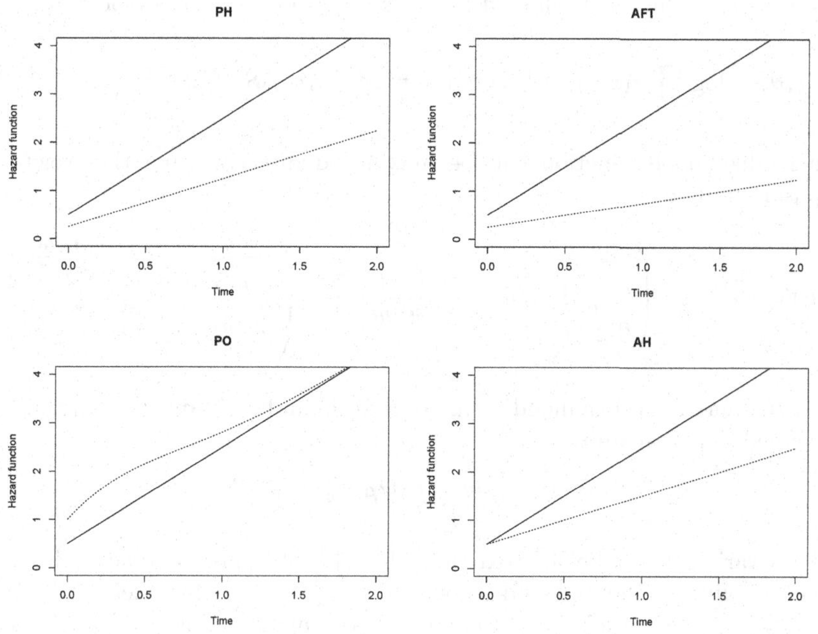

FIGURE 2.2
Examples of hazard functions of two groups under the four assumptions.

PH assumption would be appropriate. If the hazard difference between groups diminishes over time, the PO assumption may be a reasonable choice. Or one can determine a model based on whether and how the hazard functions cross. See discussions in Zhang and Peng (2009b) for some details. Unfortunately, the information about the hazard ratio for a covariate is often not available. The missing values in Y makes it infeasible to use any methods that were proposed to differentiate these models for data without cured subjects.

2.3 Model Estimation

2.3.1 Direct Maximization of Observed Likelihood Function

Suppose that the observed data of T and its censoring indicator δ, covariate $\boldsymbol{x}$, and $\boldsymbol{z}$ for n subjects are denoted as $(t_i, \delta_i, \boldsymbol{x}_i, \boldsymbol{z}_i)$, $i = 1, \ldots, n$, where $\delta_i = 1$ if t_i is uncensored and $\delta_i = 0$ if t_i is censored. Let $\boldsymbol{\alpha}$ be a vector of unknown parameters in the parametric baseline survival function $S_{u0}(\cdot)$, and

$\boldsymbol{\theta} = (\boldsymbol{\gamma}, \boldsymbol{\beta}, \boldsymbol{\alpha})'$. The log-likelihood function of the mixture cure model is

$$\ell(\boldsymbol{\theta}) = \log \prod_{i=1}^{n} [\pi(\boldsymbol{z}_i) f_u(t_i|\boldsymbol{x}_i)]^{\delta_i} [1 - \pi(\boldsymbol{z}_i) + \pi(\boldsymbol{z}_i) S_u(t_i|\boldsymbol{x}_i)]^{1-\delta_i}. \quad (2.12)$$

The log-likelihood function can be maximized directly using the Newton-Raphson method. Let

$$\boldsymbol{U}(\boldsymbol{\theta}) = \frac{\partial \ell(\boldsymbol{\theta})}{\partial \boldsymbol{\theta}} = \begin{pmatrix} \frac{\partial \ell(\boldsymbol{\theta})}{\partial \boldsymbol{\gamma}} \\ \frac{\partial \ell(\boldsymbol{\theta})}{\partial \boldsymbol{\beta}} \\ \frac{\partial \ell(\boldsymbol{\theta})}{\partial \boldsymbol{\alpha}} \end{pmatrix}, \boldsymbol{I}(\boldsymbol{\theta}) = -\frac{\partial^2 \ell(\boldsymbol{\theta})}{\partial \boldsymbol{\theta} \partial \boldsymbol{\theta}'} = -\begin{pmatrix} \frac{\partial^2 \ell(\boldsymbol{\theta})}{\partial \boldsymbol{\gamma} \partial \boldsymbol{\gamma}'} & \frac{\partial^2 \ell(\boldsymbol{\theta})}{\partial \boldsymbol{\gamma} \partial \boldsymbol{\beta}'} & \frac{\partial^2 \ell(\boldsymbol{\theta})}{\partial \boldsymbol{\gamma} \partial \boldsymbol{\alpha}'} \\ \frac{\partial^2 \ell(\boldsymbol{\theta})}{\partial \boldsymbol{\beta} \partial \boldsymbol{\gamma}'} & \frac{\partial^2 \ell(\boldsymbol{\theta})}{\partial \boldsymbol{\beta} \partial \boldsymbol{\beta}'} & \frac{\partial^2 \ell(\boldsymbol{\theta})}{\partial \boldsymbol{\beta} \partial \boldsymbol{\alpha}'} \\ \frac{\partial^2 \ell(\boldsymbol{\theta})}{\partial \boldsymbol{\alpha} \partial \boldsymbol{\gamma}'} & \frac{\partial^2 \ell(\boldsymbol{\theta})}{\partial \boldsymbol{\alpha} \partial \boldsymbol{\beta}'} & \frac{\partial^2 \ell(\boldsymbol{\theta})}{\partial \boldsymbol{\alpha} \partial \boldsymbol{\alpha}'} \end{pmatrix}.$$

Then the maximum likelihood estimate $\widehat{\boldsymbol{\theta}}$ of $\boldsymbol{\theta}$ can be obtained as a result of converged iteration steps

$$\boldsymbol{\theta}^{(k+1)} = \boldsymbol{\theta}^{(k)} + \boldsymbol{I}^{-1}(\boldsymbol{\theta}^{(k)}) \boldsymbol{U}(\boldsymbol{\theta}^{(k)}),$$

and its variance can be approximated by $\boldsymbol{I}^{-1}(\widehat{\boldsymbol{\theta}})$. This approach relies on the availability of the first and second derivatives of the log-likelihood function with respect to all the parameters in the model. This can be an issue when dealing with some multi-parameter distributions such as the generalized gamma or F distribution. Peng et al. (1998) suggested to maximize the log-likelihood function directly using the simulated annealing algorithm based on the downhill simplex method (Press et al., 1992), which does not depend on any derivatives, or use the algorithm for $\boldsymbol{\alpha}$ and the Newton-Raphson method for $\boldsymbol{\gamma}$ and $\boldsymbol{\beta}$.

2.3.2 Estimation via EM Algorithm

The EM algorithm (Dempster et al., 1977) is another method that can be conveniently used to obtain the maximum likelihood estimates of the parameters in the mixture cure models. Let y_i be the value of Y for subject i. Then $y_i = 1$ if $\delta_i = 1$, and is usually latent or unknown with $\delta_i = 0$. The unknown status of y_i is due to the fact that a subject will be censored if either the subject is cured or the subject is not cured but the subject's failure time T is greater than the censoring time C. There is no information to tell whether the subject is cured or not given the censored failure time.

If all values of y_i's are available, the corresponding complete log-likelihood function based on the complete data $(t_i, \delta_i, \boldsymbol{x}_i, \boldsymbol{z}_i, y_i)$, $i = 1, \ldots, n$ is (up to an additive constant)

$$\begin{aligned} \ell^c(\boldsymbol{\gamma}, \boldsymbol{\beta}, \boldsymbol{\alpha}) &= \log \prod_{i=1}^{n} [\pi(\boldsymbol{z}_i) f_u(t_i|\boldsymbol{x}_i)^{\delta_i} S_u(t_i|\boldsymbol{x}_i)^{1-\delta_i}]^{y_i} [1 - \pi(\boldsymbol{z}_i)]^{1-y_i} \\ &= \ell_1(\boldsymbol{\gamma}) + \ell_2(\boldsymbol{\beta}, \boldsymbol{\alpha}), \end{aligned}$$

where

$$\ell_1(\gamma) = \sum_{i=1}^{n} \{y_i \log[\pi(\boldsymbol{z}_i)] + (1 - y_i)\log[1 - \pi(\boldsymbol{z}_i)]\},$$

$$\ell_2(\boldsymbol{\beta}, \boldsymbol{\alpha}) = \sum_{i=1}^{n} y_i \{\delta_i \log[f_u(t_i|\boldsymbol{x}_i)] + (1 - \delta_i)\log[S_u(t_i|\boldsymbol{x}_i)]\}.$$

Let

$$w_{0i}(t) = \frac{\pi(\boldsymbol{z}_i)S_u(t|\boldsymbol{x}_i)}{1 - \pi(\boldsymbol{z}_i) + \pi(\boldsymbol{z}_i)S_u(t|\boldsymbol{x}_i)} \tag{2.13}$$

be the probability of a subject with covariates $\boldsymbol{x}_i$ and $\boldsymbol{z}_i$ to be uncured conditional on surviving at t under the mixture cure model (2.1). Given the estimates of $\boldsymbol{\gamma}, \boldsymbol{\beta}, \boldsymbol{\alpha}$ in the $(k-1)$th iteration of the EM algorithm, denoted as $\boldsymbol{\gamma}^{(k-1)}, \boldsymbol{\beta}^{(k-1)}, \boldsymbol{\alpha}^{(k-1)}$, the E-step in the kth iteration of the EM algorithm calculates the posterior expectation of y_i as

$$w_i^{(k)} = \delta_i + (1 - \delta_i)w_{0i}(t_i)\,\big|_{\boldsymbol{\gamma}=\boldsymbol{\gamma}^{(k-1)}, \boldsymbol{\beta}=\boldsymbol{\beta}^{(k-1)}, \boldsymbol{\alpha}=\boldsymbol{\alpha}^{(k-1)}} \tag{2.14}$$

following the property of y_i above and Bayes' theorem. It can be interpreted as the probability the subject being uncured given the observed data for that subject and current parameter estimates.

The M-step in the kth iteration of the EM algorithm maximizes ℓ_1 and ℓ_2 after replacing y_i in ℓ_1 and ℓ_2 with $w_i^{(k)}$. That is, the M-step maximizes

$$\ell_1(\gamma) = \sum_{i=1}^{n} \left\{w_i^{(k)} \log[\pi(\boldsymbol{z}_i)] + (1 - w_i^{(k)})\log[1 - \pi(\boldsymbol{z}_i)]\right\}, \tag{2.15}$$

$$\ell_2(\boldsymbol{\beta}, \boldsymbol{\alpha}) = \sum_{i=1, w_i^{(k)}>0}^{n} w_i^{(k)} \{\delta_i \log[f_u(t_i|\boldsymbol{x}_i)] + (1 - \delta_i)\log[S_u(t_i|\boldsymbol{x}_i)]\} \tag{2.16}$$

to update the estimates of $\boldsymbol{\gamma}, \boldsymbol{\beta}, \boldsymbol{\alpha}$. The updated estimates of $\boldsymbol{\gamma}, \boldsymbol{\beta}, \boldsymbol{\alpha}$, denoted as $\boldsymbol{\gamma}^{(k)}, \boldsymbol{\beta}^{(k)}, \boldsymbol{\alpha}^{(k)}$, will be compared to $\boldsymbol{\gamma}^{(k-1)}, \boldsymbol{\beta}^{(k-1)}, \boldsymbol{\alpha}^{(k-1)}$ to determine the convergence of the algorithm. If not, the E-step and M-step iterate until a convergence is achieved.

It is easy to see that (2.15) can be viewed as the log-likelihood function from a logistic regression with $(w_1^{(k)}, \ldots, w_n^{(k)})$ as values of the response variable. Thus, it can be maximized by the Newton-Raphson method or using existing software for the logistic regression (Peng, 2003b). For (2.16), it is similar to the log-likelihood function for censored data except the multiplicative term $w_i^{(k)}$. Therefore, it can be treated as a weighted log-likelihood function for censored data without a cure fraction and can be maximized by the Newton-Raphson method or by existing software for classic survival models that accept case weights. For example, one can assume that

$S_{u0}(t) = \exp(-\lambda t)$ is the survival function of the exponential distribution with rate λ in (2.5). The log-likelihood function reduces to $\ell_2(\boldsymbol{\beta}, S_{u0}) = \ell_2(\boldsymbol{\beta}, \lambda) = \sum_{i=1, w_i^{(k)}>0}^{n} \left\{ \delta_i \log \lambda + \delta_i \boldsymbol{\beta}' \boldsymbol{x}_i - \lambda t_i e^{\log w_i^{(k)} + \boldsymbol{\beta}' \boldsymbol{x}_i} \right\}$. It can be maximized by either the Newton-Raphson method or an existing software package to fit the exponential distribution to data that allows case weight.

The M-step can also be completed using the Monte Carlo EM algorithm of Tanner and Wong (1987) by simulating y_i's from w_i's in (2.14). See Lam et al. (2005) and Xu and Zhang (2010) for details.

These features demonstrate that the EM algorithm for the mixture cure model is not only an alternative method to obtain the maximum likelihood estimates of the parameters in the model, but also a bridge to connect the mixture cure models with existing classical survival models, which makes it possible to use existing methods for the classical survival models to estimate the parameters in the mixture cure models.

One challenge in using EM algorithm is that the variances of the estimates are not directly available at the convergence of the EM algorithm. For the parametric mixture cure model, the methods proposed by Louis (1982) and Oakes (1999) may be considered. These methods depend on availability of derivatives of ℓ_1 and ℓ_2 with respect to the parameters in the model, which can be challenging for some parameters in the specified distribution in ℓ_2. An alternative approach is to use the bootstrap method (Davison and Hinkley, 1997; Li and Datta, 2001) to estimate the standard errors of the estimates.

2.4 Non-Mixture Cure Models

2.4.1 Proportional Hazards Cure Model

Another approach to define a cure model is to based on a theory of tumor kinetics in cancer studies. The theory assumes (Yakovlev et al., 1996; Tsodikov, 2001) that each subject has N cancer cells at the baseline. A cured subject has $N = 0$ cancer cells while an uncured subject has $N > 0$ cancer cells, and the uncured subject will develop cancer if one of the $N > 0$ cancer cells develops a detectable cancer mass. That is,

$$T = \min\{\tilde{T}_1, \ldots, \tilde{T}_N\} = \tilde{T}_{(1)}, \tag{2.17}$$

where $\tilde{T}_i$'s are i.i.d. latent event times or activation times for cancer cells to develop a detectable cancer mass, and $\tilde{T}_{(1)}$ is the first order statistic of $\tilde{T}_1$, $\ldots, \tilde{T}_N$. This is also called the first-activation scheme and is one of a number of schemes developed in Cooner et al. (2007) that may be suitable for tumor kinetics. The schemes involve different distributions for N and $\tilde{T}_i$ and different order statistics $\tilde{T}_{(r)}$, $1 \leq r \leq N$, to define the failure time T, and they lead to different cure models. The most popular model is based on the first-activation scheme with N following a Poisson distribution with mean $\exp(\gamma_0+\boldsymbol{z}'\boldsymbol{\gamma})$ that is independent of $\tilde{T}_i$'s. If $\tilde{T}_i \sim F^H(t)$, a proper cumulative distribution function, then unconditional survival function of T is

$$\begin{aligned}P(T>t)=S(t|\boldsymbol{z}) =& P(N=0)+P(\tilde{T}_1>t,\ldots,\ldots,\tilde{T}_N>t,N\geq 1)\\ =& \exp(-e^{\gamma_0+\boldsymbol{z}'\boldsymbol{\gamma}})+\sum_{k=1}^{\infty}\frac{[S^H(t)e^{\gamma_0+\boldsymbol{z}'\boldsymbol{\gamma}}]^k}{k!}\exp(-e^{\gamma_0+\boldsymbol{z}'\boldsymbol{\gamma}})\\ =& \exp[-e^{\gamma_0+\boldsymbol{z}'\boldsymbol{\gamma}}F^H(t)], \end{aligned} \tag{2.18}$$

where $S^H(t) = 1 - F^H(t)$. The model can be rewritten as $S(t|z) = [e^{-\exp(\gamma_0)F^H(t)}]^{\exp(\boldsymbol{z}'\boldsymbol{\gamma})}$ or $h(t|\boldsymbol{z}) = [e^{\gamma_0}f^H(t)]\exp(\boldsymbol{z}'\boldsymbol{\gamma})$, where $f^H(t) = dF^H(t)/dt$. It is obviously similar to the classic PH model except that the baseline survival function counterpart of the PH model in model (2.18) is an improper survival function satisfying $\lim_{t\to\infty}\exp[-e^{\gamma_0}F^H(t)] = \exp(-e^{\gamma_0}) \in (0, 1)$. Thus, we refer to this model as the proportional hazards cure (PHC) model. Since the baseline cumulative hazard counterpart of the PH model in model (2.18), $e^{\gamma_0}F^H(t)$, is bounded, model (2.18) is also called the bounded cumulative hazard cure model.

As a comparison, the mixture cure model does not have a PH structure when the latency does not depend on any covariates. This can be seen from the fact that

$$h(t|\boldsymbol{z}) = \frac{f(t|\boldsymbol{z})}{S(t|\boldsymbol{z})} = \frac{\pi(\boldsymbol{z})f_u(t)}{\pi(\boldsymbol{z})S_u(t)+1-\pi(\boldsymbol{z})} = w_0(t,\boldsymbol{z})h_u(t).$$

As in the discussion for (2.13), $w_0(t,\boldsymbol{z})$ is a conditional probability of being uncured at t and is generally not independent of t. Thus, the model does not have the PH structure in general (the mixture cure model may behave like the PH model with $h(t|\boldsymbol{z}) = \pi(\boldsymbol{z})h_u(t)$ when $t \to 0$ or $h(t|\boldsymbol{z}) = \frac{\pi(\boldsymbol{z})}{1-\pi(\boldsymbol{z})}f_u(t)$ when $t \to \infty$).

If there is no covariate present and $F^H(t)$ is the distribution function of the exponential distribution, then $S(t|\boldsymbol{z})$ is a survival function from an improper generalized Gompertz distribution. This particular parametric PHC model was discussed in detail in the literature (Cantor and Shuster, 1992; Yakovlev et al., 1994b; Cantor, 2001).

The PHC model can be written in a form of a mixture cure model (2.1) where $\pi = 1 - \exp(-e^{\gamma_0+\boldsymbol{z}'\boldsymbol{\gamma}})$ and

$$S_u(t) = \frac{\exp[e^{\gamma_0+\boldsymbol{z}'\boldsymbol{\gamma}}F^H(t)]-1}{\exp[e^{\gamma_0+\boldsymbol{z}'\boldsymbol{\gamma}}]-1}.$$

The incidence part is essentially the complementary log-log model (2.3). However, the latency part does not have a simple interpretation of covariate effects as in the mixture cure models discussed in Section 2.2. Moreover, it is clear

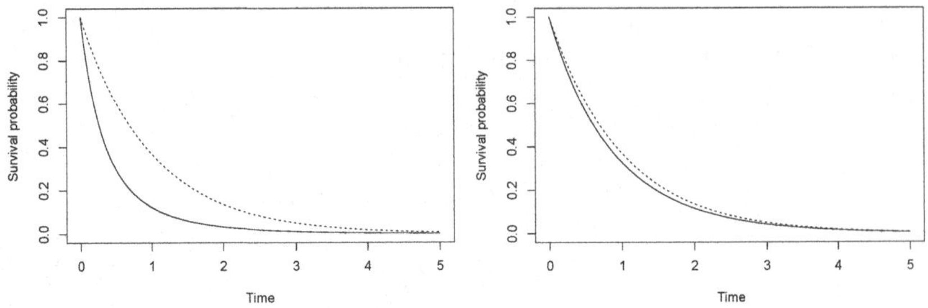

FIGURE 2.3
$S_u(t)$ (solid line) and $S^H(t)$ (dotted line) when the cure rate is 7% (left) and 69% (right).

that for any $\boldsymbol{z}$, we have $S_u(t) \leq S^H(t)$ and equality occurs when $e^{\gamma_0+\boldsymbol{z}'\boldsymbol{\gamma}} \to 0$. It implies that $S^H(t)$ cannot be viewed as a survival function for uncured subjects, unless the cure rate is close to 1. Figure 2.3 demonstrates the difference between $S_u(t)$ and $S^H(t)$ when the cure rate increases (Peng and Xu, 2012).

As an alternative to the mixture cure model, the PHC model received a great deal of interest in the last decade due to its similarity to the classical PH model. However, the proportionality restriction in $\boldsymbol{z}$ in the model also limits the wide applications of the model in practice. The restriction can be relaxed by including covariate effects in $F^H(t)$, such as under the proportional hazards assumption

$$1 - F^H(t|\boldsymbol{x}) = S^H(t|\boldsymbol{x}) = S_0^H(t)^{\exp(\boldsymbol{x}'\boldsymbol{\beta})}, \tag{2.19}$$

where $S_0^H(t)$ is a baseline survival function (Tsodikov, 2002). This is the so-called PHPH cure model. The inclusion of $\boldsymbol{x}$ in $F^H(t)$ widens the applicability of the PHC model, because there are now two sets of parameters to describe the effects of the covariates. But the covariate effects in $S_u(t)$ are difficult to interpret compared to the PH mixture cure model because both effects of $\boldsymbol{z}$ and $\boldsymbol{x}$ appear in the latency part.

Let $f(t|\boldsymbol{z}) = e^{\gamma_0+\boldsymbol{z}'\boldsymbol{\gamma}} f^H(t) \exp[-e^{\gamma_0+\boldsymbol{z}'\boldsymbol{\gamma}} F^H(t)]$ be the unconditional density function corresponding to (2.18) and $F^H(t)$ is parametrically specified up to a few unknown parameters $\boldsymbol{\alpha}$. The log-likelihood function for the model is

$$\ell(\gamma_0, \boldsymbol{\gamma}, \boldsymbol{\alpha}) = \log \prod_{i=1}^{n} [f(t_i|\boldsymbol{z}_i)]^{\delta_i} [S(t_i|\boldsymbol{z}_i)]^{1-\delta_i}.$$

The standard Newton-Raphson method discussed in Section 2.3.1 can be used to maximize the likelihood function to obtain the maximum likelihood estimates of the model parameters. See Asselain et al. (1996) and Tsodikov et al. (1998) for some details of the model estimation and applications.

2.4.2 Cure Models Based on Tumor Activation Scheme

The PHC model can be viewed as a result of the latent first-activation scheme described as (2.17), which is one of a few latent activation schemes proposed. Other latent activation schemes are discussed in detail in Section 7.2. As indicated by Tucker and Taylor (1996), however, the interpretation above may not be appropriate because tumor cells proliferate or die spontaneously and the simple Poisson model may not be appropriate to describe the kinetics. Hanin et al. (2001) proposed a new distribution for N that takes into account the spontaneous proliferation or death of tumor cells in fractionated radiotherapy. Here we will consider other distributions for N under the first-activation scheme (2.17) that lead to other cure models.

If N follows a Bernoulli distribution with the probability given in (2.2), then T defined in (2.17) will follow a mixture cure model with $S_u(t) = S^H(t)$. Thus, the mixture cure model is one of the models that can be defined using the first-activation scheme.

If N follows a binomial distribution with n and $e^{\gamma_0+\boldsymbol{\gamma}'\boldsymbol{z}}/(1+e^{\gamma_0+\boldsymbol{\gamma}'\boldsymbol{z}})$ as the probability of success, then the survival function of T defined in (2.17) is (Peng and Xu, 2012)

$$\begin{aligned} S(t|\boldsymbol{z}) &= P(N=0) + P(\tilde{T}_1 > t, \ldots, \tilde{T}_N > t, N \geq 1) = \left(1+e^{\gamma_0+\boldsymbol{\gamma}'\boldsymbol{z}}\right)^{-n} \\ &\quad + \sum_{i=1}^{n} \left[S^H(t)\right]^i \binom{n}{i} \left(\frac{e^{\gamma_0+\boldsymbol{\gamma}'\boldsymbol{z}}}{1+e^{\gamma_0+\boldsymbol{\gamma}'\boldsymbol{z}}}\right)^i \left(1+e^{\gamma_0+\boldsymbol{\gamma}'\boldsymbol{z}}\right)^{i-n} \\ &= \left(S^H(t)\frac{e^{\gamma_0+\boldsymbol{\gamma}'\boldsymbol{z}}}{1+e^{\gamma_0+\boldsymbol{\gamma}'\boldsymbol{z}}} + \frac{1}{1+e^{\gamma_0+\boldsymbol{\gamma}'\boldsymbol{z}}}\right)^n. \end{aligned} \tag{2.20}$$

This model is similar to the mixture cure model except it adds an extra parameter as the power to the unconditional survival function of the mixture cure model. This model arises when there are at most n carcinogenic cells in a patient. It is easy to see that the interpretation above reduces to the one for the mixture cure model when $n = 1$.

If N follows a geometric distribution with mean $\mu = e^{\gamma_0+\boldsymbol{\gamma}'\boldsymbol{z}}$, then the survival function of T defined in (2.17) is

$$\begin{aligned} S(t|\boldsymbol{z}) &= P(N=0) + P(\tilde{T}_1 > t, \ldots, \tilde{T}_N > t, N \geq 1) = \left(1+e^{\gamma_0+\boldsymbol{\gamma}'\boldsymbol{z}}\right)^{-1} \\ &\quad + \sum_{i=1}^{\infty} \left[S^H(t)\right]^i \left(\frac{e^{\gamma_0+\boldsymbol{\gamma}'\boldsymbol{z}}}{1+e^{\gamma_0+\boldsymbol{\gamma}'\boldsymbol{z}}}\right)^i \left(1+e^{\gamma_0+\boldsymbol{\gamma}'\boldsymbol{z}}\right)^{-1} \\ &= \left(1+F^H(t)e^{\gamma_0+\boldsymbol{\gamma}'\boldsymbol{z}}\right)^{-1}. \end{aligned} \tag{2.21}$$

This is a PO model similar to (2.11) except that the baseline odds function is $F^H(t)$, which is an improper odds function. Thus, this model is an analogy of the extension of the PH model to the PHC model by using an improper baseline odds function in the PO model. The resulting survival function $S(t|\boldsymbol{z})$ is an improper survival function and can be used to model survival data with a cured fraction. It is also called the proportional odds cure (POC) model. The POC model is considered in Tsodikov (2002); Gu et al. (2011), and covariates can also be included in $F^H(t)$ in the model.

It is clear that (2.17) always defines a cure model as long as N follows a distribution that has a probability mass at 0. We only considered discrete distributions above because of the biological interpretation attached to N. A non-discrete distribution can be considered as well, and this will be further discussed in the following section.

With the different cure models, it becomes important to choose an appropriate cure model among them for a given data set. The biological interpretation specified in (2.17) may help if it is plausible. However, the elusive nature of N and the latent variables $\tilde{T}_1, \ldots, \tilde{T}_N$ used in the biological interpretation makes this task challenging.

2.4.3 Cure Models Based on Frailty Models

A cure model can also be formed using the transformation model with a frailty (Choi et al., 2014). Given a frailty ξ, let the conditional cumulative hazard function be

$$H(t|\xi, \boldsymbol{x}) = \xi g\left(\int_0^t I(T \geq s)\exp(\boldsymbol{x}(s)'\boldsymbol{\gamma})dH_0(s)\right), \qquad (2.22)$$

where $H_0(t)$ is a proper baseline cumulative hazard function and $g(\cdot)$ is a prespecified nonnegative transformation function that is strictly increasing and continuously differentiable and satisfies $g(0) = 0$, $g(\infty) = \infty$, and $g'(0) > 0$. This model will be suitable for modeling survival data with a cured fraction if ξ follows a distribution that has a probability mass at zero since the hazard for cured subjects is zero. For example, if ξ follows a Bernoulli distribution with probability π, then the marginal survival function from model (2.22) is

$$S(t|\boldsymbol{x}) = 1 - \pi + \pi \exp\left[-g\left(\int_0^t I(T \geq s)\exp(\boldsymbol{x}(s)'\boldsymbol{\gamma})dH_0(s)\right)\right].$$

This is a mixture model discussed in Section 2.2 if π is allowed to be affected by $\boldsymbol{z}$ in the logit form.

If ξ follows a Poisson distribution with mean μ, the marginal survival function from model (2.22) is

$$S(t|\boldsymbol{x}) = \exp\left[-\left(1 - e^{-g\left(\int_0^t I(T\geq s)\exp(\boldsymbol{x}(s)'\boldsymbol{\gamma})dH_0(s)\right)}\right)\mu\right].$$

This is the PHC model discussed in Section 2.4.1 if μ is allowed to be affected by $\boldsymbol{z}$ in the complementary log-log form and $\boldsymbol{\gamma} = 0$.

If ξ follows a geometric distribution with mean μ, the marginal survival function from model (2.22) is

$$S(t|\boldsymbol{x}) = 1 \Big/ \left[1 + \left(1 - e^{-g\left(\int_0^t I(T \geq s) \exp(\boldsymbol{x}(s)'\boldsymbol{\gamma}) dH_0(s)\right)}\right) \mu\right].$$

This is essentially the POC model (2.21) if μ is allowed to be affected by $\boldsymbol{z}$ in a form of $\mu = \exp(\boldsymbol{z}'\gamma)$ and $\boldsymbol{\gamma} = 0$.

A more complicated distribution can be assumed for model (2.22) to be a cure model. In addition to discrete distributions considered above, a mixed type distribution with a continuous component and a discrete component at zero can be considered as well. One such a distribution is the compound Poisson distribution (Aalen, 1992). Such a distribution can also be formed by assuming ξ is a product of two random variables: one is a discrete with a positive probability mass at 0 and the other is a continuous distribution.

It is easy to see the cure models built on (2.22) are similar to those built on (2.17). This is not an unexpected result. Both the frailty ξ and N are latent variables and played a similar role in the models. They both cannot be observed. However, N in (2.17) provides an interpretation for ξ in (2.22).

2.4.4 Cure Models Based on Box-Cox Transformation

Another approach to build a general cure model is to use the Box-Cox transformation (Box and Cox, 1964). For example, the unconditional survival function of T may be defined as follows (Yin and Ibrahim, 2005a)

$$S(t|\boldsymbol{z}, \boldsymbol{x}) = \begin{cases} \left\{1 - \dfrac{\lambda \exp(\gamma_0 + \boldsymbol{\gamma}'\boldsymbol{z})}{1 + \lambda \exp(\gamma_0 + \boldsymbol{\gamma}'\boldsymbol{z})} F^H(t|\boldsymbol{x})\right\}^{1/\lambda} & 0 < \lambda \leq 1 \\ \exp\left[-e^{\gamma_0 + \boldsymbol{\gamma}'\boldsymbol{z}} F^H(t|\boldsymbol{x})\right] & \lambda = 0, \end{cases} \tag{2.23}$$

where λ is the transformation parameter and $F^H(t|\boldsymbol{x})$ is a proper cumulative distribution function that may depend on a vector of covariates $\boldsymbol{x}$. It is easy to see that model (2.23) becomes the mixture cure model (2.1) when $\lambda = 1$ and the PHC model (2.18) when $\lambda \to 0$. Therefore model (2.23) unifies the mixture cure model and the PHC model.

This model can also be motivated using the model (2.20) (Peng and Xu, 2012). Assume temporarily that $1/\lambda$ is a positive integer and let N be a binomial variate with $n = 1/\lambda$ and $\lambda e^{\gamma_0 + \boldsymbol{\gamma}'\boldsymbol{z}}/(1 + \lambda e^{\gamma_0 + \boldsymbol{\gamma}'\boldsymbol{z}})$ as the probability of success. Then the survival function in (2.20) can be rewritten as

$$S(t|\boldsymbol{x}, \boldsymbol{z}) = \left(1 - \frac{\lambda e^{\gamma_0 + \boldsymbol{\gamma}'\boldsymbol{z}}}{1 + \lambda e^{\gamma_0 + \boldsymbol{\gamma}'\boldsymbol{z}}} F^H(t|\boldsymbol{x})\right)^{1/\lambda},$$

which is the same as the survival function defined in (2.23). Thus, when $1/\lambda$ is a positive integer, this model arises when there are at most $1/\lambda$ carcinogenic cells in a patient, and it generalizes the tumor kinetics interpretation above by allowing the number of carcinogenic cells $1/\lambda$ to be a real valued number in $[1, \infty)$. It is easy to see that the interpretation above reduces to the one for the mixture cure model when $\lambda = 1$.

Given the interpretation of $1/\lambda$ as the real-valued maximum number of carcinogenic cells that a patient can have, Peng and Xu (2012) also suggested to relax the requirement of $1/\lambda > 1$ by assuming $1/\lambda > 0$. That is,

$$S(t|\boldsymbol{z}, \boldsymbol{x}) = \begin{cases} \left\{1 - \dfrac{\lambda \exp(\gamma_0 + \boldsymbol{\gamma}'\boldsymbol{z})}{1 + \lambda \exp(\gamma_0 + \boldsymbol{\gamma}'\boldsymbol{z})} F^H(t|\boldsymbol{x})\right\}^{1/\lambda} & \lambda > 0 \\ \exp\left[-e^{\gamma_0 + \boldsymbol{\gamma}'\boldsymbol{z}} F^H(t|\boldsymbol{x})\right] & \lambda = 0. \end{cases} \tag{2.24}$$

Treating $1/\lambda$ as a positive real number is particularly attractive in understanding tumor kinetics. For example, the positive real number $1/\lambda$ may be considered as tumor volume in a patient, which may be more practical in cancer oncology than the number of tumor cells. An immediate result of extending λ from $(0, 1]$ to $(0, \infty)$ is that $S_u(t) > S^H(t|x)$ when $\lambda > 1$, a feature that Cooner et al. (2007) tried to obtain by defining the so-called last-activation scheme $T = \max\{\tilde{T}_1, \ldots, \tilde{T}_N\}$. The model (2.24) can be viewed as a model that unifies both the first- and last-activation schemes to allow $S_u(t|\boldsymbol{x})$ to be less than or greater than $S^H(t|\boldsymbol{x})$.

Another family of cure models is given by (Taylor and Liu, 2007)

$$S(t|\boldsymbol{z}, \boldsymbol{x}) = \begin{cases} \left\{1 + \left[\left(1 + e^{\gamma_0 + \boldsymbol{\gamma}'\boldsymbol{z}}\right)^{-\lambda} - 1\right] F^H(t|\boldsymbol{x})\right\}^{\frac{1}{\lambda}} & \lambda \neq 0 \\ (1 + e^{\gamma_0 + \boldsymbol{\gamma}'\boldsymbol{z}})^{-F^H(t|\boldsymbol{x})} & \lambda = 0. \end{cases} \tag{2.25}$$

It is easy to see that model (2.25) is a mixture cure model when $\lambda = 1$ and a PHC model when $\lambda = 0$ (except that the cure rate is $(1 + e^{\gamma_0 + \boldsymbol{\gamma}'\boldsymbol{z}})^{-1}$ instead of $\exp(-e^{\gamma_0 + \boldsymbol{\gamma}'\boldsymbol{z}})$). Note also that this model has the appealing feature that the limit as $t \to \infty$ of $S(t|\boldsymbol{z}, \boldsymbol{x})$ is $(1 + e^{\gamma_0 + \boldsymbol{\gamma}'\boldsymbol{z}})^{-1}$ and it does not depend on the value of λ.

Zeng et al. (2006) proposed another cure model based on the Box-Cox transformation as follows:

$$S(t|\boldsymbol{z}) = \begin{cases} [1 + \lambda e^{\gamma_0 + \boldsymbol{z}'\boldsymbol{\gamma}} F^H(t|\boldsymbol{x})]^{-1/\lambda} & \lambda > 0 \\ \exp[-e^{\gamma_0 + \boldsymbol{z}'\boldsymbol{\gamma}} F^H(t|\boldsymbol{x})] & \lambda = 0. \end{cases} \tag{2.26}$$

It is easy to show that model (2.26) unifies the PHC model (2.18) (when $\lambda \to 0$) and the POC model (2.21) (when $\lambda = 1$).

The Box-Cox transformation can also be used to unify the PHC model with a non-cure additive model as follows (Yin and Ibrahim, 2005b):

$$h(t|\boldsymbol{z}) = \begin{cases} [f^H(t)^\lambda + \lambda(\gamma_0 + \boldsymbol{z}'\boldsymbol{\gamma})]^{1/\lambda} & 0 < \lambda \leq 1 \\ f^H(t) \exp(\gamma_0 + \boldsymbol{z}'\boldsymbol{\gamma}) & \lambda = 0, \end{cases} \tag{2.27}$$

where $f^H(t)$ is a proper probability density function. It is clear that this model reduces to the PHC model when $\lambda = 0$ and an additive hazard model $h(t|\boldsymbol{z}) = f^H(t) + \gamma_0 + \boldsymbol{z}'\boldsymbol{\gamma}$ when $\lambda = 1$. The latter is the usual additive hazard model (Lin and Ying, 1994) except that the baseline hazard function is replaced with $f^H(t)$. When estimating this model, one has to ensure that the estimated hazard function $h(t|\boldsymbol{z})$ is non-negative.

There are a variety of estimation methods proposed in the literature to estimate the parameters in the unified cure models above, including parametric, semiparametric, and Bayesian methods. Unfortunately, due to the complexity of the unified models, the estimation methods usually fix the value of λ in the Box-Cox transformation at a prespecified value and then apply the estimation methods to estimate other parameters in the models. This approach greatly limits the application of the unified cure models.

2.5 Model Assessment

2.5.1 Choosing an Appropriate Parametric Distribution

One important issue with a parametric cure model is to determine a distribution for the cure model that is most appropriate for a data set. Preferably the subject knowledge can help determine the most appropriate distribution for a particular data set. However, if such knowledge is not available, statistical methods may be used to aid the selection among a few candidate distributions.

If the candidate distributions are nested, statistical tests may be used to select a parsimonious distribution that provides a fit to data with no significant difference from a fit by a complex distribution. For example, the generalized F distribution (2.9) reduces to the generalized log-gamma distribution (2.8) if $s_1 \to \infty$ or $s_2 \to \infty$, and the latter further reduces to the normal distribution if $q \to 0$ and the extreme value distribution if $q = 1$. Thus, it is possible to test adequacy of, say lognormal distribution, using the generalized F or generalized gamma distributions. Peng et al. (2001) discussed the use of the likelihood ratio test (LRT) within the generalized gamma distribution family to select a parsimonious distribution in the family for a data set. One challenging issue with this approach is that the asymptotic null distribution of the LRT statistic is no longer chi-square distribution if a parsimonious distribution corresponds to a boundary value of a parameter in the distribution family that it belongs to, such as the generalized log-gamma distribution versus generalized F distribution.

For non-nested distributions, some information criteria may be used to compare the cure models based on the distributions. The most common criteria include the Akaike information criterion (AIC), defined as

$$\text{AIC} = 2p - 2\ell(\hat{\boldsymbol{\theta}}),$$

and the Bayesian information criterion (BIC), defined as

$$\text{BIC} = p\log(n) - 2\ell(\hat{\boldsymbol{\theta}}),$$

where p is the number of estimated parameters in the cure model. A cure model with a smaller value of AIC or BIC is preferred to a model with a larger value. This method, however, may not be useful if one is interested in the adequacy of one model relative the other model for data.

2.5.2 Mixture vs Non-Mixture Cure Models

When $\boldsymbol{z}$ is absent and $F^H(t|\boldsymbol{x})$ is unspecified, the mixture cure and PHC models are equivalent. They are simply different forms of the same model. When $\boldsymbol{z}$ is present and $\boldsymbol{x}$ is absent, the PHC model is a PH model and the mixture cure model is not, and they are clearly models for different data structures. When both $\boldsymbol{x}$ and $\boldsymbol{z}$ are present, both models are flexible and they can be considered for modeling survival data with a cure fraction. An emerging question is to determine which one of the two models is appropriate for given data, particularly when there is no convincing biological evidence to favor any of the two models. Similar questions apply to other cure models. With the unified cure models discussed in Section 2.4.4, it is possible to use statistical tests to examine the adequacy of models relative to the unified cure models and choose one that does not show a significant difference (Peng and Xu, 2012). For example, if we consider the following hypotheses under the model (2.24):

$$H_0 : \lambda = 1 \text{ vs } H_a : \lambda \neq 1, \tag{2.28}$$

$$H_0 : \lambda = 0 \text{ vs } H_a : \lambda > 0, \tag{2.29}$$

then the first set is to test the adequacy of the mixture cure model and the second set is to test the adequacy of the PHC model. Let $\boldsymbol{\theta} = (\lambda, \boldsymbol{\gamma}', \boldsymbol{\beta}', \boldsymbol{\alpha}')'$ be the parameters in model (2.24) ($\boldsymbol{\alpha}$ is a set of parameters in the baseline distribution in $F^H(t|\boldsymbol{x})$), $\ell(\lambda, \boldsymbol{\gamma}, \boldsymbol{\beta}, \boldsymbol{\alpha})$ be the log-likelihood function from the model, $\hat{\boldsymbol{\theta}} = \arg\max_{(\lambda,\boldsymbol{\gamma},\boldsymbol{\beta},\boldsymbol{\alpha})} \ell(\lambda, \boldsymbol{\gamma}, \boldsymbol{\beta}, \boldsymbol{\alpha})$, $\hat{\boldsymbol{\theta}}_0 = \arg\max_{(\lambda=0,\boldsymbol{\gamma},\boldsymbol{\beta},\boldsymbol{\alpha})} \ell(\lambda, \boldsymbol{\gamma}, \boldsymbol{\beta}, \boldsymbol{\alpha})$, and $\hat{\boldsymbol{\theta}}_1 = \arg\max_{(\lambda=1,\boldsymbol{\gamma},\boldsymbol{\beta},\boldsymbol{\alpha})} \ell(\lambda, \boldsymbol{\gamma}, \boldsymbol{\beta}, \boldsymbol{\alpha})$. The LRTs for the two sets of hypotheses are

$$X^2_{MCM} = -2[\ell(\hat{\boldsymbol{\theta}}_1) - \ell(\hat{\boldsymbol{\theta}})], \quad X^2_{PHC} = -2[\ell(\hat{\boldsymbol{\theta}}_0) - \ell(\hat{\boldsymbol{\theta}})] \tag{2.30}$$

and the score tests are

$$Z^2_{MCM} = (\partial\ell(\boldsymbol{\theta})/\partial\lambda)^2 \Big/ \left(-\partial^2\ell(\boldsymbol{\theta})/\partial\lambda^2 - AB^{-1}A^T\right)\Big|_{\boldsymbol{\theta}=\hat{\boldsymbol{\theta}}_1},$$

$$Z^2_{PHC} = (\partial\ell(\boldsymbol{\theta})/\partial\lambda)^2 \Big/ \left(-\partial^2\ell(\boldsymbol{\theta})/\partial\lambda^2 - AB^{-1}A^T\right)\Big|_{\boldsymbol{\theta}=\hat{\boldsymbol{\theta}}_0}, \tag{2.31}$$

where $A = \left(-\frac{\partial^2 \ell(\boldsymbol{\theta})}{\partial\lambda\partial\boldsymbol{\gamma}^T}, -\frac{\partial^2 \ell(\boldsymbol{\theta})}{\partial\lambda\partial\boldsymbol{\beta}^T}, -\frac{\partial^2 \ell(\boldsymbol{\theta})}{\partial\lambda\partial\boldsymbol{\alpha}^T}\right)$ and

$$B = \begin{pmatrix} -\frac{\partial^2 \ell(\boldsymbol{\theta})}{\partial\boldsymbol{\gamma}\partial\boldsymbol{\gamma}^T} & -\frac{\partial^2 \ell(\boldsymbol{\theta})}{\partial\boldsymbol{\gamma}\partial\boldsymbol{\beta}^T} & -\frac{\partial^2 \ell(\boldsymbol{\theta})}{\partial\boldsymbol{\gamma}\partial\boldsymbol{\alpha}^T} \\ -\frac{\partial^2 \ell(\boldsymbol{\theta})}{\partial\boldsymbol{\beta}\partial\boldsymbol{\gamma}^T} & -\frac{\partial^2 \ell(\boldsymbol{\theta})}{\partial\boldsymbol{\beta}\partial\boldsymbol{\beta}^T} & -\frac{\partial^2 \ell(\boldsymbol{\theta})}{\partial\boldsymbol{\beta}\partial\boldsymbol{\alpha}^T} \\ -\frac{\partial^2 \ell(\boldsymbol{\theta})}{\partial\boldsymbol{\alpha}\partial\boldsymbol{\gamma}^T} & -\frac{\partial^2 \ell(\boldsymbol{\theta})}{\partial\boldsymbol{\alpha}\partial\boldsymbol{\beta}^T} & -\frac{\partial^2 \ell(\boldsymbol{\theta})}{\partial\boldsymbol{\alpha}\partial\boldsymbol{\alpha}^T} \end{pmatrix}.$$

For H_0 in (2.28), $\lambda = 1$ is an interior point of the parameter space of λ in (2.24). Therefore, based on the standard likelihood theory both the LRTs and the score tests approximately follow the chi-square distribution with 1 degree of freedom when the H_0 is true. For H_0 in (2.29), $\lambda = 0$ is on the boundary of the parameter space of λ. The null distribution of the score test can still be approximated by the chi-square distribution with 1 degree of freedom (Rao, 2005). The null distribution of the LRT under H_0 is however nonstandard (Self and Liang, 1987). To overcome this issue, Peng and Xu (2012) suggested to extend the domain of λ in (2.24) further into negative values by $\lambda > -\exp(-\boldsymbol{\gamma z})$ so that $\lambda = 0$ is not on the boundary and the standard LRT results can apply.

The tests have reasonable power to select between the mixture cure model and the PHC model if $F^H(t)$ is parametrically specified. It is expected that other unified cure models have similar properties.

2.5.3 Goodness of Fit by Residuals

There are not many methods proposed specifically for checking the goodness of fit of parametric cure models. One method is to use a revised Schoenfeld residual (Wileyto et al., 2013) to compare different parametric mixture cure models (2.1). Assuming the same set of covariates in both the incidence and latency parts of the mixture cure model, the revised Schoenfeld residual is defined in the following form

$$\delta_i \left[\boldsymbol{x}_i - \frac{\sum_{j=1}^n Y_j(t_i)\boldsymbol{x}_j h(t_i|\boldsymbol{x}_j, \boldsymbol{z}_j)}{\sum_{j=1}^n Y_j(t_i) h(t_i|\boldsymbol{x}_j, \boldsymbol{z}_j)} \right], \quad i = 1, \ldots, n,$$

where $h(t|\boldsymbol{x}, \boldsymbol{z})$ is the unconditional hazard function corresponding to $S(t|\boldsymbol{x}, \boldsymbol{z})$ in (2.1), $Y_i(t) = I(t_i \geq t)$, and $I(A)$ is the indicator function: $I(A) = 1$ if A is true and $I(A) = 0$ otherwise. This residual measures the difference between the covariate values of a subject with uncensored times and the weighted average of the covariate values of all subjects who are still at the risk at the uncensored time, and the unconditional hazard function at the uncensored time is used as the weight. The residuals from a correctly specified mixture cure model have zero mean and they are useful to examine the overall fit of a mixture cure model (2.1). A plot of the residuals against time is useful to reveal any patterns of the fit. The patterns can also be revealed by fitting a polynomial regression to the residuals against time.

Section 3.5 will introduce methods for assessing the fit of semiparametric and nonparametric cure models. Some of them may be used for parametric cure models too.

2.6 Software and Applications

For some simple parametric cure models, special software packages may not be required and standard statistical packages often can be used to fit them with minimal coding work. For example, a simple mixture cure model without covariates such as (2.1) with $S_u(t)$ from the exponential or Weibull distribution can be easily coded in R (Ihaka and Gentleman, 1996) or SAS (SAS Institute Inc., 2011) to obtain the maximum likelihood estimates of parameters in the model. When a complicated distribution is considered for $S_u(t)$ or nonlinear covariate effects are considered in π or in $S_u(t)$, the necessary coding becomes complicated in standard statistical software packages and specialized software packages are useful to fit such models. We will show some R software packages and SAS macros for parametric cure models discussed in this chapter and illustrate their applications to real data sets for some cure models.

The real data we consider are from a comparative study of autologous and allogeneic transplantation in patients with high-risk acute lymphoblastic leukemia from March 1982 to May 1987 (Kersey et al., 1987). In this study, 46 patients who had sibling donors HLA-matched by mixed-lymphocyte culture received allogeneic marrow transplants, and 45 Patients without a matched sibling donor and with the common B-lineage phenotypes received autologous marrow purged with a mixture of the three antibodies BA-I, BA-2, and BA-3 plus complement. One objective of the study is to assess the time to leukemia recurrence in recipients of autologous and allogeneic transplants. Some patients did not experience a relapse due to either death before a relapse or insufficient follow-up before a relapse, and their observed times are censored at the time of death or at the time of last observation. There are total 22 censored times, 13 from patients with allogeneic transplants and 9 from those with autologous transplants. The data are displayed in Table 2.1. The numbers followed by a plus sign "+" are censored times.

To demonstrate the potential presence of cured subjects in this study, we estimate the survival functions of the two groups of data with the Kaplan-Meier survival estimator (Kaplan and Meier, 1958) and plot the survival curves in Figure 2.4. The small circles on the curves mark the censored times. It can be seen that most of relapses occurred within 500 days and there is no more relapse after 1256 days until 1845 days, whereas the censoring occurred only after 500 days. The obvious plateaus in their right tails and the long follow-up in the study strongly suggest the presence of cured subjects among the study subjects, and a cure model should be considered for the data. The problems of

TABLE 2.1
Time to leukemia recurrence or relapse (days) for leukemia patients with marrow transplants

Allogeneic	Autologous
11, 14, 23, 31, 32, 35, 51, 59, 62, 78, 78, 79, 87, 99, 100, 141, 160, 166, 216, 219, 235, 250, 270, 313, 332, 352, 368, 468, 491, 511, 557, 628+, 726+, 819, 915+, 966+, 1109+, 1158+, 1256, 1614+, 1619+, 1674+, 1712+, 1745+, 1820+, 1825+	21, 40, 42, 50, 53, 54, 56, 61, 64, 67, 73, 76, 79, 81, 88, 95, 98, 98, 99, 104, 105, 106, 112, 131, 147, 171, 172, 179, 189, 195, 199, 213, 223, 224, 277, 724+, 729+, 734, 1053+, 1094+, 1192+, 1475+, 1535+, 1535+, 1845+

interest for this data include estimating cure rates in the two groups and assessing the significance of the differences between the two marrow transplants in cure rates and in survival times of the uncured patients.

2.6.1 R Package gfcure

The R package `gfcure` based on the work of Peng et al. (1998) can fit various parametric AFT mixture cure models. We use `gfcure` function in the package to fit lognormal AFT mixture cure model to the leukemia data with `transplant = 1` for Autologous group and `transplant = 0` for Allogeneic group as follows:

```
> summary(gfcure(Surv(time, cens) ~ transplant,  ~ transplant, data
+ = goldman.data, dist = "lognormal"))

Lognormal mixture model

The maximum loglikelihood is -142.4011

Terms in the accelerated failure time model:
                      Coefficients   Std.err   z-score   p-value
Log(scale)               -0.034372 0.0949418 -0.362032 0.7173281
(Intercept)               4.948055 0.1758938 28.130923 0.0000000
transplantAutologous     -0.280250 0.2406373 -1.164618 0.2441738

Terms in the logistic model:
                      Coefficients   Std.err   z-score   p-value
(Intercept)               0.990842 0.3434634  2.884853 0.0039160
transplantAutologous      0.439686 0.5162291  0.851726 0.3943664
```

The syntax of `gfcure` is similar to `survreg` in R with two formula arguments, one for the latency submodel and one for the incidence submodel, and the

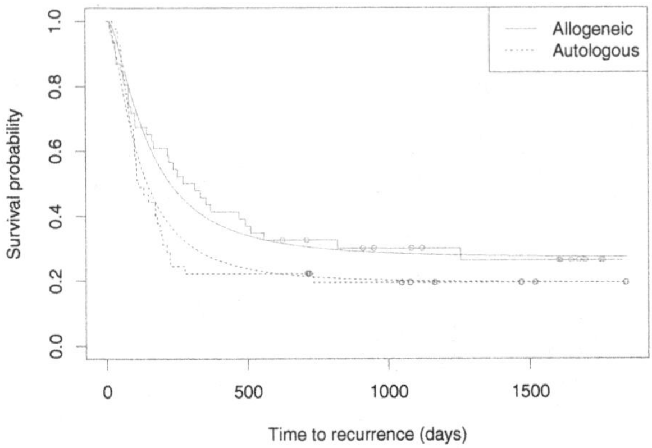

FIGURE 2.4
Estimated survival curves from the lognormal AFT mixture cure model (smooth curves) and the Kaplan-Meier method (step lines) for the two groups of leukemia patients with marrow transplants.

latter does not specify any variable to the left of ~. The estimated $\hat{\gamma} = (0.99, 0.44)'$ and $\hat{\beta} = (4.95, -0.28)'$. The estimates imply that the estimated cure rate is $1/(1 + e^{0.99}) = 0.27$ for Allogeneic group and $1/(1 + e^{0.99+0.44}) = 0.19$ for Autologous group. However, the difference in cure rate is not statistically significant. The estimated coefficient of `transplant` in the latency submodel is -0.28, which indicates that for an uncured patient, the mean log survival time in Autologous group is about 0.28 shorter than the mean log survival time in Allogeneic group, or the mean survival time of Autologous group is $e^{-0.28} = 0.76$ times of mean survival time of Allogeneic group. Again the difference in the latency submodel is not statistically significant. To examine the fit, the estimated survival curves can be obtained are plotted using `predict.gfcure` and `plot.predict.gfcure` functions as follows:

```
> z = gfcure(Surv(time, cens) ~ transplant,  ~ transplant, data =
+ goldman.data, dist = "lognormal")
> plot(survfit(Surv(time, cens) ~ transplant, data = goldman.data),
+ lty = 1:2, col = c(2,4), mark = 21, ylab = "Survival
+ probability", xlab = "Time to recurrence (days)")
> lines(predict(z, newdata = goldman.data[c(1, 91), ], newtime =
+ (1:1000)*1.845), showcure = T, col = c(2, 4))
```

The curves are plotted along with the Kaplan-Meier curves in Figure 2.4. It is easy to see that the survival curves from the lognormal AFT mixture cure models agree with the survival curves from the Kaplan-Meier survival estimator at most of time except the period around 200 to 500 days where the cure model tends to underestimate the survival probability for Allogeneic group and overestimate the survival probability for Autologous group.

Other distributions can be considered in `gfcure` for the latency part. They include `exponential`, `rayleigh`, `weibull`, `gamma`, `loglogistic`, `gll` (generalized log-logistic), `gf` (generalized F), and `egg` (extended generalized gamma). Following are `gfcure` with `exponential`, `weibull`, `gamma`, and `egg` for the leukemia data:

```
> gfcure(Surv(time, cens) ~ transplant, ~ transplant, data =
+ goldman.data, dist = "exponential")

Call:
gfcure(formula = Surv(time, cens) ~ transplant, cureform =
    ~transplant, data = goldman.data, dist = "exponential")

Distribution: Exponential

Coefficients:
         (Intercept) transplantAutologous          (Intercept)
           5.5399865           -0.6462144            0.9892163
transplantAutologous
           0.4022781

Maximized Loglikelihood: -146.0479

> gfcure(Surv(time, cens) ~ transplant, ~ transplant, data =
+ goldman.data, dist = "weibull")

Call:
gfcure(formula = Surv(time, cens) ~ transplant, cureform =
    ~transplant, data = goldman.data, dist = "weibull")

Distribution: Weibull

Coefficients:
          Log(scale)          (Intercept) transplantAutologous
          -0.1346419            5.5849274           -0.6559098
         (Intercept) transplantAutologous
           0.9708204            0.4169098

Maximized Loglikelihood: -145.0319

> gfcure(Surv(time, cens) ~ transplant, ~ transplant, data =
+ goldman.data, dist = "gamma")

Call:
gfcure(formula = Surv(time, cens) ~ transplant, cureform =
    ~transplant, data = goldman.data, dist = "gamma")

Distribution: Gamma
```

TABLE 2.2
Parametric mixture cure models with different latency distributions for the leukemia data

Latency distribution	Maximum log-likelihood	AIC	BIC	LRT	df	P-value
Generalized gamma	−142.3	296.6	311.7	-	-	-
Lognormal	−142.4	294.8	307.4	0.154	1	0.695
Weibull	−145.0	300.1	312.6	5.415	1	0.020
Gamma	−144.2	298.4	310.9	3.729	1	0.053
Exponential	−146.0	300.1	310.1	7.447	2	0.024

```
Coefficients:
              Shape           (Intercept) transplantAutologous
          0.3056717             5.2088573           -0.6249223
        (Intercept) transplantAutologous
          0.9662783             0.4216691

Maximized Loglikelihood: -144.1888

> gfcure(Surv(time, cens) ~ transplant, ~ transplant, data =
+ goldman.data, dist = "egg")

Call:
gfcure(formula = Surv(time, cens) ~ transplant, cureform =
    ~transplant, data = goldman.data, dist = "egg")

Distribution: Extended Generalized Gamma

Coefficients:
              Shape           Log(scale)          (Intercept)
         0.12433492          -0.04766131           5.03219942
transplantAutologous          (Intercept) transplantAutologous
        -0.34089158           0.98299111           0.43270369

Maximized Loglikelihood: -142.3244
```

Without a priori knowledge about the distribution, one needs to determine which parametric distribution is the most suitable as the latency distribution. One can use the methods discussed in Section 2.5 to select a distribution that provides an adequate fit to the data. Table 2.2 shows the fit of AFT mixture cure models above along with AIC and BIC values. Since the first distribution includes the rest as special cases, the LRTs to test the adequacy of the special cases relative to the first distribution are also presented in the table. It is clear that the lognormal distribution is recommended over the Weibull, gamma and the exponential distributions when used as the baseline distribution in the AFT latency submodel for the data.

2.6.2 R Package mixcure

The R package `mixcure` is designed to fit the mixture cure model by using existing R packages to fit the latency and incidence submodels of the cure model. The parametric mixture cure model can be fit by `mixcure` by using `survreg` in R package `survival` or `flexsurvreg` in R package `flexsurv` to fit the latency submodel and `glm` to fit the incidence submodel. We first use `survreg` in `mixcure` to fit the latency submodel and `glm` to fit the incidence submodel of the mixture cure model for the leukemia data. The latency distribution can be any of the distributions that are available in `survreg`. We only consider the lognormal distribution as an example.

```
> summary(mixcure(Surv(time, cens) ~ transplant, ~ transplant, data
+ = goldman.data, lmodel = list(fun = "survreg", dist =
+ "lognormal"), savedata = T))

Call:
mixcure(lformula = Surv(time, cens) ~ transplant, iformula =
    ~transplant, data = goldman.data, lmodel =
        list(fun = "survreg", dist = "lognormal"), savedata = T)

Latency model for uncured:
                      coefficient    stderr    zscore    pvalue
(Intercept)             4.9480436 0.2168121 22.821806 0.0000000
transplantAutologous   -0.2802129 0.2322965 -1.206273 0.2277124

Incidence model:
                      coefficient    stderr    zscore     pvalue
(Intercept)             0.9908102 0.3901210 2.5397510 0.01109314
transplantAutologous    0.4398913 0.5904678 0.7449878 0.45627909
```

The standard errors of the estimates are obtained by a bootstrap method when using `summary` to report the results. The results are similar to the results from `gfcure`. Note that the default model for the incidence part is `glm` with binomial distribution and `logit` link function and thus it is not specified in the above command. If one is interested in fitting a complementary log-log (2.3) instead of a logistic model (2.2) for the incidence part and the latency part stays unchanged, the model can be fitted as follows:

```
> mixcure(Surv(time, cens) ~ transplant, ~ transplant, data =
+ goldman.data, lmodel = list(fun = "survreg", dist = "lognormal"),
+ imodel = list(fun = "glm", family = binomial(link = "cloglog")),
+ savedata = T)

Call:
mixcure(lformula = Surv(time, cens) ~ transplant, iformula =
    ~transplant, data = goldman.data, lmodel =
              list(fun = "survreg", dist = "lognormal"),
    imodel = list(fun = "glm", family = binomial(link = "cloglog")),
    savedata = T)
```

```
Latency model for uncured:
                       coefficient    stderr    zscore    pvalue
(Intercept)              4.9480436 0.2270397 21.793734 0.0000000
transplantAutologous    -0.2802129 0.2659556 -1.053608 0.2920626

Incidence model:
                       coefficient    stderr    zscore    pvalue
(Intercept)              0.2673914 0.1707122 1.5663289 0.1172717
transplantAutologous     0.2304219 0.2699945 0.8534319 0.3934198
```

Other link functions, such as probit link, are also available.

`flexsurvreg` can also be used to fit parametric latency submodels with various parametric distributions in `mixcure`, including custom distributions by users. Particularly, `flexsurvspline`, a wrapper around `flexsurvreg`, can fit parametric PH, PO, and probit latency submodels with a spline-based baseline distribution by dynamically constructing a custom spline-based survival distribution. We consider to use `mixcure` to fit the PH mixture cure model (2.5) and the PO mixture cure model (2.11) for the leukemia data by using `flexsurvreg` with the log cumulative baseline hazard function and the log cumulative baseline odds function modeled by splines with 1 knot:

```
> # PH mixture cure model
> zph = mixcure(Surv(time, cens) ~ transplant, ~ transplant, data =
+ goldman.data, lmodel = list(fun = "flexsurvspline", k=1,
+ scale="hazard"))
> zph

Call:
mixcure(lformula = Surv(time, cens) ~ transplant, iformula =
    ~transplant,  data = goldman.data, lmodel = list(fun =
"flexsurvspline", k = 1, scale = "hazard"), savedata = T, debug = T)

Latency model:
Call:
flexsurvspline(formula = as.formula(ff), data = data[data$postuncure>
    0, ], weights = postuncure, k = 1, scale = "hazard")

Estimates:
                     data mean  est       L95%      U95%      se
gamma0                    NA   -10.4170  -13.4723   -7.3618    1.5588
gamma1                    NA     2.1669    1.4596    2.8742    0.3609
gamma2                    NA     0.0954    0.0403    0.1504    0.0281
transplantAutologous  0.4945     0.6656    0.1631    1.1681    0.2564
                     exp(est)  L95%      U95%
gamma0                      NA        NA        NA
gamma1                      NA        NA        NA
gamma2                      NA        NA        NA
transplantAutologous    1.9457    1.1771    3.2160
```

```
N = 91,  Events: 69,  Censored: 22
Total time at risk: 41432
Log-likelihood = -425.8415, df = 4
AIC = 859.6829

Incidence model:

Call:  structure(expression(glm(formula = postuncure ~ transplant,
data = data, ...)), srcfile = <environment>, wholeSrcref =
structure(c(1L, 0L, 2L, 0L, 0L, 0L, 1L, 2L),
srcfile = <environment>, class = "srcref"))

Coefficients:
         (Intercept)  transplantAutologous
              1.0899                0.3131

Degrees of Freedom: 90 Total (i.e. Null);  89 Residual
Null Deviance:      87.37
Residual Deviance: 86.98        AIC: 104

EM algorithm finished  59 iterations with final error 9.344802e-05

> # PO mixture cure model
> zpo = mixcure(Surv(time, cens) ~ transplant, ~ transplant, data =
+ goldman.data, lmodel = list(fun = "flexsurvspline", k=1,
+ scale="odds"))
> zpo

Call:
mixcure(lformula = Surv(time, cens) ~ transplant, iformula =
    ~transplant, data = goldman.data,
    lmodel = list(fun = "flexsurvspline", k = 1, scale = "odds"),
    savedata = T, debug = T)

Latency model:
Call:
flexsurvspline(formula = as.formula(ff),
    data = data[data$postuncure > 0, ],
    weights = postuncure, k = 1, scale = "odds")

Estimates:
                     data mean  est       L95%      U95%      se
gamma0                      NA  -11.9844  -15.4662   -8.5027   1.7764
gamma1                      NA    2.5649    1.7533    3.3765   0.4141
gamma2                      NA    0.1182    0.0541    0.1824   0.0327
transplantAutologous 0.4945     0.6525   -0.1205    1.4255   0.3944
                     exp(est)  L95%      U95%
gamma0                      NA        NA        NA
```

```
gamma1                      NA        NA        NA
gamma2                      NA        NA        NA
transplantAutologous 1.9203    0.8865    4.1599

N = 91,  Events: 69,  Censored: 22
Total time at risk: 41432
Log-likelihood = -453.9555, df = 4
AIC = 915.9111

Incidence model:

Call:  structure(expression(glm(formula = postuncure ~ transplant,
   data = data, ...)), srcfile = <environment>,
   wholeSrcref = structure(c(1L, 0L, 2L, 0L, 0L, 0L, 1L, 2L),
         srcfile = <environment>, class = "srcref"))

Coefficients:
         (Intercept)  transplantAutologous
             1.99655               0.08252

Degrees of Freedom: 90 Total (i.e. Null);  89 Residual
Null Deviance:       35.17
Residual Deviance: 35.15        AIC: 55.43

EM algorithm finished  6 iterations with final error 5.917918e-05
```

Note the standard errors and confidence intervals reported above are directly from `flexsurvspline` and `glm` and they do not provide correct standard errors and confidence intervals for the estimates in the mixture cure models. Correct standard errors and confidence intervals should be obtained using `summary` as we did above. The fit of the two models to the data can be examined by estimating the unconditional survival functions $S(t)$ from the models and plot them as follows:

```
> plot(survfit(Surv(time, cens) ~ transplant, data = goldman.data),
+ mark = 21, ylab = "Survival probability", xlab = "Time to
+ recurrence (days)")
> plot(predict(zph, newdata = goldman.data[c(1, 91), ], times =
+ 1:2000), add = T, lty = c(2,2))
> plot(predict(zpo, newdata = goldman.data[c(1, 91), ], times =
+ 1:2000), add = T, lty = c(3,3))
> legend("topright", legend = c("KM", "PH mixture cure", "PO
+ mixture cure"), lty = 1:3)
```

Figure 2.5 shows the estimated survival functions. It is clear that the PH mixture cure model fits the data better than the PO mixture cure model.

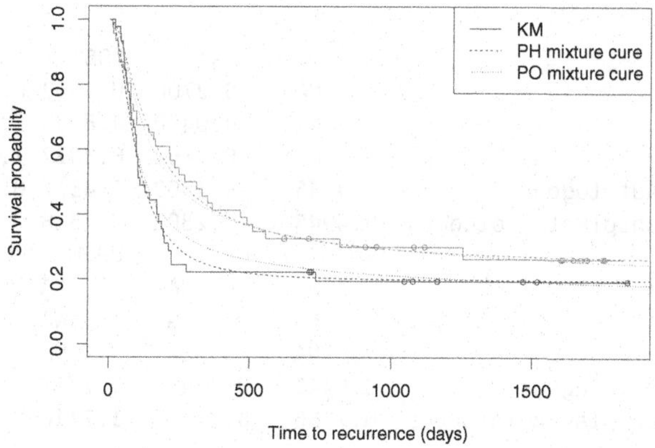

FIGURE 2.5
Estimated survival curves from the PH and PO mixture cure models with spline-based baseline distributions (smooth curves) and the Kaplan-Meier method (step lines) for the two groups (top: Allogeneic, bottom: Autologous) of leukemia patients with marrow transplants.

In addition to `survival` and `flexsurv`, it is possible to consider other R packages that can fit parametric survival models in `mixcure`. Check the manual of `mixcure` for details.

2.6.3 R Package flexsurvcure

The R package `flexsurvcure` is a wrapper for R package `flexsurv` to fit various parametric cure models, including both mixture and non-mixture cure models. It achieves this by providing custom distributions that correspond to cure models and supplying them to `flexsurv`. The feature of `flexsurv` to allow arbitrary-dimension distributions, such as spline-based hazard functions, can also be used in cure models when using `flexsurvcure`. The other feature of `flexsurv` to allow other parameters in a distribution to depend on covariates makes the resulting cure models more flexible than the parametric cure models discussed in previous sections. We first demonstrate how `flexsurvcure` can fit the lognormal mixture cure model to the leukemia data as follows:

```
> zm = flexsurvcure(Surv(time,cens) ~ transplant +
+ meanlog(transplant), data = goldman.data, dist = "lnorm", link =
+ "logistic")
> zm

Call:
flexsurvcure(formula = Surv(time, cens) ~ transplant +
    meanlog(transplant), data = goldman.data,
                dist = "lnorm", link = "logistic")
```

```
Estimates:
                                data mean  est      L95%    U95%    se
theta                                NA    0.2708   0.1592  0.4212      NA
meanlog                              NA    4.9480   4.6033  5.2928  0.1759
sdlog                                NA    0.9662   0.8022  1.1638  0.0917
transplantAutologous             0.4945   -0.4399  -1.4517  0.5719  0.5162
meanlog(transplantAutologous)    0.4945   -0.2802  -0.7518  0.1914  0.2406
                                exp(est)  L95%     U95%
theta                                NA       NA       NA
meanlog                              NA       NA       NA
sdlog                                NA       NA       NA
transplantAutologous             0.6441   0.2342   1.7717
meanlog(transplantAutologous)    0.7556   0.4715   1.2110

N = 91,  Events: 69,  Censored: 22
Total time at risk: 41432
Log-likelihood = -471.7213, df = 5
AIC = 953.4426
```

The results are similar to the results from gfcure. However, the reported maximum likelihood, AIC and BIC values are different due to different parameterization.

We then consider to fit the data with the PHC model (2.18), a non-mixture cure model. To make the model more comparable with the mixture cure model above, we assume that $F^H(t)$ is from the lognormal distribution and the location parameter in the lognormal distribution is a linear function of the treatment group variable.

```
> znm = flexsurvcure(Surv(time, cens) ~ transplant +
+ meanlog(transplant), data = goldman.data, dist = "lnorm", link =
+ "loglog", mixture = FALSE)
> znm

Call:
flexsurvcure(formula = Surv(time, cens) ~ transplant +
    meanlog(transplant), data = goldman.data,
                dist = "lnorm", link = "loglog", mixture = FALSE)

Estimates:
                                data mean est      L95%    U95%    se
theta                                NA   0.2840   0.4211  0.1601      NA
meanlog                              NA   5.2861   4.8583  5.7140  0.2183
sdlog                                NA   1.0285   0.8350  1.2669  0.1094
transplantAutologous             0.4945   0.3712  -0.1631  0.9056  0.2726
meanlog(transplantAutologous)    0.4945  -0.0425  -0.5786  0.4936  0.2735
                                exp(est)  L95%     U95%
theta                                NA       NA       NA
meanlog                              NA       NA       NA
sdlog                                NA       NA       NA
```

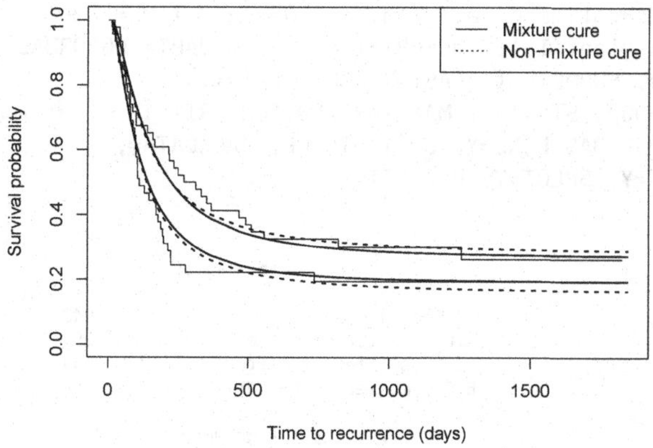

FIGURE 2.6
Estimated survival curves from the mixture cure and non-mixture cure models with lognormal distributions (smooth curves) and the Kaplan-Meier method (step lines) for the two groups (top: Allogeneic, bottom: Autologous) of leukemia patients with marrow transplants.

```
transplantAutologous            1.4495   0.8495  2.4733
meanlog(transplantAutologous) 0.9584   0.5607  1.6383

N = 91,  Events: 69,  Censored: 22
Total time at risk: 41432
Log-likelihood = -471.2055, df = 5
AIC = 952.411
```

The fit of the two models can be compared by plotting the estimated survival functions from the two models as follows:

```
> plot(zm, col = 1, ylab = "Survival probability", xlab = "Time to
+ recurrence (days)")
> plot(znm, add = T, lty = 2, col = 1)
> legend("topright", legend = c("Mixture cure", "Non-mixture
+ cure"), lty = 1:2)
```

The fitted survival curves are shown in Figure 2.6. It appears that the mixture model shows a slightly better fit to the right tail of the Kaplan-Meier survival curves than the non-mixture cure model.

2.6.4 SAS Macro PSPMCM

The SAS macro `PSPMCM` (Corbiere and Joly, 2007) implements the parametric AFT mixture cure model with the several distributions as the latency distribution, including `EXP` (exponential), `WEIBULL`, `LLOGISTIC`, and `LOGNORMAL`. We use the macro to fit the lognormal mixture cure model to the leukemia data:

```
%pspmcm(DATA=goldmandata,ID=id,CENSCOD=cens,TIME=time,
  VAR= transplant(IS), INCPART=logit, SURVPART=LOGNORMAL,
  TAIL=zero, SU0MET=pl, FAST=Y,BOOTSTRAP=Y,
  NSAMPLE=2000, STRATA=, MAXITER=200,CONVCRIT=1e-5,
  ALPHA=0.05, BASELINE=Y, BOOTMET=ALL, JACKDATA=,
  GESTIMATE=Y, SPLOT=Y, PLOTFIT=Y);
run;
```

```
                              Fit Statistics

          -2 Log Likelihood                    943.4
          AIC (smaller is better)              953.4
          AICC (smaller is better)             954.1
          BIC (smaller is better)              966.0

                         results for goldmandata
                    distribution LOGNORMAL, link=LOGIT

                           Parameter Estimates

                      Standard                               95% Confidence
Parameter     Estimate    Error  DF  t Value  Pr > |t|          Limits        Gradient
L_int           0.9908   0.3435  91     2.88    0.0049   0.3086   1.6730  -0.00003
L_TRANSPLANT    0.4399   0.5162  91     0.85    0.3964  -0.5856   1.4654  -8.49E-6
_scale          4.9480   0.1759  91    28.13    <.0001   4.5986   5.2974  -0.00002
S_TRANSPLANT    0.2900   0.2499  91     1.16    0.2489  -0.2064   0.7864     -8E-6
_shape          0.9662  0.09174  91    10.53    <.0001   0.7840   1.1485  0.000029
```

The results are similar to the results from `gfcure`. Again, the reported maximum likelihood, AIC and BIC values are different due to different parameterization.

2.7 Summary

In this chapter, we presented the basics of parametric mixture cure models and their estimation methods. Because of the finite number of parameters in the models, the maximum likelihood estimation method can be readily used to estimate the parameters in the models. In particular, we showed in detail how the EM algorithm is used to obtain the maximum likelihood estimates of the parameters in the parametric models. The EM algorithm is an important estimation method for mixture models and is widely used for cure models. The chapter also described some parametric non-mixture cure models and the cure models that unify the mixture cure models and non-mixture cure models. Some methods for model selection and goodness-of-fit assessment were also introduced. Finally, we demonstrated 3 R packages and 1 SAS macro that can be used to fit some parametric cure models. This chapter provides the foundation of cure models for the remaining chapters.

The mixture cure model is also known as a mover-stayer model in some fields. See Yamaguchi (2003) and Shen and Cook (2014) for some further discussions under the mover-stayer model.

Even though the application of parametric cure models may be limited by their strong parametric assumptions, they are still widely used because of their simple estimation methods and smoothed estimates of the latency survival functions that allow extrapolation.

We did not include any discussions on the asymptotic properties in this chapter because the asymptotic properties of the maximum likelihood estimates usually follow from the large sample likelihood theory.

3

The Semiparametric and Nonparametric Cure Models

3.1 Introduction

Parametric cure models introduced in the last chapter are attractive in their relatively simple estimation methods, and they are usually very efficient and allow for extrapolation if the parametric assumptions are acceptable. However, verifying the parametric assumptions, particularly the assumptions for the latency distribution, can be challenging. The strong parametric assumptions increase the risk of misspecification of the cure model for a given data, which can lead to biased estimates. Semiparametric and nonparametric cure models are proposed to relax the assumptions so that the results are less sensitive to the model assumptions. We first introduce semiparametric mixture cure models in Section 3.2, which do not make parametric assumptions in the baseline distribution of the latency submodel. Fully nonparametric approaches are introduced in Section 3.3. Section 3.4 presents semiparametric estimation methods for some non-mixture cure models. Section 3.5 discusses some model assessment methods for semiparametric and nonparametric cure methods, followed by Section 3.6 on available software for the some discussed models and their applications to real data. This chapter also primarily focuses on independent and right-censored data.

3.2 Semiparametric Mixture Cure Models

Both the incidence and latency parts of a mixture cure model can be modeled with weaker and semiparametric or nonparametric assumptions. In this section, we focus on the latency part of the mixture model only and introduce a few semiparametric approaches. The incidence part of the mixture cure model is specified in the same way as described in Section 2.2.1.

3.2.1 Semiparametric PH Latency Submodel

If the effects of $\boldsymbol{x}$ on $S_u(t)$ is modeled using the PH assumption in (2.5) and the baseline survival function $S_u(\cdot)$ is not parametrically specified, we have a semiparametric PH model for the latency part. Due to the unspecified baseline survival function, the direct maximization of the likelihood function (2.12) in Section 2.3.1 becomes challenging (Lu, 2008). We demonstrate how the EM algorithm in Section 2.3.2 becomes a better way to estimate the model, as proposed by many researchers (Peng and Dear, 2000; Sy and Taylor, 2000; Peng, 2003b).

Under the PH latency submodel (2.5), the corresponding hazard function is $h_u(t|\boldsymbol{x}) = h_{u0}(t)e^{\boldsymbol{\beta}'\boldsymbol{x}}$, and (2.16) becomes

$$\ell_2(\boldsymbol{\beta}, S_{u0}) = \sum_{i=1}^{n} w_i \left\{\delta_i \log h_{u0}(t_i) + \delta_i \boldsymbol{\beta}'\boldsymbol{x}_i + e^{\boldsymbol{\beta}'\boldsymbol{x}_i} \log[S_{u0}(t_i)]\right\} \tag{3.1}$$

$$= \sum_{i=1}^{n} \left\{\delta_i \log h_{u0}(t_i) + \delta_i \boldsymbol{\beta}'\boldsymbol{x}_i + e^{\log w_i + \boldsymbol{\beta}'\boldsymbol{x}_i} \log[S_{u0}(t_i)]\right\} \tag{3.2}$$

where the fact that $w_i = 1$ and $\log w_i = 0$ for $\delta_i = 1$ is used to obtain (3.2). As discussed in Section 2.3.2, (3.1) can be viewed as a weighted likelihood function from a PH model for all the subjects with $w_i > 0$. On the other hand, (3.2) can be viewed as the log-likelihood function from the PH model with $\log w_i$ as an offset term. Therefore, $\boldsymbol{\beta}$ and $S_{u0}(\cdot)$ can be updated either by the Newton-Raphson method or by an existing software package for the classical PH model that accepts either case weights or offset terms.

If $S_{u0}(t)$ is unspecified or nonparametrically specified, it is easy to see that (3.1) or (3.2) becomes the log-likelihood function considered in the context of the Cox PH model with the weights w_i or the offset terms $\log w_i$, which suggests that $\boldsymbol{\beta}$ and S_{u0} be updated separately as in Cox's PH model (Peng and Dear, 2000), where $\boldsymbol{\beta}$ is updated via the following partial log-likelihood function corresponding to (3.2)

$$\log \prod_{j=1}^{k} \frac{\exp(\boldsymbol{\beta}'\boldsymbol{s}_j)}{\left\{\sum_{i\in R_j} \exp(\log w_i + \boldsymbol{\beta}'\boldsymbol{x}_i)\right\}^{d_j}},$$

k is the number of distinct uncensored times $\tau_1 < \tau_2 < \cdots \tau_k$ in the data, $\boldsymbol{s}_j = \sum_{i:t_i=\tau_j} \delta_i \boldsymbol{x}_i$, d_j is the number of uncensored times equal to τ_j, and R_j is the risk set at τ_j. With updated $\hat{\boldsymbol{\beta}}$, the baseline survival function $S_{u0}(t)$ can be estimated with the Nelson-Aalen estimator

$$\hat{S}_{u0}(t) = \exp\left(-\sum_{j:\tau_j<t} \frac{d_j}{\sum_{i\in R_j} \exp(\log w_i + \hat{\boldsymbol{\beta}}'\boldsymbol{x}_i)}\right). \tag{3.3}$$

This approach can be easily implemented using existing software for Cox's

PH model. The M-step also maximizes (2.15), which can be carried out as described in Section 2.3.2.

Another approach is to use a discrete distribution that has probability mass on the distinct uncensored times only to approximate the failure time distribution of $T|Y = 1$ (Sy and Taylor, 2000). The likelihood function (3.2) reduces to

$$\log \prod_{j=1}^{k} \left[\prod_{i \in D_j} h_{u0}(\tau_j) e^{\boldsymbol{\beta}'\boldsymbol{x}_i} S_{u0}(\tau_j -)^{\exp(\boldsymbol{\beta}'\boldsymbol{x}_i)} \prod_{i \in C_j} S_{u0}(\tau_j)^{w_i \exp(\boldsymbol{\beta}'\boldsymbol{x}_i)} \right]$$

which can be readily maximized using the Newton-Raphson method. However few existing programs for Cox's PH model are readily available to maximize this log likelihood and a specialized software program is required.

The standard errors of the estimates can be obtained using the method of Louis (1982) after the EM algorithm converges if the approach of Sy and Taylor (2000) is used in the M-step. See Sy and Taylor (2001) for details. If the approach of Peng and Dear (2000) is used in the M-step, a bootstrap method may be used to estimate the standard errors of the estimates.

The methods above only produce a nonparametric non-smooth estimate of the baseline survival function $S_{u0}(t)$. If a smooth baseline survival function is preferred, the PH mixture cure model can be estimated by allowing flexible modeling of the hazard function $h_{u0}(t)$ using M-splines (Corbiere et al., 2009). The smoothing parameter in the M-splines can be determined using cross-validation.

3.2.1.1 Restrictions on the Upper Tail of the Baseline Distribution

Due to the presence of substantial censoring after τ_k, the nonparametric estimate of the baseline survival function $\hat{S}_{u0}(t) \not\to 0$ when $t \geq \tau_k$. Even though this is not an issue in the standard PH model, it causes an identifiability issue in the cure model context: It essentially implies that there is a non-zero probability for an uncured subject to never have any event. To alleviate this identifiability issue, $\hat{S}_{u0}(t)$ should go to 0 soon after τ_k if there is sufficient follow-up in a study. A popular approach is to impose a zero tail restriction on the survival estimate (Taylor, 1995). That is, $\hat{S}_{u0}(t) = 0$ for any $t \geq \tau_k$. This approach is simple to use, supported by other studies such as Maller and Zhou (1992, 1994), and is widely used in other semiparametric cure models in the following sections. Other more complicated approaches can be considered to allow $\hat{S}_{u0}(t)$ to go to zero gradually from $\hat{S}_{u0}(\tau_k)$, for example, at the same rate as an exponential survival function (ETAIL) or as a Weibull survival function (WTAIL) (Peng, 2003a), an idea similar to that used by Moeschberger and Klein (1985) for the Kaplan-Meier survival estimator.

3.2.1.2 Time-Dependent Covariates in the Latency Submodel

Time-dependent covariates can be conveniently included in Cox's PH model. They can also be considered in the latency submodel of the semiparametric PH mixture cure model (Dirick et al., 2017). Assume that the covariates in $\boldsymbol{x}$ are allowed to be time-dependent and denoted as $\boldsymbol{x}(t)$. Then the latency submodel can be written as

$$h_u(t|\boldsymbol{x}) = h_{u0}(t)e^{\boldsymbol{x}(t)'\boldsymbol{\beta}}$$

The corresponding cumulative hazard function is:

$$H_u(t|\boldsymbol{x}\{t\}) = \int_0^t h_{u0}(s)e^{\boldsymbol{\beta}'\boldsymbol{x}(s)}ds \tag{3.4}$$

where $\boldsymbol{x}\{t\} = \{\boldsymbol{x}(s); 0 < s \leq t\}$ is the history of $\boldsymbol{x}$ up to t. It is worth to point out that $S_u(t|\boldsymbol{x}\{t\}) = \exp[-H_u(t|\boldsymbol{x}\{t\})]$ and the effects of $\boldsymbol{x}$ cannot be factored out from the integration as in the usual PH model due to the presence of the time-dependent covariates, and estimating the baseline hazard function $h_{u0}(t)$ or the cumulative baseline hazard function $H_{u0}(t)$ is no longer useful. Given the current estimates $\hat{\boldsymbol{\beta}}$, a Nelson-Aalen estimator of the cumulative hazard function $H_u(t|\boldsymbol{x}\{t\})$ can be considered as follows (Dong et al., 2020):

$$\hat{H}_u(t|\boldsymbol{x}\{t\}) = \sum_{i=1}^{n} \int_0^t \frac{e^{\hat{\boldsymbol{\beta}}'\boldsymbol{x}(s)}dN_i(s)}{\sum_{j=1}^{n} Y_j(s)w_j e^{\hat{\boldsymbol{\beta}}'\boldsymbol{x}_j(s)}} \tag{3.5}$$

and the corresponding survival estimator is $\hat{S}_u(t|\boldsymbol{x}\{t\}) = \exp[-\hat{H}_u(t|\boldsymbol{x}\{t\})]$. As suggested by Thomas and Reyes (2014) for the PH model, the cumulative hazard function above can be readily obtained using `PHREG` in SAS if the following form is considered:

$$\hat{H}_u(t|\boldsymbol{x}\{t\}) = \sum_{i=1}^{n} \int_0^t \frac{dN_i(s)}{\sum_{j=1}^{n} Y_j(s)w_j e^{\hat{\boldsymbol{\beta}}'[\boldsymbol{x}_j(s)-\boldsymbol{x}(s)]}} \tag{3.6}$$

which implies that the cumulative hazard function can be obtained if $\boldsymbol{x}_j(t)$ is replaced with $\boldsymbol{x}_j(t) - \boldsymbol{x}(t)$.

Generally, there are two classes of time-dependent covariates, internal time-dependent covariates and external time-dependent covariates (Kalbfleisch and Prentice, 2002). The observation of an internal time-dependent covariates requires that the study subject be at risk while this is not required for an external time-dependent covariate. Thus, caution should be exercised when using internal time-dependent covariates in the latency submodel.

3.2.2 Semiparametric AFT Latency Submodel

If the effects of $\boldsymbol{x}$ on $S_u(t)$ is specified under the AFT in (2.6) and the baseline survival function $S_{u0}(t)$ is not parametrically specified, we have a semiparametric AFT model for the latency part. Similarly, due to the unspecified baseline survival function, the direct maximization of the likelihood function (2.12) in Section 2.3.1 becomes infeasible and the EM algorithm in Section 2.3.2 is often used to estimate the model, as suggested by many researchers (Li and Taylor, 2002a,b; Zhang and Peng, 2007; Lu, 2010). Even though (2.16) in theory can be updated with a program for the semiparametric AFT model that takes case weights, such a program, unlike those for the semiparametric PH model, is still rare and not available in mainstream statistical software packages. We will introduce a few proposed semiparametric methods to update $\boldsymbol{\beta}$ and $S_{u0}(t)$ in the AFT latency submodel.

3.2.2.1 Linear Rank Method

Let $f_0(\cdot)$, $h_0(\cdot)$, and $S_0(\cdot)$ be the density, hazard, and survival functions of ϵ in (2.7). The log-likelihood function (2.16) can be written as a function of $f_0(\cdot)$, $h_0(\cdot)$, and $S_0(\cdot)$ as follows:

$$\begin{aligned}\ell_2(\boldsymbol{\beta},\boldsymbol{\alpha}) &= \sum_{i=1,w_i>0}^{n}\{\delta_i \log f_0(\log t_i - \boldsymbol{\beta}'\boldsymbol{x}_i) + w_i(1-\delta_i)\log[S_0(\log t_i - \boldsymbol{\beta}'\boldsymbol{x}_i)]\}\\ &= \sum_{i=1,w_i>0}^{n}\{\delta_i \log h_0(\log t_i - \boldsymbol{\beta}'\boldsymbol{x}_i) + w_i\log[S_0(\log t_i - \boldsymbol{\beta}'\boldsymbol{x}_i)]\} \quad (3.7)\end{aligned}$$

The following rank-like estimating function can be used to update $\boldsymbol{\beta}$ in the above likelihood function (Zhang and Peng, 2007):

$$\sum_{i=1}^{n}\delta_i g(\epsilon_i)\left(\boldsymbol{x}_i - \frac{\sum_{j=1}^{n}\boldsymbol{x}_j w_j I(\epsilon_j \ge \epsilon_i)}{\sum_{j=1}^{n} w_j I(\epsilon_j \ge \epsilon_i)}\right),$$

where $\epsilon_i = \log t_i - \boldsymbol{\beta}'\boldsymbol{x}_i$ and $g(\cdot)$ is a weight function. A Gehan-type weight function $g(u) = \sum_{j=1}^{n} I(\epsilon_j \ge u)w_j/n$ will further simplify the above estimating function into

$$n^{-1}\sum_{i=1}^{n}\sum_{j=1}^{n}\delta_i(\boldsymbol{x}_i - \boldsymbol{x}_j)w_j I(\epsilon_j \ge \epsilon_i),$$

which can be viewed as a gradient of a convex function that can be minimized by the linear programming method (Jin et al., 2003).

Given estimated $\hat{\boldsymbol{\beta}}$, the survival function of ϵ can also be estimated nonparametrically using the Nelson-Aalen estimator:

$$\hat{S}_0(\epsilon) = \exp\left(-\sum_{j:\tau_j^* < \epsilon}\frac{d_j}{\sum_{i\in R_j} w_i}\right), \quad (3.8)$$

where $\tau_1^* < \tau_2^* < \cdots < \tau_k^*$ are distinct uncensored values of $\log t_i - \boldsymbol{\beta}'\boldsymbol{x}_i$ and d_j and R_j are the corresponding number of uncensored times and the risk set at τ_j^*. A zero-tail restriction discussed in Section 3.2.1.1 is recommended for this estimator to alleviate the identifiability issue. An estimate of $S_{u0}(t)$ can be obtained easily from $\hat{S}_0(\epsilon)$.

3.2.2.2 M-Estimation Method

Another semiparametric approach for the semiparametric model in the AFT latency part is based on the score function of the likelihood function (3.7) (Li and Taylor, 2002b):

$$\sum_{i=1,w_i>0}^{n} \boldsymbol{x}_i \left\{ -\delta_i \frac{f_0'}{f_0}(\log t_i - \boldsymbol{\beta}'\boldsymbol{x}_i) + w_i(1-\delta_i)\frac{f_0}{S_0}(\log t_i - \boldsymbol{\beta}'\boldsymbol{x}_i) \right\},$$

which can be written into the following general estimating equation for $\boldsymbol{\beta}$:

$$\sum_{i=1,w_i>0}^{n} \boldsymbol{x}_i \left\{ -\delta_i s(\log t_i - \boldsymbol{\beta}'\boldsymbol{x}_i) - w_i(1-\delta_i)\frac{\int_{\log t_i - \boldsymbol{\beta}'\boldsymbol{x}_i}^{\infty} s(u)dS_0(u)}{S_0(\log t_i - \boldsymbol{\beta}'\boldsymbol{x}_i)} \right\},$$

where $s(u)$ is a reasonable score function, such as $s(u) = u$. For the unknown survival function $S_0(t)$, it can be estimated by (3.8).

This method and the linear rank method in the last section can be viewed as extensions of the semiparametric methods proposed for the AFT model (Ritov, 1990), and the two methods are asymptotically equivalent (Zhang and Peng, 2012). However, both methods involve non-smooth estimating equations, which can be challenging in implementing the methods. The following method will address this issue directly.

3.2.2.3 Kernel Smoothing Method

To avoid the non-smoothed likelihood functions and estimating equations, a semiparametric kernel smoothed likelihood function can be used to approximate the likelihood function (2.16) (Lu, 2010; Zeng and Lin, 2007), which leads to the following likelihood function for $\boldsymbol{\beta}$:

$$\frac{1}{n}\sum_{i=1}^{n} \delta_i \log\left[\frac{1}{n}\sum_{j=1}^{n} \delta_j K_h(\log t_j - \log t_i + \boldsymbol{\beta}'\boldsymbol{x}_i - \boldsymbol{\beta}'\boldsymbol{x}_j)\right]$$
$$- \frac{1}{n}\sum_{i=1}^{n} \delta_i \log\left[\frac{1}{n}\sum_{j=1}^{n} w_j \int_{-\infty}^{\log t_j - \log t_i + \boldsymbol{\beta}'\boldsymbol{x}_i - \boldsymbol{\beta}'\boldsymbol{x}_j} K_h(u)du\right],$$

where $K_h(u) = K(u/h)/h$ is a kernel function with bandwidth h and a symmetric function $K(u)$. The examples of the kernel function include (Härdle et al., 2004):

- Gaussian density kernel: $K(x) = \frac{1}{\sqrt{2\pi}}\exp\left(-\frac{1}{2}x^2\right)$,
- cosine kernel: $K(x) = \frac{\pi}{4}\cos\left(\frac{\pi}{2}x\right)$ for $|x| \leq 1$,
- tri-weight kernel: $K(x) = \frac{35}{32}(1-x^2)^3$ for $|x| \leq 1$,

- triangular kernel: $K(x) = (1 - |x|)$ for $|x| \leq 1$.

The resulting likelihood function is a smooth function of $\boldsymbol{\beta}$ and can be maximized readily using the Newton-Raphson method. With the estimated $\hat{\boldsymbol{\beta}}$, the baseline hazard function can be estimated by a smoothed estimator

$$\hat{h}_{u0}(t) = \frac{t^{-1}\sum_{i=1}^{n} \delta_i K_h(\log t_i - \hat{\boldsymbol{\beta}}'\boldsymbol{x}_i - \log t)}{\sum_{i=1}^{n} w_i \int_{-\infty}^{\log t_i - \hat{\boldsymbol{\beta}}'\boldsymbol{x}_i - \log t} K_h(u)du}.$$

The estimates from the smoothed likelihood function can achieve semiparametric efficiency bound for $\boldsymbol{\beta}$ and $\boldsymbol{\gamma}$ in theory. Practically, the results of the kernel method depend on the value of the bandwidth h. Lu (2010) suggested two optimal bandwidth formulas: $(8\sqrt{2}/3)^{1/5}\sigma_1 n^{-1/5}$ and $4^{1/3}\sigma_2 n^{-1/3}$, where σ_1 is the sample standard deviation of the $(\log t_i - \boldsymbol{\beta}_{1,ls}'\boldsymbol{x}_i)$ for uncensored data with $\boldsymbol{\beta}_{1,ls}$ the least square estimate of $\boldsymbol{\beta}$ using only uncensored data, while σ_2 is the sample standard deviation of the $(\log t_i - \boldsymbol{\beta}_{2,ls}'\boldsymbol{x}_i)$ for all the data with $\boldsymbol{\beta}_{2,ls}$ the corresponding least square estimate of $\boldsymbol{\beta}$.

It is worth to note that the zero-tail restriction discussed in Section 3.2.1.1 should be considered for all the methods proposed for the semiparametric AFT mixture cure model to reduce the identifiability issue.

3.2.3 Semiparametric AH Latency Submodel

When the latency survival function $S_u(t|\boldsymbol{x})$ follows the AH model (2.10) and the baseline survival function is not parametrically specified, the direct maximization method is not easy to use as in the previous semiparametric models, and the EM algorithm is preferred. We introduce two semiparametric methods based on the EM algorithm to estimate the parameters in the latency submodel.

3.2.3.1 Linear Rank Method

One method is to use a rank-type estimating equation to update $\boldsymbol{\beta}$ (Zhang and Peng, 2009a). This method is based on the fact that under the AH model, (2.16) can be written as

$$\ell_2(\boldsymbol{\beta}, \boldsymbol{\alpha}) = \sum_{i=1, w_i>0}^{n} \left\{ \delta_i \log \left[w_i h_{u0}(t_i e^{\boldsymbol{\beta}'\boldsymbol{x}_i}) \right] + \log \left[S_{u0}(t_i e^{\boldsymbol{\beta}'\boldsymbol{x}_i})^{w_i \exp(-\boldsymbol{\beta}'\boldsymbol{x}_i)} \right] \right\}, \tag{3.9}$$

which can be viewed as the log-likelihood function of the AH model with the hazard function $w_i h_{u0}(t_i e^{\boldsymbol{\beta}'\boldsymbol{x}_i})$. Thus following Chen and Wang (2000) and Chen (2001), a rank-type estimating equation for $\boldsymbol{\beta}$ can be constructed as follows:

$$\sum_{i=1}^{n} \delta_i g(t_i e^{\boldsymbol{\beta}'\boldsymbol{x}_i}) \left(\boldsymbol{x}_i - \frac{\sum_{j=1}^{n} \boldsymbol{x}_j w_j e^{-\boldsymbol{\beta}'\boldsymbol{x}_j} I(t_j e^{\boldsymbol{\beta}'\boldsymbol{x}_j} \geq t_i e^{\boldsymbol{\beta}'\boldsymbol{x}_i})}{\sum_{j=1}^{n} w_j e^{-\boldsymbol{\beta}'\boldsymbol{x}_j} I(t_j e^{\boldsymbol{\beta}'\boldsymbol{x}_j} \geq t_i e^{\boldsymbol{\beta}'\boldsymbol{x}_i})} \right), \tag{3.10}$$

with $g(\cdot)$ as a weight function. It can be further simplified as

$$\frac{1}{n}\sum_{i=1}^{n}\sum_{j=1}^{n}\delta_i(\boldsymbol{x}_i-\boldsymbol{x}_j)w_je^{-\boldsymbol{\beta}'\boldsymbol{x}_j}I(t_je^{\boldsymbol{\beta}'\boldsymbol{x}_j}\geq t_ie^{\boldsymbol{\beta}'\boldsymbol{x}_i}),$$

if $g(u)=\frac{1}{n}\sum_{j=1}^{n}w_je^{-\boldsymbol{\beta}'\boldsymbol{x}_j}I(t_je^{\boldsymbol{\beta}'\boldsymbol{x}_j}\geq u)$. With an updated $\hat{\boldsymbol{\beta}}$ from the estimating equation, the baseline cumulative hazard function estimate can be obtained as

$$\hat{H}_{u0}(t)=\sum_{j:\tau_j<t}\frac{d_j}{\sum_{i\in R_j}w_i\exp(-\hat{\boldsymbol{\beta}}'\boldsymbol{x}_i)}.$$

This will complete the M-step and the EM algorithm in Section 2.3.2 can proceed.

3.2.3.2 Kernel Smoothing Method

The linear rank method suffers the same computational issues as the one for the AFT mixture cure model due to the non-smooth estimating equation (3.10). One can use a kernel smoothing method similar to the one considered for the AFT mixture cure model in Section 3.2.2.3 to estimate the parameters in the semiparametric AH mixture cure model (Zhang et al., 2013). Under this method, a kernel smoothed likelihood function that approximates (3.9) is

$$-\frac{1}{n}\sum_{i=1}^{n}\delta_i\boldsymbol{\beta}'\boldsymbol{x}_i+\frac{1}{n}\sum_{i=1}^{n}\delta_i\log\left[\frac{1}{n}\sum_{j=1}^{n}\delta_jK_h(\log t_j-\log t_i+\boldsymbol{\beta}'\boldsymbol{x}_j-\boldsymbol{\beta}'\boldsymbol{x}_i)\right]$$
$$-\frac{1}{n}\sum_{i=1}^{n}\delta_i\log\left[\frac{1}{n}\sum_{j=1}^{n}w_j\int_{-\infty}^{\log t_j-\log t_i+\boldsymbol{\beta}'\boldsymbol{x}_j-\boldsymbol{\beta}'\boldsymbol{x}_i}e^{-\boldsymbol{\beta}'\boldsymbol{x}_j}K_h(u)du\right].$$

This function can be maximized via the Newton-Raphson method to obtain an updated estimate $\hat{\boldsymbol{\beta}}$, with which the baseline hazard function can be estimated by

$$\hat{h}_{u0}(t)=\frac{t^{-1}\sum_{i=1}^{n}\delta_iK_h(\log t_i+\hat{\boldsymbol{\beta}}'\boldsymbol{x}_i-\log t)}{\sum_{i=1}^{n}w_ie^{-\hat{\boldsymbol{\beta}}'\boldsymbol{x}_i}\int_{-\infty}^{\log t_i+\hat{\boldsymbol{\beta}}'\boldsymbol{x}_i-\log t}K_h(u)du}.$$

The bandwidth h can be chosen from $\sigma n^{-1/3}$, $\sigma n^{-1/5}$ and $\sigma n^{-1/7}$, where σ is the sample standard deviation of $\log t_i$.

Similar to the semiparametric AFT mixture cure model, when obtaining the corresponding baseline survival function $S_{u0}(t)$ in all the methods above, the zero-tail restriction as in Section 3.2.1.1 should be considered to alleviate the identifiability issue.

3.2.4 Semiparametric Transformation Latency Submodels

The latency submodel can also be specified using the linear transformation model as follows (Lu and Ying, 2004):

$$g(T) = -\boldsymbol{\beta}'\boldsymbol{x} + \epsilon \tag{3.11}$$

where $g(\cdot)$ is a monotone increasing function with $g(0) = -\infty$ and ϵ is the error term with a known continuous distribution that is independent of $\boldsymbol{x}$ and survival time. Let the survival function of ϵ be $S_\epsilon(t)$. This latency submodel is equivalent to

$$S_u(t|\boldsymbol{x}) = S_\epsilon[g(t) + \boldsymbol{\beta}'\boldsymbol{x}]. \tag{3.12}$$

If ϵ is chosen to follow the extreme value distribution with the survival function $S_\epsilon(t) = \exp(-e^t)$, then $S_u(t|\boldsymbol{x}) = \exp(-e^{g(t)}e^{\boldsymbol{\beta}'\boldsymbol{x}})$. This is a PH model (2.5) with $e^{g(t)}$ as the baseline cumulative hazard function for uncured subjects. On the other hand, if ϵ follows the logistic distribution with the survival function $S_\epsilon(t) = 1/(1+e^t)$, then $S_u(t|\boldsymbol{x}) = 1/(1+e^{g(t)}e^{\boldsymbol{x}'\boldsymbol{\beta}})$. This is a PO model (2.11) with $e^{g(t)}$ as the baseline odds function.

This model can be estimated semiparametrically without making a parametric assumption for $g(\cdot)$. The following estimating equations can be used to estimate $\boldsymbol{\gamma}$, $\boldsymbol{\beta}$ and $g(t)$ respectively (Lu and Ying, 2004)

$$\sum_{i=1}^{n} \boldsymbol{z}_i \left\{\delta_i + (1-\delta_i)w_{0i}(t_i) - \pi(\boldsymbol{z}_i)\right\} = 0 \tag{3.13}$$

$$\sum_{i=1}^{n} \int_0^\infty \boldsymbol{x}_i[dN_i(t) - Y_i(t)d\log(1-w_{0i}(t))] = 0 \tag{3.14}$$

$$\sum_{i=1}^{n} [dN_i(t) - Y_i(t)d\log(1-w_{0i}(t))] = 0 \tag{3.15}$$

where $N_i(t) = \delta_i I(t_i \le t)$, $Y_i(t) = I(t_i \ge t)$, and $w_{0i}(t)$ is defined in (2.13). It is easy to see that (3.13) is equivalent to the estimating equation for (2.15), and (3.14) and (3.15) are obtained from the fact that a process defined as

$$M(t) = N(t) + \int_0^t Y(s)d\log\left[1 + e^{\boldsymbol{\gamma}'\boldsymbol{z} - H_u(s|\boldsymbol{x})}\right] \tag{3.16}$$

is a martingale process. The transformation function $g(\cdot)$ can be estimated within a class of nondecreasing step functions on $[0, \infty)$ with $g(0) = -\infty$ and with jumps only at the observed failure times $\tau_1, \ldots, \tau_k$. In this case, the estimating equations for $\boldsymbol{\beta}$ and $g(\tau_j)$, $j = 1, \ldots, k$, can be further simplified into

$$\sum_{i=1}^{n} \boldsymbol{x}_i[\delta_i - \log(1 - w_{0i}(\min(t_i, \tau_k)))] = 0 \tag{3.17}$$

$$d_j + \sum_{i=1}^{n} Y_i(\tau_j) \log \frac{1 - w_{0i}(\tau_j -)}{1 - w_{0i}(\tau_j)} = 0, \quad j = 1, \ldots, k \tag{3.18}$$

For any specific distribution of ϵ, $\boldsymbol{\gamma}$, $\boldsymbol{\beta}$ and $g(\tau_j)$, $j = 1, \ldots, k$, can be estimated by solving (3.13), (3.17), and (3.18) iteratively.

This model was further considered for a case with time-dependent covariates and dependent censoring (Othus et al., 2009). They proposed to use an inverse censoring probability reweighting scheme to deal with the dependent censoring and to construct unbiased estimating equations to estimate the parameters.

Furthermore, it is possible to specify the distribution of ϵ in (3.11) with an additional parameter so that the resulting latency submodel can unify the PH and PO latency submodels that are produced by $S_\epsilon(t) = \exp(-e^t)$ and $S_\epsilon(t) = 1/(1 + e^t)$ respectively. For example, if

$$S_\epsilon(t) = \exp([1 - (1 + e^t)^\rho]/\rho) \tag{3.19}$$

for $\rho \geq 0$ or if

$$S_\epsilon(t) = (1 + \rho e^t)^{-1/\rho} \tag{3.20}$$

for $\rho \geq 0$, then $S_\epsilon(t) = 1/(1 + e^t)$ when $\rho = 0$ in (3.19) (or $\rho = 1$ in (3.20)) and $S_\epsilon(t) = \exp(-e^t)$ when $\rho = 1$ in (3.19) (or $\rho = 0$ in (3.20)). Thus, the corresponding latency submodel unifies the PH and the PO latency submodels. Suppose that $S_\epsilon(t)$ is given in (3.20). Following (3.12), the latency survival function is

$$S_u(t|\boldsymbol{x}) = \left(1 + \rho e^{g(t) + \boldsymbol{\beta}'\boldsymbol{x}}\right)^{-1/\rho}.$$

Mao and Wang (2010) refers to this class of latency submodels as the generalized proportional odds models.

For a prespecified ρ, if a nonparametric estimate of $g(t)$ is desired, the likelihood function (2.16) can be maximized within a class of nondecreasing step functions on $[0, \infty)$ with $g(0) = -\infty$ and with jumps only at the observed failure times $\tau_1, \ldots, \tau_k$. It is convenient to reparametrize the step function $g(t)$ as $\exp[g(t)] = \sum_{j:\tau_j \leq t} \exp(\alpha_j)$. Let $j_i = \max\{j : \tau_j \leq t_i\}$. Then (2.16) can be written as

$$\begin{aligned} \ell_2(\boldsymbol{\beta}, \boldsymbol{\alpha}, \rho) = \sum_{i=1, w_i^{(k)} > 0}^{n} w_i^{(k)} \Bigg\{ \delta_i \left[\alpha_{j_i} - \log\left(\rho \sum_{j=1}^{j_i - 1} e^{\alpha_j} + e^{-\boldsymbol{\beta}'\boldsymbol{x}_i} \right) \right] \\ - \frac{1}{\rho} \left[\boldsymbol{\beta}'\boldsymbol{x}_i + \log\left(\rho \sum_{j=1}^{j_i} e^{\alpha_j} + e^{-\boldsymbol{\beta}'\boldsymbol{x}_i} \right) \right] \Bigg\}. \end{aligned} \tag{3.21}$$

A Newton-Raphson method may be used to maximize this function to update $\boldsymbol{\beta}$ and $\boldsymbol{\alpha}$.

Since k is in the same order as n and is potentially large, the high-dimensional $\boldsymbol{\alpha}$ may cause some numerical issues when directly apply the Newton-Raphson method to maximize (3.21). To overcome the issues, Mao and Wang (2010) suggested to use the minimization-maximization algorithm (Hunter and Lange, 2002). The minimization-maximization algorithm requires the construction for a simpler surrogate function than (3.21) to be maximized and is thus more computationally stable. However, it is not clear whether or not the surrogate function used in their work could be extended to semiparametric transformation models that are not the generalized proportional odds models.

The estimation method above requires a prespecified value for ρ. Unlike the parametric cases discussed in Section 2.5.2, there is little work on the inference of ρ in this semiparametric transformation model. Mao and Wang (2010) selected a grid of candidate values for ρ and chose the one that maximizes the profile likelihood function. Interval estimation of ρ and tests for a specific value of ρ for model selection may require a large sample size, and details remain to be worked out.

3.2.5 Semiparametric Incidence Submodel

Above semiparametric cure models assume a nonparametric baseline distribution for the latency submodels but leave the parametric logistic incidence submodels intact. To relax the parametric assumption in the incidence submodel, Li et al. (2020) suggested a more flexible support vector machine (SVM) approach to obtain $\pi(\boldsymbol{z}_i)$ in the M-step of the EM algorithm. That is, instead of maximizing (2.15) based on a parametric link such as the logit link or the complementary log-log link, an SVM method is considered here to update $\pi(\boldsymbol{z}_i)$.

If y_i's are all available, the SVM aims to build an optimal classification rule $g(\boldsymbol{z}) = \sum_{i=1}^n a_i(2y_i - 1)K(\boldsymbol{z}, \boldsymbol{z}_i) + b$ where $K(\cdot,\cdot)$ is a kernel function, a_i's and b are the solution of the following optimization problem:

$$\max_{a_1,\ldots,a_n,b} -\frac{1}{2}\sum_{i,j=1}^{n} a_i a_j(2y_i - 1)(2y_j - 1)K(\boldsymbol{z}_i, \boldsymbol{z}_j) + \sum_{i=1}^{n} a_i \tag{3.22}$$

subject to $\sum_{i=1}^n a_i(2y_i - 1) = 0$ and $0 \le a_i \le c$, $i = 1, 2, \ldots, n$, and c is a tuning parameter that controls the degree of the model overfitting. The kernel function $K(\cdot,\cdot)$ should be a symmetric positive (semi-) definite function. An example of this kernel function is the radial basis function $K(\boldsymbol{z}, \mathbf{v}) = e^{-\sigma(\boldsymbol{z}-\mathbf{v})'(\boldsymbol{z}-\mathbf{v})}$ where σ is the kernel width. Both c and σ can be estimated using the cross-validation method (Chang and Lin, 2011). The sequential minimal optimization method (Platt, 1998) can be used to solve (3.22). With the estimated function $g(\boldsymbol{z})$, an update of $\pi(\boldsymbol{z}_i)$ can be obtained using the Platt scaling method (Platt et al., 1999). Let N_+ and N_- be the numbers of uncured and cured subjects in the data respectively, $\tilde{y}_i = \frac{N_+ + 1}{N_+ + 2}$ if $y_i = 1$ and $\tilde{y}_i = \frac{1}{N_- + 2}$ if $y_i = 0$, and $p_i = g(\boldsymbol{z}_i)$. The Platt scaling method estimates $\pi(\boldsymbol{z}_i)$ as $[1 + \exp(Ap_i + B)]^{-1}$ where A and B minimize

$$-\sum_{i=1}^{n} \{(1 - \tilde{y}_i)(Ap_i + B) - \log[1 + \exp(Ap_i + B)]\}. \tag{3.23}$$

Since y_i's are usually unknown for subjects with $\delta_i = 0$, a multiple imputation method can be used to obtain the values of y_i's with $\delta_i = 0$ based on the current $w_i^{(r)}$. That is, multiple imputed values of y_i from a Bernoulli distribution with probability $w_i^{(r)}$ are obtained. Then the rth update $\pi^{(r)}(\boldsymbol{z}_i)$ is obtained as the average of the estimates of $\pi(\boldsymbol{z}_i)$ from the multiple imputed samples, and the M-step is completed. The E-step and the M-step iterate until the EM algorithm converges.

It is recommended that covariates $\boldsymbol{x}_i$ and $\boldsymbol{z}_i$ be normalized when using the SVM method, that is, for the jth covariate x_{ij} in $\boldsymbol{x}_i$ or z_{ij} in $\boldsymbol{z}_i$, use $\frac{x_{ij} - \min_i(x_{ij})}{\max_i(x_{ij}) - \min_i(x_{ij})}$ instead of x_{ij} and use $\frac{z_{ij} - \min_i(z_{ij})}{\max_i(z_{ij}) - \min_i(z_{ij})}$ instead of z_{ij} in the model fitting.

As other semiparametric cure models, directly estimating the standard errors of estimates from the EM algorithm can be difficult. The bootstrap method should be employed to obtain the standard errors.

3.2.6 Semiparametric Spline-Based Cure Models

It is also possible to relax parametric assumptions in both parts of the semiparametric mixture cure models by using additive effects of the covariates in the two submodels. This idea was first discussed in Peng (2003b) by employing the generalized additive model for the incidence part provided in R function `gam` and additive effects in the Cox PH latency submodel provided in R function `coxph`. This method can be further extended to include interactions between two and more covariates in the two submodels (Wang et al., 2012a). Specifically, if $\boldsymbol{x} = (x_1, \ldots, x_{p_x})'$ and $\boldsymbol{z} = (z_1, \ldots, z_{p_z})'$, then the incidence part is modeled by

$$\pi(\boldsymbol{z}) = \frac{e^{\varsigma(\boldsymbol{z})}}{1 + e^{\varsigma(\boldsymbol{z})}}, \tag{3.24}$$

and the latency part is modeled by

$$h_u(t|\boldsymbol{x}) = e^{\eta(t,\boldsymbol{x})}. \tag{3.25}$$

where

$$\begin{aligned}\zeta(\boldsymbol{z}) =& \zeta_0 + \sum_{i=1}^{p_z} \zeta_i(z_i) + \sum_{ij} \zeta_{ij}(z_i, z_j) + \cdots \\ &+ \zeta_{1\cdots p_z}(z_1, \ldots, z_{p_z}) = \psi_\zeta(\boldsymbol{z})'\boldsymbol{\gamma}, \end{aligned} \tag{3.26}$$

$$\begin{aligned}\eta(t, \boldsymbol{x}) =& \eta_0 + \eta_t(t) + \sum_{i=1}^{p_x} \eta_i(x_i) + \sum_{ij} \eta_{ij}(x_i, x_j) + \cdots \\ &+ \eta_{1\cdots p_x}(x_1, \ldots, x_{p_x}) = \psi_\eta(t, \boldsymbol{x})'\boldsymbol{\beta}, \end{aligned} \tag{3.27}$$

and ψ_ζ and ψ_η are chosen spline basis functions. It can be seen that this approach uses splines, instead of specific linear or nonlinear effects, to model the main effects, two-way interaction effects, and high order interaction effects of x_i's in the latency part and similar effects of z_i's in the incidence part. The flexibility of splines reduces the dependence of the covariate effects on any particular parametric form. To reduce the dimensionality of $\boldsymbol{\beta}$ and $\boldsymbol{\gamma}$, the time–covariate interaction in the latency part, and higher-order interactions than two-way interactions in $\boldsymbol{x}$ and $\boldsymbol{z}$ may be excluded.

To estimate $\boldsymbol{\beta}$ and $\boldsymbol{\gamma}$, a penalized version of the EM algorithm in Section 2.3.2 can be used. That is, the likelihoods in (2.15) and (2.16) are replaced with their penalized versions:

$$\ell_1^P(\boldsymbol{\gamma}) = -\frac{1}{n}\ell_1(\boldsymbol{\gamma}) + \frac{\lambda_1}{2}J_1(\zeta), \tag{3.28}$$

$$\ell_2^P(\boldsymbol{\beta}, \boldsymbol{\alpha}) = -\frac{1}{n}\ell_2(\boldsymbol{\beta}, \boldsymbol{\alpha}) + \frac{\lambda_2}{2}J_2(\eta), \tag{3.29}$$

where $J_1(\zeta) = \sum_j \theta_{1j}^{-1}\|P_j(\zeta)\|^2$ is the roughness penalty with additional smoothing parameters θ_{1j} measuring the smoothness of ζ, and the smoothing parameter $\lambda_1 (> 0)$ controls the tradeoff between bias and variance. Similarly $J_2(\eta) = \sum_j \theta_{2j}^{-1}\|P_j(\eta)\|^2$ is the roughness penalty with additional smoothing parameters θ_{2j} measuring the smoothness of η, and the smoothing parameter $\lambda_2 (> 0)$ controls the tradeoff. Cubic and tensor cubic smoothing splines can be used in (3.26) and (3.27). The number of knots is suggested to be $10n^{2/9}$. The Newton-Raphson method can be used to minimize $\ell_1^P(\boldsymbol{\gamma})$ and $\ell_2^P(\boldsymbol{\beta}, \boldsymbol{\alpha})$, and the cross-validation scores are used in selecting smoothing parameters. Once $\boldsymbol{\beta}$ and $\boldsymbol{\gamma}$ are updated in the M-step, the E-step can proceed and the two steps iterate until the EM algorithm converges. The standard errors of estimated $\boldsymbol{\beta}$ and $\boldsymbol{\gamma}$ can be obtained using Louis (1982) method.

3.3 Nonparametric Mixture Cure Models

The semiparametric methods discussed in previous sections focus on semiparametric estimation in the latency part of the mixture cure models. The incidence part and the latency part beyond the baseline distribution are still parametrically specified. That is, the covariate effects on cure rate is modeled by specific link functions such as the logit link $\pi(\boldsymbol{z}) = \exp(\boldsymbol{\beta}'\boldsymbol{z})/(1+\exp(\boldsymbol{\beta}'\boldsymbol{z}))$ or the complementary log-log link $\pi(\boldsymbol{z}) = \exp(-\exp(\boldsymbol{\beta}'\boldsymbol{z}))$, and the covariate effects in the latency part is always in the form of $\exp(\boldsymbol{\beta}'\boldsymbol{x})$. When the underlying covariate effects in the cure model cannot be well approximated by the parametric assumptions in any of the two parts, applying the semiparametric models can still lead to biased estimates. In this section, we introduce nonparametric methods to estimate the effects of covariates in the latency part that do not require any parametric assumptions. We will also introduce methods to nonparametrically estimate covariate effects in the latency part.

3.3.1 Nonparametric Incidence Submodels

3.3.1.1 Kaplan-Meier Estimator

We start with a nonparametric estimation of cure rate for a single sample without covariates. Let $\hat{S}^{\text{KM}}(t)$ be the Kaplan-Meier survival estimate of $S(t)$ based on data $\{(t_i, \delta_i), i = 1, \ldots, n\}$, and $t_{(n)} = \max\{t_i\colon i = 1, \ldots, n\}$. Since $1 - \pi = \lim_{t\to\infty} S(t)$ in (2.1), the simplest cure rate estimate is the lowest value of $\hat{S}^{\text{KM}}(t)$. That is, a nonparametric estimate of π is

$$\hat{\pi} = 1 - \hat{S}^{\text{KM}}(t_{(n)}). \tag{3.30}$$

It can be shown that $\hat{\pi}$ in (3.30) is a consistent estimator of π and is asymptotically normal with the variance that can be estimated by (Maller and Zhou, 1992)

$$\hat{\pi}^2 \sum_{j=1}^{k} \frac{d_j}{n_j(n_j - d_j)},$$

where k and d_j are defined as in Section 3.2 and $n_j = \sum_{i=1}^{n} Y_i(\tau_j)$ is the number of subjects at risk at τ_j. Let $\tau_u = \inf\{t\colon S_u(t) = 0\}$ and $\tau_G = \inf\{t\colon G(t) = 0\}$ where $G(t)$ is the survival function of the censoring distribution. That is, τ_u and τ_G are the right extremes of the supports of the latency distribution and the censoring distribution respectively. The main condition for the asymptotic properties is that $\tau_u \leq \tau_G$, which implies that a sufficient follow-up is required for a nonparametric cure rate estimation.

This method can be generalized to multiple sample cases (Laska and Meisner, 1992; Tsodikov, 2001). For the two-sample leukemia data set with the

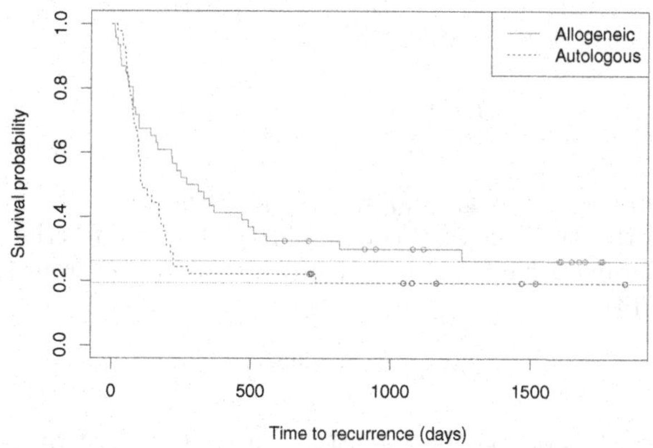

FIGURE 3.1
Nonparametric cure rate estimates indicated by the horizontal lines at the heights of the right tails of the Kaplan-Meier survival curves for the two groups of leukemia patients with marrow transplants.

Kaplan-Meier survival estimates in Figure 2.4, the corresponding nonparametric estimates of the cure rates $1 - \hat{\pi}$ from the two groups are marked in Figure 3.1.

3.3.1.2 Generalized Kaplan-Meier Estimator

The above method can be viewed as a method to model the incidence part with a single categorical variable z. The method however cannot handle continuous covariates in data. To model the effect of a continuous covariate z nonparametrically in the incidence part, the generalized Kaplan-Meier estimator of Beran (1981) can be considered. For survival data $(t_i, \delta_i, z_i), i = 1, \ldots, n$, the generalized Kaplan-Meier estimator for $S(t|z)$ is given by

$$\hat{S}^{\text{GKM}}(t|z) = I(t \leq t_{(n)}) \prod_{j=1}^{n} \left[\frac{1 - \sum_{r=1}^{n} I(t_r \leq t_j) B_r(z)}{1 - \sum_{r=1}^{n} I(t_r < t_j) B_r(z)} \right]^{I(t_j \leq t; \delta_j = 1)}, \quad (3.31)$$

where $B_j(z)$ is a proper weight function satisfying $B_j(z) \geq 0$ and $\sum_{j=1}^{n} B_j(z) = 1$. As a generalization of the prominent Kaplan-Meier survival estimator, the generalized Kaplan-Meier estimator (3.31) has been widely used to estimate the survival function with covariates. The weight function $B_j(z)$ can be the Nadaraya-Watson weight (Nadaraya, 1964; Watson, 1964) function

$$B_j(z) = \frac{K_h(z_j - z)}{\sum_{r=1}^{n} K_h(z_r - z)}, \quad (3.32)$$

where $K_h(\cdot)$ is a kernel density function as defined in Section 3.2.2.3. If the covariate z is continuous, the following Gasser-Müller weight (Gasser and Müller,

1979) function can also be used in (3.31),

$$B_j(z) = \int_{s_{j-1}}^{s_j} K_h(z-u)du,$$

where $s_0 = 0, s_j = \frac{1}{2}(z_j + z_{j+1}), j = 1, \ldots, n-1$ and $s_n = 1$.

Following the same idea in Section 3.3.1.1, if a cure fraction is present in data, a nonparametric estimate of $\pi(z)$ can be obtained from (3.31) by (Xu and Peng, 2014)

$$\hat{\pi}(z) = \hat{S}^{\text{GKM}}(t^1_{(n)}|z), \tag{3.33}$$

where $t^1_{(n)} = \max_{i:\, \delta_i=1}(t_i)$ is the largest uncensored failure time. Under mild conditions, it can be shown that the estimator (3.33) is a consistent estimator of $\pi(z)$, where $0 < \pi(z) < 1$ for any interior point z, and the estimator is asymptotically normal with the variance estimated by $\hat{\pi}^2(z)\hat{\sigma}^2(z)$, where

$$\hat{\sigma}^2(z) = \int K^2(t)dt \sum_{j=1}^{n} \frac{\delta_j B_j(z)}{\hat{H}(t_j|z)\hat{H}(t_j-|z)},$$

and $H(t|z) = P[\min(T, C) > t|z]$ and

$$\hat{H}(t|z) = 1 - \sum_{j=1}^{n} I(t_j \leq t)B_j(z).$$

The conditions required for the asymptotic properties include those typically for smooth nonparametric estimators, kernel function, Gasser-Müller weight function, and the bandwidth h. The most prominent condition is that for any z

$$\tau_u < \tau_G(z) \tag{3.34}$$

with probability 1, where $\tau_u = \sup_{z \in D} \tau_{S_u}(z)$, $\tau_{S_u}(z) = \inf\{t\colon S_u(t|z) = 0\}$, D is the support of z, and $\tau_G(z) = \inf\{t\colon G(t|z) = 0\}$. This condition guarantees a sufficient follow-up so that censored subjects beyond the largest observed failure time are most likely to be cured and hence our estimator does not overestimate the true cure rate. Amico and Van Keilegom (2018) suggested that this condition be further relaxed into

$$\tau_u(z) < \tau_G(z) \tag{3.35}$$

where $\tau_u(z) = \inf\{t\colon S_u(t|z) = 0\}$. In practice, we find that as long as the censoring distribution $G(t|z)$ has a heavier tail than $S_u(t|z)$, $\hat{\pi}(z)$ in (3.33) will tend to have smaller biases regardless of the value of $\tau_{S_u(z)}$.

The convergence rate of (3.33) to $\pi(z)$ is related to the convergence rate of the convergence of generalized Kaplan-Meier survival estimator to $S(t)$, which is generally slower than $n^{-1/2}$ compared to the Kaplan-Meier survival estimate because it only uses a portion of data. The actual rate of convergence depends on how fast h goes to 0 as well as on the smoothness of $S(t)$. A decrease in the bandwidth would reduce the bias but, on the other hand, increase the variance of the estimate, and vice versa. An optimal bandwidth that minimizes the asymptotic mean square error is given by (López-Cheda et al., 2017a)

$$h = \left(\frac{c_K \tilde{\sigma}^2(z)}{d_K^2 \mu^2(z)} \right)^{1/5} n^{-1/5} \tag{3.36}$$

where c_K, $\tilde{\sigma}^2(z)$, d_K^2, and $\mu(z)$ depend on the kernel function $K_h(\cdot)$, the density of the covariate z, and $H(t|z)$. Thus, (3.36) is not very useful to determine the value of h in practice. A more practical method to determine the bandwidth is to use a bootstrap method. Details can be found in López-Cheda et al. (2017a).

When there is no covariate, $B_j(\cdot) = 1/n$ for $j = 1, \ldots, n$ by (3.32) and hence the estimator (3.33) reduces to the single sample cure rate estimator (3.30).

The proposed method can be extended to multiple covariates. If $\boldsymbol{z} = (z_1, \ldots, z_{p_z})'$, one may use the product kernel (Simonoff, 2012), i.e., $K(\boldsymbol{z}) = \prod_{i=1}^{p_z} K(z_i)$, in (3.33) to estimate $\pi(\boldsymbol{z})$.

3.3.2 Nonparametric Latency Submodels

If the same covariate affects both the latency and the incidence parts of the mixture cure model as follows

$$S(t|x) = \pi(x) S_u(t|x) + 1 - \pi(x)$$

then given nonparametric estimates of $S(t|x)$ and $\pi(x)$, such as (3.31) and (3.33), a nonparametric estimate of the latency part can be obtained as follows (López-Cheda et al., 2017b):

$$\hat{S}_u(t|x) = \frac{\hat{S}^{\text{GKM}}(t|x) - 1 + \hat{\pi}(x)}{\hat{\pi}(x)} \tag{3.37}$$

One issue with this estimator is the bandwidth selection. The optimal bandwidths for $\hat{S}^{\text{GKM}}(t|x)$ and $\hat{\pi}(x)$ can be different. However, different bandwidths may not yield a proper survival function estimate for $S_u(t|x)$ since the limit of $\hat{S}^{\text{GKM}}(t|x)$ as $t \to \infty$ needs not to be $\hat{\pi}(x)$ with different bandwidths. Therefore the same bandwidth is recommended in (3.37). Under similar conditions and a suitable bandwidth h, it can be shown that $\hat{S}_u(t|x)$ is a consistent estimate of $S_u(t|x)$ and is asymptotically normal with variance $V(t, z)c_K$, where $V(t, z)$ depends on $\pi(x)$, $S(t|x)$, $H(t|x)$, and the density of x. The bandwidth can be selected using the bootstrap method. See details in López-Cheda et al. (2017b).

One obvious limitation of the estimator (3.37) is that it requires the two parts of the mixture cure model share the same covariate. If different covariates are required in the two parts, the method will not be appropriate to estimate $S_u(t|x)$ directly. One could allow all covariates to appear in both parts so that (3.37) can be used. However, the estimator may produce a spurious relationship between some covariates and the two submodels of the mixture cure model, and the estimation may not be efficient.

Even though the generalized Kaplan-Meier survival estimator can be used with more than one covariate by choosing appropriate kernel functions that can work with multiple covariates, the application of the method in practice can be challenging with more than one covariate.

3.4 Semiparametric Non-Mixture Cure Models

3.4.1 Semiparametric PHC Model

In addition to the parametric approaches to estimate non-mixture cure models discussed in Section 2.4, there are also semiparametric approaches to estimate the non-mixture cure models if a parametric distributional assumption is not desirable. For the PHC model in (2.18), given its similarity to the PH model, a similar semiparametric estimation method to the PH model can be used to estimate the PHC model (Tsodikov, 1998b). Particularly, estimating γ in (2.18) can be obtained using the partial log-likelihood function:

$$\log \prod_{j=1}^{k} \frac{\exp(\gamma' \boldsymbol{s}_j)}{\left\{\sum_{i \in R_j} \exp(\gamma' \boldsymbol{z}_i)\right\}^{d_j}},$$

following the notations in Section 3.2, where $\boldsymbol{s}_j = \sum_{i:t_i=\tau_j} \delta_i \boldsymbol{z}_i$. However, if γ_0 or $F^H(t)$ is of interest, the partial likelihood function is not very useful, and a usual nonparametric baseline survival function estimation method for Cox's PH model can be used to estimate $\exp[-e^{\gamma_0} F^H(t)]$. For example, given $\hat{\gamma}$, the estimate of γ from the partial log-likelihood function, a Nelson-Aalen estimator of the baseline survival function is given by

$$\widehat{S}_0(t) = \exp\left(-\sum_{j:\tau_j<t} \frac{d_j}{\sum_{i \in R_j} \exp(\hat{\gamma}' \boldsymbol{z}_i)}\right).$$

Then following the idea in Section 3.3.1.1, γ_0 can be estimated by $\hat{\gamma}_0 = \log[-\log(\widehat{S}_0(\tau_k))]$, and $F^H(t)$ can be estimated by $\widehat{F^H(t)} = -\log[\widehat{S}_0(t)^{\exp(-\hat{\gamma}_0)}]$ (Tsodikov et al., 2003), which essentially implies that $\widehat{F^H(\tau_k)} \equiv 1$ and any subjects with censored times greater than τ_k is deemed cured. Assuming the censored subjects with survival times greater than the largest uncensored time as cured is often necessary in semiparametric estimation methods to ensure the PHC model is identifiable, similar to what is discussed in Section 3.2.1.1 for semiparametric mixture cure models.

Other approaches, such as the marginal likelihood approach of the PH model (Kalbfleisch and Prentice, 2002), can also be extended to estimate the PHC model semiparametrically (Tsodikov, 1998b). Asymptotic properties of the estimates and a comparison with a parametric PHC model are discussed in detail in Tsodikov (1998a, 2001).

3.4.2 General Non-Mixture Cure Models

The general non-mixture cure models based on Box-Cox transformation in Section 2.4.4 can be estimated semiparametrically as well. Let $g(\cdot|\lambda)$ denote the transformation and the corresponding survival function of the cure model is $S(t|\boldsymbol{z}) = g[e^{\gamma_0+\boldsymbol{\gamma}'\boldsymbol{z}}F^H(t)]$. For example, model (2.26) corresponds to

$$g(x|\lambda) = \begin{cases} (1+\lambda x)^{-1/\lambda} & \lambda > 0 \\ e^{-x} & \lambda = 0. \end{cases}$$

Without making any parametric assumption for $F^H(t)$, we consider a non-parametric maximum likelihood estimation approach, where $F^H(t)$ is allowed to be a right-continuous function. Let $\boldsymbol{\alpha}' = (\alpha_1, \ldots, \alpha_n)$, where α_i be the jump size of $F^H(t)$ at t_i. The observed likelihood function is

$$\prod_{i=1}^{n} \left\{ \left(-g'[e^{\gamma_0+\boldsymbol{\gamma}'\boldsymbol{z}_i}F^H(t_i)]e^{\gamma_0+\boldsymbol{\gamma}'\boldsymbol{z}_i}\alpha_i \right)^{\delta_i} \left(g[e^{\gamma_0+\boldsymbol{\gamma}'\boldsymbol{z}_i}F^H(t_i)] \right)^{1-\delta_i} \right\}$$

subject to $\sum_i \delta_i\alpha_i = 1$, where $F^H(t_i) = \sum_{j:t_j \le t_i} \delta_j\alpha_j$. Suppose that t_i's are arranged from smallest to largest and $m = \sum_i I(t_i \le \tau_k)$. Because of the identifiability requirement as discussed earlier, it is easy to see that $\alpha_i \equiv 0$ for $i > m$. For the remaining α_i, $i = 1, \ldots, m$, γ_0 and $\boldsymbol{\gamma}$, it can be shown (Zeng et al., 2006) that their constrained maximum likelihood estimates can be obtained from the following equations:

$$
\begin{aligned}
0 = & \sum_{i=1}^{m} \frac{1}{\alpha_i} \frac{\partial \alpha_i}{\partial(\gamma_0, \boldsymbol{\gamma}')'} + \sum_{i=1}^{n} \delta_i \boldsymbol{z}_i - C \sum_{i=1}^{m} \frac{\partial \alpha_i}{\partial(\gamma_0, \boldsymbol{\gamma}')'} \\
& + \sum_{i=m+1}^{n} \frac{g'[e^{\gamma_0+\boldsymbol{\gamma}'\boldsymbol{z}_i}]}{g[e^{\gamma_0+\boldsymbol{\gamma}'\boldsymbol{z}_i}]} e^{\gamma_0+\boldsymbol{\gamma}'\boldsymbol{z}_i} \boldsymbol{z}_i \\
& + \sum_{i=1}^{m} \frac{g''[e^{\gamma_0+\boldsymbol{\gamma}'\boldsymbol{z}_i} F^H(t_i)]}{g'[e^{\gamma_0+\boldsymbol{\gamma}'\boldsymbol{z}_i} F^H(t_i)]} \left[\boldsymbol{z}_i F^H(t_i) + \frac{\partial F^H(t_i)}{\partial(\gamma_0, \boldsymbol{\gamma}')'} \right] e^{\gamma_0+\boldsymbol{\gamma}'\boldsymbol{z}_i} \\
& + \sum_{i=1}^{m} \sum_{t_i < t_j \le t_{i+1}} \frac{g'[e^{\gamma_0+\boldsymbol{\gamma}'\boldsymbol{z}_j} F^H(t_i)]}{g[e^{\gamma_0+\boldsymbol{\gamma}'\boldsymbol{z}_j} F^H(t_i)]} \left[\boldsymbol{z}_j F^H(t_i) + \frac{\partial F^H(t_i)}{\partial(\gamma_0, \boldsymbol{\gamma}')'} \right] e^{\gamma_0+\boldsymbol{\gamma}'\boldsymbol{z}_j} \\
0 = & \sum_{i=1}^{m} \frac{1}{\alpha_i} \frac{\partial \alpha_i}{\partial \alpha} - C \sum_{i=1}^{m} \frac{\partial \alpha_i}{\partial \alpha} + \sum_{i=1}^{m} \frac{g''[e^{\gamma_0+\boldsymbol{\gamma}'\boldsymbol{z}_i} F^H(t_i)]}{g'[e^{\gamma_0+\boldsymbol{\gamma}'\boldsymbol{z}_i} F^H(t_i)]} \frac{\partial F^H(t_i)}{\partial \alpha} e^{\gamma_0+\boldsymbol{\gamma}'\boldsymbol{z}_i} \\
& + \sum_{i=1}^{m} \sum_{t_i < t_j \le t_{i+1}} \frac{g'[e^{\gamma_0+\boldsymbol{\gamma}'\boldsymbol{z}_j} F^H(t_i)]}{g[e^{\gamma_0+\boldsymbol{\gamma}'\boldsymbol{z}_j} F^H(t_i)]} \frac{\partial F^H(t_i)}{\partial \alpha} e^{\gamma_0+\boldsymbol{\gamma}'\boldsymbol{z}_j} \\
0 = & \sum_{i=1}^{m} \alpha_i - 1.
\end{aligned}
$$

where $\alpha \equiv \alpha_m$ and C is the Lagrange multiplier. The derivative of α_i with respect to γ_0, $\boldsymbol{\gamma}$ and α can be obtain from a recursive formula between α_i and α_{i+1}:

$$
\begin{aligned}
\frac{1}{\alpha_i} = \frac{1}{\alpha_{i+1}} - & \frac{g''[e^{\gamma_0+\boldsymbol{\gamma}'\boldsymbol{z}_i} F^H(t_i)] e^{\gamma_0+\boldsymbol{\gamma}'\boldsymbol{z}_i}}{g'[e^{\gamma_0+\boldsymbol{\gamma}'\boldsymbol{z}_i} F^H(t_i)]} \\
& - \sum_{t_i < t_j \le t_{i+1}} \frac{g'[e^{\gamma_0+\boldsymbol{\gamma}'\boldsymbol{z}_j} F^H(t_i)] e^{\gamma_0+\boldsymbol{\gamma}'\boldsymbol{z}_j}}{g[e^{\gamma_0+\boldsymbol{\gamma}'\boldsymbol{z}_j} F^H(t_i)]}.
\end{aligned}
$$

The semiparametric method above is for a fixed value of λ in $g(\cdot|\lambda)$. If one is interested in estimating the value of λ using data, one has to ensure that λ is identifiable. For model (2.26), it can be shown that if $\boldsymbol{\gamma}'\boldsymbol{z} \neq 0$, then γ_0, $F^H(t)$ and λ are identifiable. In this case, λ_0 can be jointly estimated with other parameters in the model. Or one can use the AIC or BIC to select λ from preselected candidate values.

Another generalization of the semiparametric PHC model is the nonlinear transformation model (NTM) (Tsodikov et al., 2003), in which the survival function of T^* is given by

$$S(t|\boldsymbol{z}) = g[S^H(t)|\boldsymbol{z}], \tag{3.38}$$

where $g(\cdot|\boldsymbol{z})$ some parametrically specified cumulative distribution function with support on [0, 1]. The model can also be defined in survival function as

$$S(t|\boldsymbol{z}) = E[S^H(t)^M|\boldsymbol{z}], \tag{3.39}$$

where M is a distribution that has a probability mass at 0 and the expectation is with respect to M. If $g(x|\boldsymbol{z}) = \exp(-e^{\gamma_0+\boldsymbol{\gamma}'\boldsymbol{z}}(1-x))$ or if M follows a Poisson distribution with mean $e^{\gamma_0+\boldsymbol{\gamma}'\boldsymbol{z}}$, the above models reduce to the PHC model (2.18). If $M = \exp(\boldsymbol{\beta}'\boldsymbol{x})v$ and v follows a Poisson distribution with mean $e^{\gamma_0+\boldsymbol{\gamma}'\boldsymbol{z}}$, then the above model reduces to the PHPH cure model (2.19). If $M = \exp(\boldsymbol{\beta}'\boldsymbol{x})v$ and v follows a Bernoulli distribution with mean $1/[1+\exp(-\boldsymbol{\gamma}'\boldsymbol{z})]$, the above model reduces the PH mixture cure model (2.5). A necessary and sufficient condition for the two forms (3.38) and (3.39) to be equivalent is that the function $\psi(t) = g(e^{-t})$ has $(-1)^n\psi^{(n)}(t) \geq 0$ for any n.

Given observed data $(t_i, \delta_i, \boldsymbol{x}_i, \boldsymbol{z}_i)$, $i = 1, \ldots, n$, the likelihood function can be written as

$$\ell = \sum_{i=1}^{n} \left\{\delta_i \log\left(g[S^H(t_i-)] - g[S^H(t_i)]\right) + (1-\delta_i)\log g[S^H(t_i)]\right\}.$$

A semiparametric estimation method often maximizes the likelihood function for a step function $S^H(t)$ with steps at the uncensored times. It is also necessary to require that $\lim_{t\to\infty} \widehat{S^H}(t) = 0$ for $\widehat{S^H}(t)$ as an estimate of $S^H(t)$ and there is no intercept term in $\boldsymbol{\beta}$. The unknown parameters in this model include $\boldsymbol{\gamma}$ and the steps in $S^H(t)$ (and $\boldsymbol{\beta}$ if covariates $\boldsymbol{x}$ are considered as in the PHPH model).

The likelihood function can be maximized using the Newton-Raphson method or the profile likelihood method. However, these methods may fail sometimes due to the high dimensional steps in $S^H(t)$. Alternative approaches include a restricted nonparametric maximum likelihood estimation method (RNPMLE) (Tsodikov, 2002) and a quasi-EM (QEM) algorithm (Tsodikov, 2003) can be considered. In the RNPMLE method, the estimates of the unknown parameters are obtained from the following estimating functions

$$0 = \frac{\partial \ell}{\partial \gamma}$$

$$0 = \frac{\partial \ell}{\partial F^H(t_j)} = g_i(F^H(t_{j-1}), F^H(t_j), F^H(t_{j+1})), \quad j = 1, \ldots, n.$$

The last equation can be solved recurrently given $F^H(t_0) = 0$ and $F^H(t_n) = 1$.

The QEM algorithm is similar to the EM algorithm except that it uses a distribution-free E-step in the EM algorithm where M in (3.39) is treated as the latent variable. The distribution-free method for the E-step is to update the conditional expectation of M by

$$E[M(\cdot)|t_i, \delta_i] = \widetilde{M}[S^H(t_i)|\cdot, \delta_i],$$

where

$$\widetilde{M}[x|\cdot, \delta] = \delta + \frac{g^{(\delta+1)}(x|\cdot)}{g^{(\delta)}(x|\cdot)}.$$

For the PHC model (2.18), $\widetilde{M}[x|\cdot,\delta] = \delta + xe^{\gamma_0+\gamma'\boldsymbol{z}}$, and for the PHPH cure model (2.19), $\widetilde{M}[x|\cdot,\delta] = \delta e^{\boldsymbol{\beta}'\boldsymbol{x}} + x^{\exp(\boldsymbol{\beta}'\boldsymbol{x})}e^{\boldsymbol{\beta}'\boldsymbol{x}+\gamma_0+\gamma'\boldsymbol{z}}$. The estimate of the step of the corresponding cumulative hazard function of $F^H(t)$ at the jth uncensored time is given by $d_j \Big/ \sum_{l\in R_j} \widetilde{M}[S^H(t_l)|\gamma,\delta_l,\boldsymbol{z}_l]$. Details of the QEM algorithm can be found in Tsodikov et al. (2003) and Tsodikov (2003).

3.5 Model Assessment

3.5.1 Residuals for Overall Model Fitting

Residuals are often used in statistical models to examine the overall model fitting. The generalized residuals considered in Section 2.5.3, however, are primarily used for parametric mixture cure models because of their dependence on the hazard functions. Their use for semiparametric mixture cure models is limited because the estimated hazard function is usually not directly available in most semiparametric mixture cure models.

For semiparametric mixture cure models, some residual-based methods for standard survival models may be used to assess the fit of the model. For example, based on (3.16), the martingale residual for model (2.5) can be defined as

$$M_i = \delta_i + \log\left[1 + e^{\boldsymbol{\gamma}'\boldsymbol{z}_i - H_{u0}(t_i)\exp(\boldsymbol{\beta}'\boldsymbol{x}_i)}\right] - \log[1 + e^{\boldsymbol{\gamma}'\boldsymbol{z}_i}]. \tag{3.40}$$

Let $\hat{M}_i$ be the estimated M_i when $\boldsymbol{\beta}$, $H_{u0}(t)$ and $\boldsymbol{\gamma}$ are replaced with their estimates. The martingale residual can be viewed as a difference between the observed number of events for an individual and the conditionally expected number given the fitted mixture cure model, follow-up time, and covariates. It shares some of the properties of the martingale residuals for classical survival models, such as $M_i \leq 1$, $E(M_i) = 0$, $\sum \hat{M}_i = 0$, $Cov(M_i, M_j) = 0$, and $Cov(\hat{M}_i, \hat{M}_j) < 0$. However, the martingale residual in (3.40) has a lower bound $\log[1-\pi(z_i)]$ while in the classical survival models the martingale residual does not have a lower bound (Peng and Taylor, 2017). The presence of the lower bound may limit the use of the martingale residuals to detect outliers. Numerical studies also show that the martingale residuals are insensitive to the covariate effects in the incidence part of the cure model.

With the martingale residuals M_i in (3.40), the Cox-Snell residuals can be defined by

$$r_i = \delta_i - M_i, \quad i = 1, \ldots, n, \tag{3.41}$$

for the mixture cure model (2.1). Under a standard survival model, if the model is correctly specified and is consistently estimated, then the Cox-Snell residuals can be viewed as a censored sample from a unit exponential distribution. However, under the mixture cure model (2.1), the Cox-Snell residuals

(r_i, δ_i), $i = 1, \ldots, n$ can no longer be viewed as a sample from a unit exponential distribution when the cure model is correctly specified. This can be seen from the fact that

$$P[-\log S(T|\boldsymbol{x}, \boldsymbol{z}) > t] = \begin{cases} e^{-t} & \text{if } t < -\log[1 - \pi(\boldsymbol{z})] \\ 0 & \text{if } t \geq -\log[1 - \pi(\boldsymbol{z})] \end{cases}.$$

It is a mixed type distribution with a unit exponential distribution as the continuous component between 0 and $-\log[1-\pi(\boldsymbol{z})]$ and a probability mass $1-\pi(\boldsymbol{z})$ at $-\log[1 - \pi(\boldsymbol{z})]$ as the discrete component. Despite this fact, the usual approach of checking the estimated cumulative hazard rate of the (r_i, δ_i)'s against the cumulative hazard function of the unit exponential distribution is still appropriate because the residuals that are equal to $-\log[1 - \pi(\boldsymbol{z})]$ are always censored and thus the entire residuals still can be treated as a censored sample from the unit exponential distribution.

When the mixture cure model (2.1) is misspecified, the Cox-Snell residuals (3.41) will still follow a mixed type distribution. Suppose that the incidence submodel of the mixture cure model (2.1) is misspecified, but the latency submodel is still correct. Let $\pi^*(\boldsymbol{z})$ be the incorrect model for the uncure rate and $\pi(\boldsymbol{z})$ be the true model for the uncure rate. Then the survival function of the Cox-Snell residuals is

$$P[-\log S(T|\boldsymbol{x}, \boldsymbol{z}) > t] = \begin{cases} 1 - \frac{\pi(\boldsymbol{z})}{\pi^*(\boldsymbol{z})} + \frac{\pi(\boldsymbol{z})}{\pi^*(\boldsymbol{z})} e^{-t} & \text{if } t < -\log[1 - \pi^*(\boldsymbol{z})] \\ 0 & \text{if } t \geq -\log[1 - \pi^*(\boldsymbol{z})] \end{cases}.$$

It is a mixed type distribution with a non-unit exponential distribution as the continuous component between 0 and $-\log[1 - \pi^*(\boldsymbol{z})]$ and a probability mass $1 - \pi(\boldsymbol{z})$ at $-\log[1 - \pi^*(\boldsymbol{z})]$ as the discrete component. If the incidence part is correct but the latency part is misspecified, and the misspecified latency submodel is $S_u^*(t|\boldsymbol{x})$, the survival function of the Cox-Snell residuals is

$$\begin{cases} 1 - \pi(\boldsymbol{z}) + \pi(\boldsymbol{z}) S_u \left[S_u^{*-1} \left(\frac{e^{-t}}{\pi(\boldsymbol{z})} - \frac{1-\pi(\boldsymbol{z})}{\pi(\boldsymbol{z})} \right) \right] & \text{if } t < -\log[1 - \pi(\boldsymbol{z})] \\ 0 & \text{if } t \geq -\log[1 - \pi(\boldsymbol{z})] \end{cases}.$$

It is again a mixed type distribution with a distribution of a mixture cure model with an unknown distribution as the continuous component between 0 and $-\log[1 - \pi(\boldsymbol{z})]$ and a probability mass $1 - \pi(\boldsymbol{z})$ at $-\log[1 - \pi(\boldsymbol{z})]$ as the discrete component.

Similar to martingale residuals, numerical studies show that the Cox-Snell residuals in the mixture cure models are sensitive to the choice of the model assumption in the latency submodel but less sensitive to the misspecification in the incidence submodel.

3.5.2 Residuals for Latency Submodels

Residuals are also available for examining the fit of the latency submodel in the semiparametric mixture cure model. If the latency submodel is correctly specified for $T|Y = 1$, the martingale residuals for the fitted latency submodel for uncured subjects can be defined as

$$M_i^{(u)} = \delta_i - y_i H_u(t_i|\boldsymbol{x}_i). \tag{3.42}$$

The estimated $\hat{M}_i^{(u)}$ can be obtained by replacing y_i with w_i in (2.14), and H_u with its estimate from the EM algorithm at convergence. For the PH mixture cure model (2.1) and (2.5), the estimated martingale residual for an uncured subject i is (Peng and Taylor, 2017)

$$\hat{M}_i^{(u)} = \delta_i - w_i \hat{H}_{u0}(t_i) \exp(\hat{\boldsymbol{\beta}}' \boldsymbol{x}_i). \tag{3.43}$$

This modified martingale residual shares similar properties as the martingale residual for the standard PH model. For example, if the baseline distribution is estimated by a Nelson-Aalen estimator (3.3), it can be shown that $\sum_{i=1}^n \hat{M}_i^{(u)} = 0$. Because of this condition, $\hat{M}_i^{(u)}$ and $\hat{M}_j^{(u)}$ will be slightly negatively correlated even though $Cov[M_i^{(u)}(t), M_j^{(u)}(t)] = 0$. The modified martingale residuals (3.43) may be used to examine the functional forms of covariates in x in the latency PH model in the same way as in the standard PH model (Therneau and Grambsch, 2000).

Similarly, a score process as a function of the modified martingale process can be defined as

$$U(\hat{\boldsymbol{\beta}}, t) = \sum_{i=1}^n \int_0^t [\boldsymbol{x}_i - \bar{\boldsymbol{x}}(u)]\, d\hat{M}_i^{(u)}(u) = \sum_{i=1}^n \boldsymbol{x}_i \hat{M}_i^{(u)}(t), \tag{3.44}$$

where $\bar{\boldsymbol{x}}(u) = \frac{\sum_{i=1}^n Y_i(u) w_i \boldsymbol{x}_i e^{\hat{\boldsymbol{\beta}}' \boldsymbol{x}_i}}{\sum_{i=1}^n Y_i(u) w_i e^{\hat{\boldsymbol{\beta}}' \boldsymbol{x}_i}}$. It is a special case of a cumulative sum $W_x(t, \boldsymbol{x}) = \sum_{i=1}^n g(\boldsymbol{x}_i) I(\boldsymbol{x}_i \leq \boldsymbol{x}) \hat{M}_i^{(u)}(t)$, where $g(\cdot)$ is a known smooth function. The cumulative sums from the Cox's PH model converge to a zero-mean Gaussian process if the PH model is correctly specified and consistently estimated, a property that can be used to check the functional form of a covariate, the exponential link function, and the PH assumption in the Cox's PH model. And $U(\hat{\boldsymbol{\beta}}, t)$ is asymptotically equivalent to a function of independent standard normal random variables, which facilitates a resampling approach to approximate the distribution of $U(\hat{\boldsymbol{\beta}}, t)$ (Lin et al., 1993). A similar property can be obtained for the latency PH submodel following the fact that w_i can be treated as an offset term in the latency PH submodel. Thus, the fit of the latency PH submodel can be examined based on $W_x(t, \boldsymbol{x})$ in a similar way as Cox's PH model without a cure fraction. For example, let $U_j(\hat{\boldsymbol{\beta}}, t)$ be the jth component of $U(\hat{\boldsymbol{\beta}}, t)$, $\mathscr{I}(\hat{\boldsymbol{\beta}})$ be minus the derivative matrix of $U(\hat{\boldsymbol{\beta}}, \infty)$, and $\mathscr{I}^{-1}(\hat{\boldsymbol{\beta}})_{jj}$ be the element of the inverse of the matrix at the jth row and jth column. A visual examination of $U_j(\hat{\boldsymbol{\beta}}, t)$ versus t against simulated zero-mean Gaussian processes will reveal a departure from the assumptions in the latency PH submodel. The departure from the PH assumption for covariate $\boldsymbol{x}_j$ can be tested based on the Kolmogorov-type supremum test:

$$\sup_{t\in[0,\tau]} \|U_j(\hat{\boldsymbol{\beta}},t)\| \quad \text{or} \quad \sup_{t\in[0,\tau]} \left\| \sqrt{\mathscr{I}^{-1}(\hat{\boldsymbol{\beta}})_{jj}} U_j(\hat{\boldsymbol{\beta}},t) \right\|. \tag{3.45}$$

The p-value of the test can be obtained as the proportion of the values of (3.45) based on the simulated processes that are greater than the values of (3.45) based on the observed process.

A Schoenfeld residuals for the latency part can also be defined as

$$\delta_i[\boldsymbol{x}_i - \bar{\boldsymbol{x}}(t_i)], \tag{3.46}$$

which corresponds to the first part of $\int_0^t [\boldsymbol{x}_i - \bar{\boldsymbol{x}}(u)]\, d\hat{M}_i^{(u)}(u)$ in (3.44) evaluated at $t = \infty$. In comparison, the modified Schoenfeld residuals discussed in Section (2.5.3) is not appropriate for assessing the latency part because it depends on $h(t|\boldsymbol{x},\boldsymbol{z})$. If $h(t|\boldsymbol{x},\boldsymbol{z})$ is replaced with $h_{u0}(t)\exp(\boldsymbol{\beta}'\boldsymbol{x})$ under the PH mixture cure model, the residual in Section (2.5.3) is reduced to the modified Schoenfeld residual for the latency part in (3.46).

A Cox-Snell residual for the latency submodel for subjects with $u_i = 1$ can also be defined as follows (Peng and Taylor, 2017)

$$r_i^u = -\log S_u(t_i|\boldsymbol{x}_i). \tag{3.47}$$

To examine the distribution of r_i^u, the survival function of the distribution can be estimated using a weighted Kaplan-Meier survival estimator (Lumley, 2010) with weight $P(u_i = 1)$. In practice, $\hat{r}_i^u = -\log \hat{S}_u(t_i|x_i)$ and the weight $P(u_i = 1)$ is estimated by w_i in (2.14). The estimated cumulative hazard function can be compared with the 45° line as the usual way for Cox-Snell residuals to examine the goodness-of-fit of the latency submodel in the mixture cure model.

To assist the comparison between the estimated distribution of modified Cox-Snell residuals (with its estimated cumulative distribution function denoted as $\hat{F}_n^{CS}(t)$) and the unit exponential distribution (with the cumulative distribution function denoted as $F_0^{CS}(t) = 1 - e^{-t}$), the Cramér–von Mises criterion (Anderson, 1962) may be used to quantify the distance between the two distributions: $D(\hat{F}_n^{CS}) = \int_0^\infty \left[\hat{F}_n^{CS}(t) - F_0^{CS}(t)\right]^2 dF_0^{CS}(t)$. A smaller $D(\hat{F}_n^{CS})$ indicates a better approximation of the distribution of the modified Cox-Snell residuals by the unit exponential distribution.

3.5.3 Assessing Cure Rate Prediction

The residual approaches discussed above are either not designed to check the model fit of the incidence submodel or less sensitive to departures in the incidence submodel. To examine the performance of the incidence submodel, one can directly compare the cure status y with the predicted value of $\pi(\boldsymbol{z})$ from a cure model. Let $\hat{\pi}_{d_n}(\boldsymbol{z})$ be the estimator from a cure model based on data $d_n = \{(t_i, \delta_i, y_i, \boldsymbol{x}_i, \boldsymbol{z}_i), i = 1, \ldots, n\}$, and $\{(t_j, \delta_i, y_j, \boldsymbol{x}_j, \boldsymbol{z}_j), j = 1, \ldots, m\}$ are data from m new subjects. The so-called Brier score (Brier, 1950) to measure the discrepancy between y_j and $\hat{\pi}_{d_n}(\boldsymbol{z}_j)$, $j = 1, \ldots, m$ is given by

$$\tilde{e}(\hat{\pi}_{d_n}) = \frac{1}{m} \sum_{j=1}^{m} \{y_j - \hat{\pi}_{d_n}(\boldsymbol{z}_j)\}^2. \tag{3.48}$$

In practice, the cure status is only known for a subject either with $\delta = 1$ and thus uncured ($y = 1$), or with $\delta = 0$ but $t \geq \tau$ and thus cured ($y = 0$). For a subject with $\delta = 0$ and $t < \tau$, the cure status is unknown and cannot be used in (3.48). To correct biases due to the missing values of some y_j's, an inverse probability of censoring weights (IPCW) estimator of $\tilde{e}(\hat{\pi}_{d_n})$ can be calculated (Jiang et al., 2017; Gerds and Schumacher, 2006):

$$\tilde{e}(\hat{\pi}_{d_n}, \hat{G}_n) = \frac{1}{m} \sum_{j=1}^{m} \frac{1 - I(t_j < \tau, \delta_j = 0)}{\hat{G}_n(t_j \wedge \tau)} \{y_j - \hat{\pi}_{d_n}(\boldsymbol{z}_j)\}^2, \tag{3.49}$$

where $\hat{G}_n(\cdot)$ is the Kaplan-Meier estimate of the survival function for censoring times based on d_n and $t_j \wedge \tau = \min(t_j, \tau)$. There are three different weights assigned according to the IPCW scheme in (3.49):

- For a subject with $\delta_j = 1$, the assigned weight is $1/\{m\hat{G}_n(t_j)\}$ based on the fact that $C \geq t_j$ with probability $P(C \geq t_j) = G(t_j)$.
- For a subject with $\delta_j = 0$ and $t_j \geq \tau$, the assigned weight is $1/\{m\hat{G}_n(\tau)\}$ based on the fact that $C \geq \tau$ with probability $P(C \geq \tau) = G(\tau)$.
- For a subject with $\delta_j = 0$ and $t_j < \tau$, the cure status is unknown and the assigned weight is 0. This subject is excluded in the calculation of (3.49).

Let $e(\pi) = \mathrm{E}_F\{Y - \pi(\boldsymbol{z})\}^2$, and suppose that $\hat{\pi}_{d_n}(\boldsymbol{z})$ is a consistent estimator of $\pi(\boldsymbol{z})$. It can be shown that $\tilde{e}(\hat{\pi}_{d_n}, \hat{G}_n)$ of (3.49) is a consistent estimator of $e(\pi)$, and asymptotically equivalent to $\tilde{e}(\hat{\pi}_{d_n})$ of (3.48). The property holds when the censoring distribution depends on covariates $\tilde{\boldsymbol{x}}$. In this case, the survival estimate $\hat{G}_n(\cdot)$ needs to be replaced by the conditional estimate $\hat{G}_n(\cdot|\tilde{\boldsymbol{x}}_j)$, which can be obtained using the method discussed in Section 3.3.1.2, a kernel-type nonparametric regression (Dabrowska, 1987, 1989) for discrete and continuous covariates, or by a grouped Kaplan-Meier estimate for discrete covariates.

Calculating $\tilde{e}(\hat{\pi}_{d_n}, \hat{G}_n)$ in (3.49) requires a large independent test set from new subjects. In practice, however, the large independent test set is usually not available. In this case, one can use the resubstitution method to estimate $\tilde{e}(\hat{\pi}_{d_n}, \hat{G}_n)$ by using d_n both as the training set to build the cure model and as the test set to estimate $\tilde{e}(\hat{\pi}_{d_n}, \hat{G}_n)$:

$$\hat{e}^{\text{rs}}(\hat{\pi}_{d_n}, \hat{G}_n) = \frac{1}{n}\sum_{i=1}^{n} \frac{1 - I(t_i < \tau, \delta_i = 0)}{\hat{G}_n(t_i \wedge \tau)}\{y_i - \hat{\pi}_{d_n}(\boldsymbol{z}_i)\}^2.$$

The resubstitution method tends to have $\hat{e}^{\text{rs}}(\hat{\pi}_{d_n}, \hat{G}_n)$ that is smaller than $\tilde{e}(\hat{\pi}_{d_n}, \hat{G}_n)$. A better approach is the cross-validation method that splits the observed data set d_n into K folds, denoted by $f_1, \ldots, f_K$, with approximately the same number of subjects, and leaves one fold out as the test set at a time while taking the remaining $K-1$ folds as the training set. The K-fold cross-validation estimate takes the following form

$$\hat{e}^{\text{Kcv}}(\hat{\pi}_{d_n}, \hat{G}_n) = \frac{1}{n}\sum_{k=1}^{K}\sum_{l \in f_k} \frac{1 - I(t_l < \tau, \delta_l = 0)}{\hat{G}_n(t_l \wedge \tau)}\{y_l - \hat{\pi}_{f_{-k}}(\boldsymbol{z}_l)\}^2,$$

where $\hat{\pi}_{f_{-k}}(\boldsymbol{z}_l)$ is an estimator of π based on the observed data set d_n with f_k removed. In this method, $\hat{G}_n(\cdot)$ can be estimated based on all training data d_n instead of all but f_k fold in estimating the IPCW weights because the former is expected to provide more accurate estimates of the weights than the latter.

3.5.4 Concordance Measures for Cure Models

Concordance measures are often used to assess a model fit. For example, area under the curve (AUC) is a concordance measure for logistic regression. Consider the logistic regression in the incidence submodel of the mixture cure model. If all y_i's are available, the AUC is defined as the area under the receiver operating characteristic (ROC) curve, which is a plot of sensitivity

$$\frac{\sum_{i=1}^{n} I(\hat{\pi}(\boldsymbol{z}_i) \geq c) y_i}{\sum_{i=1}^{n} y_i}$$

against 1− specificity

$$\frac{\sum_{i=1}^{n} I(\hat{\pi}(\boldsymbol{z}_i) \geq c)(1 - y_i)}{\sum_{i=1}^{n}(1 - y_i)}$$

for all possible values of c. However, this measure cannot be used directly for the logistic regression in the incidence submodel of the mixture cure model due to the unknown cure status y_i for some subjects. A workaround approach is to replace y_i's by $\hat{\pi}(\boldsymbol{z}_i)$'s for all subjects or only for those subjects with unknown y_i's (Asano et al., 2014). The bootstrap method can be used to estimate the standard error of the AUC, which allows inferences based on the AUC.

A concordance measure can also be defined for the failure times. Zhang and Shao (2017) considered a slightly more general transformation model than (3.12) for the latency part of the mixture cure model

$$S_u(t|\boldsymbol{x}) = S_\epsilon[g(t) + \phi(\boldsymbol{x}'\boldsymbol{\beta})],$$

where $\phi(\cdot)$ is a known function, and suggested a k-index concordance measure

$$K(\hat{\boldsymbol{\beta}}, \hat{\gamma}) = \frac{\sum_{i \neq j} G(\boldsymbol{x}_i'\hat{\boldsymbol{\beta}}, \boldsymbol{x}_j'\hat{\boldsymbol{\beta}}) I(\boldsymbol{x}_i'\hat{\boldsymbol{\beta}} < \boldsymbol{x}_j'\hat{\boldsymbol{\beta}}) \hat{\pi}(\boldsymbol{z}_i) \hat{\pi}(\boldsymbol{z}_j)}{\sum_{i \neq j} I(\boldsymbol{x}_i'\hat{\boldsymbol{\beta}} < \boldsymbol{x}_j'\hat{\boldsymbol{\beta}}) \hat{\pi}(\boldsymbol{z}_i) \hat{\pi}(\boldsymbol{z}_j)}$$

where

$$G(u_1, u_2) = \int_{-\infty}^{u_2} [S_\epsilon(u_1 - u_2 + u) - S_\epsilon(u_1)] dS_\epsilon(u)$$

This measure extends Harrell's c-index for PH model and can be shown to be asymptotically normal. A bootstrap method can be employed to estimate the standard error of the estimate of the measure, which allows inferences based on the k-index. A similar measure can also be defined for the transformation model for the non-mixture cure model discussed in Section 2.4.4.

3.5.5 Testing Goodness-of-Fit of Parametric Cure Rate Estimation

The proposed nonparametric estimation method for $\pi(z)$ in Section 3.3.1 is flexible to accommodate different effects of z on π than the parametric estimation methods based on logistic models or parametric models based on the complementary log-log link function discussed in Section 2.2.1. However, the parametric methods are more efficient if the parametric assumptions are correct and the results from the parametric methods are easier to interpret. Therefore, it is of interest to examine the goodness-of-fit of the parametric estimates for $\pi(z)$ relative to the flexible nonparametric estimate for $\pi(z)$ to determine any significant difference between them. This is similar to the question about comparing nonparametric versus parametric regression fits (Hardle and Mammen, 1993).

Let $\hat{\pi}(z)$ be the nonparametric estimate in (3.33) and $\pi_{\hat{\gamma}}(z)$ be the parametric estimate in (2.2) or (2.3). The hypotheses for the goodness-of-fit question can be expressed as follows:

$$H_0\colon \pi(z) = \pi_{\boldsymbol{\gamma}}(z) \text{ for some } \boldsymbol{\gamma} \in \boldsymbol{\Gamma} \text{ vs } H_1\colon \pi(z) \neq \pi_{\boldsymbol{\gamma}}(z) \text{ for all } \boldsymbol{\gamma} \in \boldsymbol{\Gamma} \quad (3.50)$$

where $\boldsymbol{\Gamma}$ is a finite-dimensional parameter space of $\boldsymbol{\gamma}$ and the function $\pi_{\boldsymbol{\gamma}}(z)$ is a known function up to a parameter vector $\boldsymbol{\gamma} \in \boldsymbol{\Gamma}$. A goodness-of-fit test to test above hypotheses can be constructed based on the following distance measure between the two estimates (Müller and van Keilegom, 2019)

$$\mathcal{T}_n = nh^{1/2} \int \{\hat{\pi}(z) - \pi_{\hat{\gamma}}(z)\}^2 p(z) dz$$

or its empirical version

$$\tilde{\mathcal{T}}_n = nh^{1/2} \frac{1}{n} \sum_{i=1}^{n} \{\hat{\pi}(z_i) - \pi_{\hat{\gamma}}(z_i)\}^2,$$

where $p(z)$ is the density function of z and h is the bandwidth used in the nonparametric estimate $\hat{\pi}(z)$. Let $H(t|z) = P(\min(T,C) \leq t|z)$, $H_1(t|z) = P(\min(T,C) \leq t, \delta = 1|z)$, $\zeta(t|z) = \frac{I(T\leq t, T\leq C)}{1-H(\min(T,C)|z)} - \int_0^t \frac{I(\min(T,C)\geq s)}{[1-H(s|z)]^2} dH_1(s|z)$, $\tau_u(z) = \inf\{t\colon S_u(t|z) = 0\}$ and $\tau_G(z) = \inf\{t\colon G(t|z) = 0\}$. Under the sufficient follow-up condition $\tau_u(z) < \tau_G(z)$ and some mild conditions for $p(z)$, $\pi(z)$, the kernel function in the nonparametric estimate $\hat{\pi}(z)$, the latency survival time distribution and the censoring time distribution, if $nh^3(\log n)^{-5} \to \infty$ and $nh^5/(\log n) = O(1)$ as $n \to \infty$, the two distance measures are asymptotically equivalent and $\mathcal{T}_n$ is asymptotically normally distributed under the null hypothesis in (3.50) with

$$\mathcal{T}_n - b_h \to N(0, V),$$

where $b_h = h^{-1/2} \int K^2(s)ds \int_0^1 [1 - \pi(z)]^2 \mu(z)dz = O(h^{-1/2})$, $V = 2K^{(4)}(0) \int_0^1 [(1-\pi(z))^2 \mu(z)]^2 dz$, $K^{(4)}$ denotes the fourth convolution product of K and $\mu(z) = E[\zeta^2(\tau_u(z)|z)|Z = z]$. Under a local alternative of the form $\pi(z) = \pi_\gamma(z) + n^{-1/2}h^{-1/4}\Delta_n(z)$ with $\Delta_n(z)$ bounded uniformly in z and n, $\mathcal{T}_n$ is also asymptotically normally distributed

$$\mathcal{T}_n - b_h - \int \Delta_n(z)^2 p(z)dz \to N(0, V),$$

which enables power and sample size estimation. However, due to slow convergence rates, the normal distribution does not provide an accurate approximation to the null distribution of $\mathcal{T}_n$ or $\tilde{\mathcal{T}}_n$ under finite sample sizes, and a bootstrap method is suggested to better approximate the distribution (Müller and van Keilegom, 2019). A proposed algorithm for the bootstrap method to approximate the null distribution is given below:

Step 1 Use the data, a pilot bandwidth h_0 and the estimator in Section 3.3.1 to obtain $\hat{\pi}_{h_0}(z_i)$, $\hat{S}_{h_0}(t|z_i)$ and $\hat{G}_{h_0}(t|z_i)$.

Step 2 Fit a logistic model to data $\{(z_i, \hat{\pi}_{h_0}(z_i)), i = 1, \ldots, n\}$ to obtain $\hat{\gamma}$. That is, $\hat{\gamma} = \arg\max_\gamma \sum_{i=1}^n [\hat{\pi}_{h_0}(z_i) \log(\pi_\gamma(z_i) + (1 - \hat{\pi}_{h_0}(z_i)) \log(1 - \pi_\gamma(z_i))]$. The corresponding parametric estimator is denoted as $\hat{\pi}_{h_0,\hat{\gamma}}(z_i)$.

Step 3 Generate the bth of B bootstrap samples data $\{(z_i, t^*_{i,b}, \delta^*_{i,b}), i = 1\ldots, n\}$ from the mixture cure model with the latency uncured survival function $[\hat{S}_{h_0}(t|z_i) - 1 + \hat{\pi}_{h_0}(z_i)]/\hat{\pi}_{h_0}(z_i)$ and incidence uncure rate $\hat{\pi}_{h_0,\hat{\gamma}}(z_i)$. The censoring distribution is set to $\hat{G}_{h_0}(t|z_i)$.

Step 4 For the bth bootstrap sample and a bandwidth h, use the method of Section 3.3.1 to obtain a nonparametric estimate $\hat{\pi}^*_{hh_0,b}(z_i)$, and then use $(z_i, \hat{\pi}^*_{hh_0,b}(z_i))$ and the method in Step 2 to obtain a parametric estimate $\hat{\pi}_{hh_0,\hat{\gamma}^*,b}(z_i)$.

Step 5 Find the $(1-\alpha)\times 100$th percentile of $\{\mathcal{T}^*_{n,b}, b = 1, \ldots, B\}$ as the critical value of the test, where

$$\mathcal{T}^*_{n,b} = nh^{-1/2}\frac{1}{n}\sum_{i=1}^{n}\left[\hat{\pi}^*_{hh_0,b}(z_i) - \hat{\pi}_{hh_0,\hat{\gamma}^*,b}(z_i)\right]^2.$$

3.5.6 Variable Selection

Similar to other regression models, variable selection is an important issue in the mixture cure model, particularly when there are a large number of covariates available for the two regression submodels involved in a mixture cure model. The AIC discussed in Section 2.5.1 has long been used to select a parsimonious model among candidate models. For a parametric mixture cure model with observed maximum likelihood function (2.12) available, it is not difficult to use this method to select covariates and models in the mixture cure model context, as discussed in Section 2.5.1.

For semiparametric mixture cure models, since most of the models are estimated using the EM algorithm, the observed maximum likelihood function is not readily available, which makes AIC calculation difficult. Dirick et al. (2015) proposed an approach to calculate the AIC values based on the maximum complete likelihood function (2.15) and (2.16).

A popular and modern approach to select covariates in regression models is via penalization, such as LASSO (Tibshirani, 1996) or SCAD (Fan and Li, 2001) methods. We demonstrate in this section how these methods can be implemented for mixture cure models under the EM framework (Liu et al., 2012). Consider the semiparametric PH model in Section 3.2.1. If the EM algorithm is used to estimate the parameters in the model, then the M-step maximizes (2.15) and (3.2). The penalized method suggests replacing the two functions by their corresponding penalized versions:

$$\ell_1^P(\gamma) = \log\prod_{i=1}^{n}\left\{\pi(\boldsymbol{z}_i)^{w_i^{(k)}}[1-\pi(\boldsymbol{z}_i)]^{1-w_i^{(k)}}\right\} - n\sum_{j=1}^{p_z} P_{\lambda_{1j}}(|\gamma_j|) \tag{3.51}$$

$$\ell_2^P(\boldsymbol{\beta},\boldsymbol{\alpha}) = \log\prod_{i=1,w_i^{(k)}>0}^{n}\left\{h_u(t_i|\boldsymbol{x}_i)^{\delta_i}S_u(t_i|\boldsymbol{x}_i)^{w_i^{(k)}}\right\} - n\sum_{j=1}^{p_x} P_{\lambda_{2j}}(|\beta_j|) \tag{3.52}$$

where $P_\lambda(|\cdot|)$ is a penalty function and $\boldsymbol{\lambda} = (\lambda_{11}, \ldots, \lambda_{1p_z}, \lambda_{21}, \ldots, \lambda_{1p_x})$ are tuning parameters, which may be chosen by a data-driven method, such as generalized cross validation (GCV). The penalty function can be either the LASSO penalty $P_\lambda(|x|) = \lambda|x|$ or the SCAD penalty

$$P_\lambda(|x|) = \begin{cases} \lambda|x| & \text{if } 0 \le |x| < \lambda \\ \frac{(a^2-1)\lambda^2-(|x|-a\lambda)^2}{2(a-1)} & \text{if } \lambda \le |x| < a\lambda \\ \frac{(a+1)\lambda^2}{2} & \text{if } |x| \ge a\lambda. \end{cases}$$

The penalized likelihood (3.51) can be maximized by the Newton-Raphson method or by a program that can handle penalized logistic regression analysis. The penalized likelihood (3.52) can be replaced with a penalized partial likelihood discussed in (Fan and Li, 2002) to obtain an update of $\boldsymbol{\beta}$ and the baseline survival function can be estimated by the Nelson-Aalen estimator (3.3). Since the added penalty terms do not depend on y_i, the E-step does not change and (2.14) is calculated to complete the E-step.

To speed up the estimation, instead of minimizing GCV with respect to the $p_x + p_z$-dimensional parameter $\boldsymbol{\lambda}$, one can set $\lambda_{1j} = \lambda_1 \mathrm{SE}(\hat{\gamma}_j^u)$ and $\lambda_{2j} = \lambda_2 \mathrm{SE}(\hat{\beta}_j^u)$ where λ_1 and λ_2 are tuning parameters and $\mathrm{SE}(\hat{\gamma}_j^u)$ and $\mathrm{SE}(\hat{\beta}_j^u)$ are the standard errors of the estimates from semiparametric PH model in Section 3.2.1 without the penalties. The tuning parameters λ_1 and λ_2 can be selected by minimizing GCVs from the logistic regression model and the Cox's PH model in the M-step. If some variable is believed to be or must be in the model, the corresponding tuning parameter in $\boldsymbol{\lambda}$ can be set to zero, that is, the penalty on the variable's coefficient is zero. For example, we do not put any penalty on the intercept because the intercept is always in the logistic regression part.

A similar idea can also be applied to other semiparametric cure models, such as the semiparametric PHC model (Masud et al., 2018). For parametric cure models, due to the availability of the observed likelihood function, it is possible to penalize the observed likelihood function directly instead of the complete likelihood function in the M-step (Scolas et al., 2016).

For semiparametric spline-based additive effects mixture cure model discussed in Section 3.2.6, the penalized likelihood approach above does not work since the effects of covariates are in the form of functionals rather than in a form of coefficients. Variable selection can be carried out using the Kullback-Leibler distance (Gu, 2013). For two estimates ζ_1 and ζ_2 of ζ in (3.24), the Kullback-Leibler distance between them is defined as

$$\mathrm{KL}(\zeta_1, \zeta_2) = \frac{1}{n}\sum_{i=1}^{n}\left[\frac{e^{\zeta_1(\boldsymbol{z}_i)}}{1+e^{\zeta_1(\boldsymbol{z}_i)}}\{\zeta_1(\boldsymbol{z}_i) - \zeta_2(\boldsymbol{z}_i)\} \right. \\ \left. - \{\log(1+\zeta_1(\boldsymbol{z}_i)) - \log(1+\zeta_2(\boldsymbol{z}_i))\}\right]$$

For two estimates η_1 and η_2 of η in (3.25), the Kullback-Leibler distance between them is defined as

$$\mathrm{KL}(\eta_1, \eta_2) = \frac{1}{n}\sum_{i=1}^{n}\int_0^{t_i}\left[e^{\eta_1(t,\boldsymbol{x}_i)}\{\eta_1(t,\boldsymbol{x}_i) - \eta_2(t,\boldsymbol{x}_i)\} \right. \\ \left. - \{e^{\eta_1(t,\boldsymbol{x}_i)} - e^{\eta_2(t,\boldsymbol{x}_i)}\}\right].$$

Let $\hat{\zeta}$ be an estimate of ζ in a space $\mathcal{H}_1$ for a full model, $\hat{\zeta}^*$ be an estimate of ζ in a subspace $\mathcal{H}_2 \subset \mathcal{H}_1$ for a reduced model, and $\hat{\zeta}_c$ be an estimate of ζ from a constant model. Then $\mathrm{KL}(\hat{\zeta}, \hat{\zeta}^*)/\mathrm{KL}(\hat{\zeta}, \hat{\zeta}_c) \leq 0.05$ can be used to favor the reduced model. A similar criterion can be obtained for $\hat{\eta}$ (Wang et al., 2012a).

3.6 Software and Applications

There are several R and SAS packages that can be used to fit the semiparametric and nonparametric cure models. We will show some software packages and use them to illustrate the applications of some cure models discussed in early sections to real data sets.

3.6.1 R Package mixcure

The R package `mixcure` can fit the semiparametric PH mixture cure model in addition to the parametric mixture cure models discussed in Section 2.6.2. We demonstrate the use of this package to fit the model to the leukemia data introduced in Section 2.6 as follows. The treatment group variable `transplant` enters both parts of the mixture cure model.

```
> summary(mixcure(Surv(time, cens) ~ transplant, ~ transplant, data
+ = goldman.data, savedata = T), R = 300)

Call:
mixcure(lformula = Surv(time, cens) ~ transplant, iformula =
    ~transplant, data = goldman.data, savedata = T)

Latency model for uncured:
                     coefficient    stderr   zscore     pvalue
transplantAutologous   0.6332632 0.3085259 2.052545 0.04011672

Incidence model:
                     coefficient    stderr    zscore      pvalue
(Intercept)            1.0283684 0.3703484 2.7767593 0.005490381
transplantAutologous   0.3769905 0.7157321 0.5267202 0.598387918
```

Under this model, the two treatment groups are not statistically significant in cure rates. However, the Autologous group does show significantly higher hazards than the Allogeneic group with an estimated hazard ratio of 1.88 and 95% confidence interval (1.03, 3.45). The fitted survival curves are plotted against the Kaplan-Meier survival curves in Figure 3.2. It is clear that the semiparametric PH mixture cure model provides a better fit to the data than the previous parametric mixture cure models, and the improved fit leads to a significant effect of the treatment in the latency part.

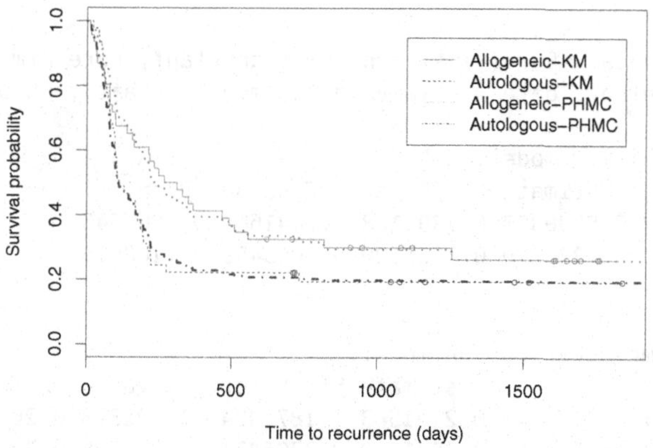

FIGURE 3.2
Estimated survival curves (dotted lines) from the semiparametric PH mixture cure model for the leukemia data.

3.6.2 R Package smcure

The R package `smcure` can also fit the semiparametric PH mixture cure model as follows

```
> smcure(Surv(time, cens) ~ transplant, ~ transplant, data =
+ goldman.data, model = "ph", nboot = 500)

Call:
smcure(formula = Surv(time, cens) ~ transplant, cureform =
    ~transplant, data = goldman.data, model = "ph", nboot = 500)

Cure probability model:
             Estimate Std.Error   Z value  Pr(>|Z|)
(Intercept) 0.6986655 0.8792946 0.7945750 0.4268608
transplant  0.3579095 0.6011734 0.5953516 0.5516085

Failure time distribution model:
                     Estimate Std.Error  Z value   Pr(>|Z|)
transplantAutologous 0.6363645 0.3314896 1.919712 0.05489429
```

There are some differences in the estimates of incidence parameters between `mixcure` and `smcure`. The differences may be due to the quasi-binomial-logit link instead of the binomial-logit link used in `smcure`.

Another model `smcure` can fit is the semiparametric AFT mixture cure model discussed in Section 3.2.2. We can use it to fit the leukemia data as follows:

```
> smcure(Surv(time, cens) ~ transplant, ~ transplant, data =
+ goldman.data, model = "aft", nboot = 500)
```

```
Call:
smcure(formula = Surv(time, cens) ~ transplant, cureform =
    ~transplant, data = goldman.data, model = "aft", nboot = 500)

Cure probability model:
             Estimate Std.Error   Z value  Pr(>|Z|)
(Intercept) 0.5800933 0.7795188 0.7441684 0.4567746
transplant  0.4273070 0.5286190 0.8083459 0.4188915


Failure time distribution model:
                        Estimate Std.Error   Z value  Pr(>|Z|)
(Intercept)            0.2101563 0.1872494  1.122333 0.2617208
transplantAutologous -0.3531250 0.2706421 -1.304768 0.1919720
```

The results show that the two treatment groups are not statistically significant in either of the incidence and latency part. The differences in results between the semiparametric PH model and the semiparametric AFT model may partly be due to the poor fit of the AFT model to the data.

3.6.3 SAS Macro PSPMCM

The SAS macro `PSPMCM` (Corbiere and Joly, 2007) can fit the semiparametric PH model as follows

```
%pspmcm(DATA=goldmandata,ID=id,CENSCOD=cens,TIME=time,
  VAR= transplant(IS), INCPART=logit, SURVPART=cox,
  TAIL=zero, SU0MET=pl, FAST=Y,BOOTSTRAP=Y,
  NSAMPLE=2000, STRATA=, MAXITER=200,CONVCRIT=1e-5,
  ALPHA=0.05, BASELINE=Y, BOOTMET=ALL, JACKDATA=,
  GESTIMATE=Y, SPLOT=Y, PLOTFIT=Y);
run;
```

```
                    FAST RESULTS FOR THE LOGIT PART (goldmandata)
                       Analysis of Maximum Likelihood Estimates

                                  Standard      Wald        Pr >      Estimation
      Variable    DF  Estimate     Error    Chi-Square  Chi-Square      Type
      Intercept    1    1.0283    0.3347       9.4373     0.0021        MLE
      transplant   1    0.3770    0.5025       0.5629     0.4531        MLE

                   FAST RESULTS FOR THE SURVIVAL PART (goldmandata)
                       Analysis of Maximum Likelihood Estimates

                                                                  95% Lower
                                                                 Confidence
                 Parameter  Standard                Pr >   Hazard    Limit for
Parameter   DF   Estimate      Error Chi-Square    ChiSq    Ratio Hazard Ratio
transplant   1    0.63323    0.26031     5.9175   0.0150    1.884        1.131
lpi          0    1.00000          0          .        .        .            .

               95% Upper
              Confidence
               Limit for
Parameter   Hazard Ratio
```

```
transplant      3.138
lpi               .

                       BOOTSTRAP CONFIDENCE INTERVAL FOR PARAMETERS ESTIMATES
                         (confidence level=95%, 2000 bootstrap resamples)

                       Method=BC  Method=BC Method=BCA Method=BCA
                         Lower      Upper     Lower      Upper      Method=    Method=
          Observed Confidence Confidence Confidence Confidence PCTL Lower PCTL Upper
Variable Statistic    Limit      Limit      Limit      Limit   percentile percentile
L_Int     1.02808    0.35720    1.89458    0.33647    1.83466    0.34868    1.85686
L_TRANSP  0.37722   -0.82064    1.46265   -0.86845    1.44908   -0.67219    1.56175
S_TRANSP  0.63323    0.03407    1.26047   -0.02173    1.22178    0.05280    1.30678

          Method=HYB
             Lower
Variable  percentile
L_Int       0.19930
L_TRANSP   -0.80732
S_TRANSP   -0.04032

                                   Method=BOOTN Method=BOOTN Method=JACK Method=JACK
                       Method=HYB     Lower        Upper        Lower       Upper
           Observed      Upper     Confidence   Confidence   Confidence  Confidence
Variable   Statistic  percentile      Limit        Limit        Limit       Limit
L_Int       1.02808     1.70748      0.26070      1.76367      0.27630     1.72789
L_TRANSP    0.37722     1.42663     -0.77328      1.44392     -0.71742     1.40118
S_TRANSP    0.63323     1.21366     -0.00909      1.23399     -0.05167     1.27977
```

The results are very similar to the results from `mixcure`.

The SAS macro `PSPMCM` also provides `WTAIL` and `ETAIL` options in addition to `ZERO` when estimating the upper tail of the baseline distribution in the latency submodel. See more detailed discussions of the tail completion methods in Section 3.2.1.1.

3.6.4 R Package Survival

The R package `survival` can be used to fit a mixture cure model and estimate cure rate nonparametrically with one categorical variable or discrete variable using the method discussed in Section 3.3.1. Using the leukemia data introduced in Section 2.6 as an example, we first obtain the nonparametric survival estimates of the two treatment groups using `survfit` function in `survival` package as follows:

```
> z = survfit(Surv(time, cens) ~ transplant, data = goldman.data)
> summary(z)

Call: survfit(formula = Surv(time, cens) ~ transplant,
      data = goldman.data)

                transplant=Allogeneic
 time n.risk n.event survival std.err lower 95% CI upper 95% CI
   11     46       1    0.978  0.0215        0.937        1.000
   14     45       1    0.957  0.0301        0.899        1.000
   23     44       1    0.935  0.0364        0.866        1.000
    .      .       .        .       .            .            .
```

```
   .      .        .        .        .             .             .
   .      .        .        .        .             .             .
 557     16        1    0.326   0.0691         0.215         0.494
 819     13        1    0.301   0.0682         0.193         0.469
1256      8        1    0.263   0.0693         0.157         0.441

                transplant=Autologous
time n.risk n.event survival std.err lower 95% CI upper 95% CI
  21     45       1    0.978  0.0220        0.936        1.000
  40     44       1    0.956  0.0307        0.897        1.000
  42     43       1    0.933  0.0372        0.863        1.000
   .      .       .        .       .            .            .
   .      .       .        .       .            .            .
   .      .       .        .       .            .            .
 224     12       1    0.244  0.0641        0.146        0.409
 277     11       1    0.222  0.0620        0.129        0.384
 734      8       1    0.194  0.0601        0.106        0.356
```

Following (3.30), the cure rate estimates for the two treatment groups are given by the last lines of the survival output for the two groups as follows

```
> summary(z[1], time = 1256)

Call: survfit(formula = Surv(time, cens) ~ transplant,
      data = goldman.data)

 time n.risk n.event survival std.err lower 95% CI upper 95% CI
 1256      8      33    0.263  0.0693        0.157        0.441
> summary(z[2], time = 734)
Call: survfit(formula = Surv(time, cens) ~ transplant,
      data = goldman.data)

 time n.risk n.event survival std.err lower 95% CI upper 95% CI
  734      8      36    0.194  0.0601        0.106        0.356
```

That is, the cure rate and its 95% confidence intervals are 0.263 and (0.157, 0.441) for Allogeneic group and 0.194 and (0.106, 0.356) for Autologous group. The latency survival functions of the two groups can be obtained using the method of (3.37). For example, the estimated latency survival function for the Allogeneic group is

```
> cbind(time = z[1]$time, surv = (z[1]$surv - cure1)/(1-cure1))

      time       surv
 [1,]   11 0.97048808
 [2,]   14 0.94097616
 [3,]   23 0.91146425
    .    .          .
    .    .          .
    .    .          .
```

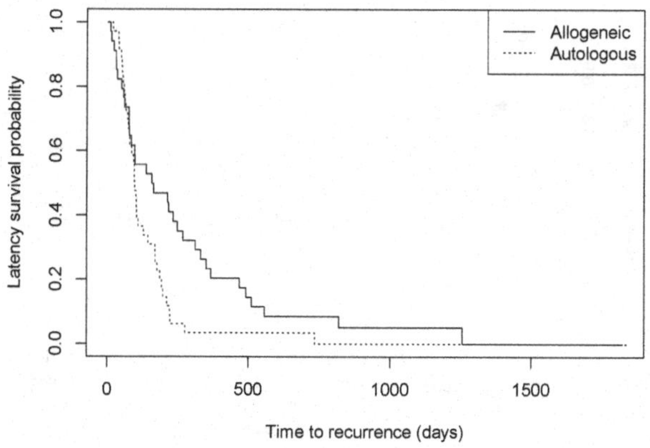

FIGURE 3.3
Estimated latency survival curves from the nonparametric mixture cure model for the leukemia data.

```
[36,] 1109 0.05107832
[37,] 1158 0.05107832
[38,] 1256 0.00000000
```

Similar estimation can be done for Autologous group. The estimated survival curves can be obtained as follows and plotted in Figure 3.3:

```
> cure1 = summary(z[1], time = 1256)$surv
> cure2 = summary(z[2], time = 734)$surv
> plot(cbind(time = c(0, z[1]$time), surv = c(1, (z[1]$surv -
+ cure1)/(1-cure1))), type = "s", ylab = "Latency survival
+ probability", xlab = "Time to recurrence (days)")
> lines(cbind(time = c(0, z[2]$time), surv = c(1, (z[2]$surv -
+ cure2)/(1-cure2))), type = "s", lty = 2)
> legend("topright", legend = c("Allogeneic","Autologous"), lty=1:2)
```

3.6.5 R Package npcure

To fit a nonparametric cure rate model with a continuous covariate, one can use an R package `npcure`. We consider the data from a study of bone marrow transplant for leukemia patients reported by Copelan et al. (1991) (the data is available in Klein and Moeschberger (2003)). The study included 137 leukemia patients from hospitals in the United States and Australia, and they were followed up to 2,640 days. There are 42 patients relapsed, 41 died in remission and 54 censored at the end of the study (the overall censoring percentage was 39.4%). The event of interest is relapse or death due to leukemia following bone marrow transplantation. Figure 3.4 shows the Kaplan-Meier survival function estimate for the data. The curve shows a long plateau that levels off

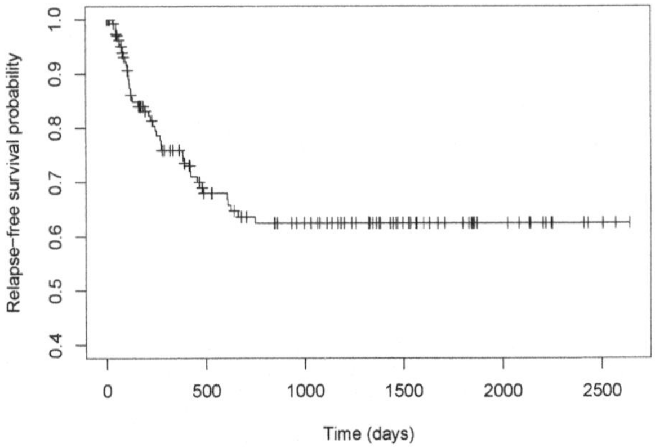

FIGURE 3.4
The Kaplan-Meier survival curve of time to relapse or death due to leukemia after bone marrow transplant.

substantially above zero. It indicates that a substantial fraction of patients may be viewed as cured after a sufficiently long follow-up, and cure models may be suitable to analyze the data.

Following the work of Xu and Peng (2014), we consider patient's age effect in the cure model in the following analysis. The data are stored in `bmt`.

```
> str(bmt)

'data.frame':    137 obs. of  4 variables:
 $ time: int  2081 1602 1496 1462 1433 1377 1330 996 226 1199 ...
 $ cens: int  0 0 0 0 0 0 0 0 0 0 ...
 $ pAge: int  26 21 26 17 32 22 20 22 18 24 ...
 $ dAge: int  33 37 35 21 36 31 17 24 21 40 ...
```

The function `probcure` in `npcure` can be used to obtain a nonparametric estimate of the effect of `pAge` on cure rate and its 95% confidence interval as follows. A plot of the estimated effect and its confidence interval is given in Figure 3.5. The figure is slightly different from Figure 3 in Xu and Peng (2014) due to local optimal bandwidths are used at different values of `pAge`.

```
> z = probcure(pAge, time, cens, data = bmt, x0 = 7:52,   conflevel
+ = 0.95)
> plot(with(z, cbind(x0, q)), type = "l", ylim = c(0, 1), xlab =
+ "Patient's age", ylab = "Cure rate")
> lines(with(z, cbind(x0, conf$lower)), lty = 2)
> lines(with(z, cbind(x0, conf$upper)), lty = 2)
```

The package also provides a function `latency` to estimate the latency survival function using the method of Section 3.3.2. We use the function to estimate the latency survival functions for patient's age from 7 to 52 and plot them in Figure 3.6 as follows.

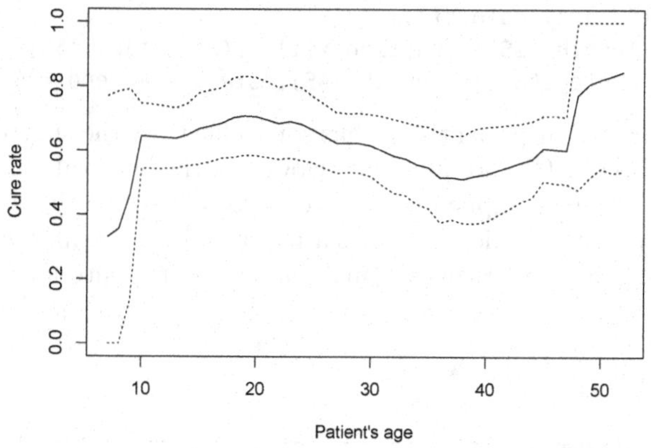

FIGURE 3.5
The estimated patient's age effect on cure rate and its 95% confidence interval for leukemia patients after bone marrow transplant.

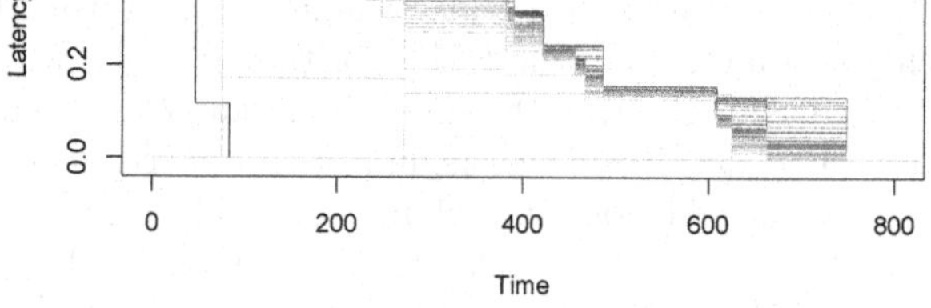

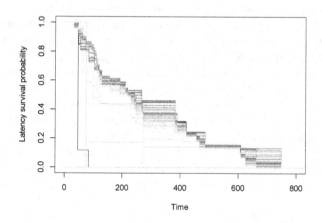

FIGURE 3.6
The estimated latency survival functions for leukemia patients with age 7 (darkest line) to 52 (lightest line) after bone marrow transplant.

```
> z = latency(pAge, time, cens, data = bmt, x0 = 7:52)
> plot(with(z, cbind(testim, S[[1]])), type = "s", ylim = c(0, 1),
+ xlab = "Time", ylab = "Latency survival probability", xlim = c(0,
+ 800), col = gray.colors(1))
> lapply(1:length(z$S), function(x)lines(z$testim, z$S[[x]], type =
+ "s", col = gray.colors(length(z$S), start = 0, end = 0.9)[x]))
```

The figure shows that patient's age has some effects on the survival within 100 days and between 200 and 400 days. However, the survival curves cross and show some potential complicated effect of patient's age on the survival time of the uncured patients, which indicates a parametric or semiparametric latency submodel, such as the PH model, may not be appropriate for modeling such an effect.

3.7 Summary

Semiparametric cure models are the models with unspecified baseline distributions that are usually estimated by a nonparametric method. Other parts of the models are parametrically specified, such as the incidence submodel and the covariate effects in the latency submodel of the mixture cure models. This chapter presented details of the semiparametric mixture cure models under various assumptions in the latency submodels and their estimation methods. In particular, we demonstrated that the EM algorithm can simplify the estimation process and connect the cure models with standard cure models. We also showed the semiparametric non-mixture cure models and their estimation methods. Cure models without any parametric assumptions are referred to as nonparametric cure models. We introduced two methods to estimate the incidence submodel and the latency submodel under the nonparametric mixture cure model based on the generalized Kaplan-Meier estimator. We also discussed some model diagnosis methods based on mixture cure models, including residuals, good-of-fit measures, and variable selection using the penalized complete likelihood functions in the EM algorithm. Finally, we demonstrated 4 R packages and 1 SAS macro to fit some semiparametric cure models.

We skipped some details of the asymptotic properties of the estimates of the semiparametric and nonparametric cure models. For semiparametric mixture cure models, we refer readers to Fang et al. (2005), Lu and Ying (2004), and Zeng et al. (2006) among others for further details.

One consequence of using semiparametric and nonparametric cure models versus parametric cure models is that the nonparametric latency distribution estimate cannot be extrapolated beyond the last observed data, which results in an identifiability issue. We introduced a few methods in this chapter to overcome the identifiability issue. One popular remedy is to set the estimated latency survival function to zero after the largest uncensored time, which essentially assumes that the largest uncensored time is the threshold for cure. The single cure threshold for every subject may not applicable in other situations, and Betensky and Schoenfeld (2001) proposed a method to deal with random cure threshold. Wu et al. (2014) further considered a situation where the cure status can be detected with a diagnostic procedure with prespecified sensitivity and specificity and adapted the EM algorithm for the semiparametric mixture cure model to include the information in the estimation.

We only considered covariate effects in the latency submodel in the semi parametric cure models via hazard functions or the mean of log survival time in this chapter. Semiparametric mixture cure models with quantile regression as the latency submodel have also been proposed, where the covariate effects in the latency submodel is via the quantile of the latency distribution. See Wu and Yin (2013) and Wu and Yin (2017a,b) for details.

Covariates with measurement errors or mismeasured covariates and partially missed covariates in cure models are also well studied in the literature. In the context of semiparametric and nonparametric cure models, we refer readers to Bertrand et al. (2017) and Beesley et al. (2016) for details.

4

Cure Models for Multivariate Survival Data and Competing Risks

4.1 Introduction

Multivariate survival data are abundant in sociological studies and biomedical research. For example, clustered survival data often arise when failure times from the homogeneous groups are correlated, e.g., overall survival times for patients from the same clinical center in a multicenter clinical trial, the disease onset time for subjects from the same family. Recurrent event data may happen when a subject experiences events of the same type more than once, e.g., cancer recurrences. There has been extensive research on the analysis of multivariate survival data. Crowder (2012) provided a comprehensive overview of various distributions and models that have been proposed for multivariate survival data and competing risks data. Hougaard (2000) presented four approaches to the analysis of multivariate survival data, i.e., the multi-state model, the frailty model, the marginal modeling approach, and the nonparametric approach.

When positively correlated failure times are treated as if they were independent, it may lead to confidence intervals with incorrect coverage probabilities. Two common approaches have been developed to handle multivariate survival data. The random-effects (frailty) model treats the cluster-specific effects as random effects (Hougaard, 2000). The marginal model estimates the marginal population-averaged fixed effects (Lin, 1994). When the joint survival distribution is correctly specified, the random effect frailty model is more appropriate to capture the association between the correlated survival times, whereas the marginal model may yield biased estimates. The popularity of the marginal approach can be attributed in part to their robustness against misspecification of the correlation structure and their relative ease of use.

Like univariate survival data, correlated survival data and competing risk data may also include a cure fraction in the data. Thus, both the cure fraction and the correlation/competing risks among the survival times have to be considered in modeling such data. In this chapter, we show how the random-effects frailty models and marginal survival models can be adapted to accommodate correlated survival times with a possible cure fraction (Section 4.2 and Section 4.3) and recurrent survival data with a cure fraction (Section 4.4).

Competing risks data with a cure fraction are discussed in Section 4.5. Finally, the chapter is concluded with a demonstration of the applications of some of the cure models to real data set (Section 4.6).

4.2 Marginal Cure Models

4.2.1 Marginal Models with Working Independence

We assume that the survival data from n clusters and there are n_i subjects in the ith cluster. The observed failure time, censoring indicator and two sets of covariates for the jth individual in the ith cluster are denoted as $t_{ij} = \min(t^*_{ij}, c_{ij})$, $\delta_{ij} = I(t^*_{ij} \leq c_{ij})$, $\boldsymbol{x}_{ij}$, $\boldsymbol{z}_{ij}$ respectively, where $I(\cdot)$ is the indicator function, t^*_{ij} and c_{ij} are the true underlying failure and censoring times. We assume that the censoring time c_{ij} and failure time t^*_{ij} are independent conditional on the observed covariates. Due to the presence of cured subjects, we also define y_{ij} as the cure status for subject j in cluster i with $y_{ij} = 0$ if this subject is cured and $y_{ij} = 1$ otherwise. Similarly, y_{ij} is usually observed with $y_{ij} = 1$ if $\delta_{ij} = 1$ and unknown otherwise. Because of shared environmental or genetic factors, the failure times t^*_{ij} and the cure status y_{ij} from the same cluster may be correlated. The setting above also includes recurrent times by considering t^*_{ij} as the jth recurrent time for subject i. However, the cure status is usually defined at the subject level, not at the individual recurrent time level. A more detailed discussion on recurrent survival times is given in Section 4.4.

The marginal cure model focuses on the population average survival distribution of clustered survival data. The survival function of the marginal mixture cure model of T^*_{ij} is given as follows:

$$S(t|\boldsymbol{x}_{ij}, \boldsymbol{z}_{ij}) = 1 - \pi(\boldsymbol{z}_{ij}) + \pi(\boldsymbol{z}_{ij})S_u(t|\boldsymbol{x}_{ij}), \tag{4.1}$$

where

$$\pi(\boldsymbol{z}_{ij}) = P(Y_{ij} = 1) = \frac{\exp(\boldsymbol{\gamma}'\boldsymbol{z}_{ij})}{1 + \exp(\boldsymbol{\gamma}'\boldsymbol{z}_{ij})} \tag{4.2}$$

is the probability of the jth subject in the ith cluster being cured, and $S_u(t|x_{ij}) = P(T^*_{ij} > t|Y_{ij} = 1, \boldsymbol{x}_{ij})$ is the survival function of T^*_{ij} if the subject is not cured. As noted before, $\boldsymbol{x}_{ij}$ and $\boldsymbol{x}_{ij}$ may share the same covariates. The effects of the covariate $\boldsymbol{x}_{ij}$ on the survival function $S_u(t|\boldsymbol{x}_{ij})$ may take the form of the PH model or the accelerated failure time model, to name a few, as discussed in Chapter 2 and 3. For example, the Weibull distribution can be considered for the marginal survival function $S_u(t|\boldsymbol{x}_{ij})$ as follows (Yu and Peng, 2008):

$$S_u(t|\boldsymbol{x}_{ij}) = \exp\left\{-\exp\left(\frac{\log t - \mu_{ij}}{\sigma}\right)\right\}, \tag{4.3}$$

where the location parameter μ_{ij} is related to covariates $\mu_{ij} = \exp(\boldsymbol{\beta}'\boldsymbol{x}_{ij})$ and the scale parameter σ is the common for all individuals. If a semiparametric model is preferred, the marginal survival function $S_u(t|\boldsymbol{x}_{ij})$ can be modeled as a PH model

$$S_u(t|\boldsymbol{x}_{ij}) = S_{u0}(t|\boldsymbol{\alpha})^{\exp(\boldsymbol{\beta}'\boldsymbol{x}_{ij})}, \tag{4.4}$$

with the baseline survival function $S_{u0}(t|\boldsymbol{\alpha})$ specified nonparametrically as (Peng et al., 2007b)

$$S_{u0}(t|\boldsymbol{\alpha}) = \exp\left(-\sum_{s:\tau_s \le t} \alpha_s\right), \tag{4.5}$$

where $0 = \tau_0 < \tau_1 < \cdots < \tau_k < \infty$ are k distinct uncensored failure times, $\alpha_0 = 0$, and $\boldsymbol{\alpha} = (\alpha_1, \ldots, \alpha_k)$ is the vector of k nonnegative parameters. The parameters to be estimated in the marginal mixture cure model are $\boldsymbol{\theta} = (\boldsymbol{\alpha}, \boldsymbol{\beta}, \boldsymbol{\gamma})$.

Under the working independence assumption, the likelihood function is

$$L(\boldsymbol{\theta}) = \prod_{i=1}^{n} L_i(\boldsymbol{\theta}) = \prod_{i=1}^{n}\prod_{j=1}^{n_i} \{f(t_{ij}|\boldsymbol{x}_{ij}, \boldsymbol{z}_{ij})\}^{\delta_{ij}} \{S(t_{ij}|\boldsymbol{x}_{ij}, \boldsymbol{x}_{ij})\}^{1-\delta_{ij}}, \tag{4.6}$$

where $f(\cdot)$ is the density function corresponding to $S(\cdot)$. An estimate $\hat{\boldsymbol{\theta}}$ can be obtained based on the likelihood, which treats the correlation between individuals as nuisance parameters, using the methods discussed in Chapter 2 and 3 for non-clustered survival data. If the marginal mixture cure model is correctly specified, the estimate $\hat{\boldsymbol{\theta}}$ that maximizes likelihood (4.6) usually provides a consistent estimate of $\boldsymbol{\theta}$. However, the Hessian matrix from the likelihood function does not provide a valid variance-covariance estimate of $\hat{\boldsymbol{\theta}}$. A robust and consistent estimate of the variance-covariance matrix is usually given by the so-called "sandwich" variance estimator (Lipsitz et al., 1994)

$$\left[\sum_{i=1}^{n} I_i(\hat{\boldsymbol{\theta}})\right]^{-1} \left[\sum_{i=1}^{n} U_i(\hat{\boldsymbol{\theta}})U_i(\hat{\boldsymbol{\theta}})'\right] \left[\sum_{i=1}^{n} I_i(\hat{\boldsymbol{\theta}})\right]^{-1},$$

where $U_i(\boldsymbol{\theta}) = \frac{\partial \log L_i(\boldsymbol{\theta})}{\partial \boldsymbol{\theta}}$ is the score vector and $I_i(\boldsymbol{\theta}) = -\frac{\partial U_i(\boldsymbol{\theta})}{\partial \boldsymbol{\theta}}$ is the information matrix for the ith cluster. The variance of the parameters in the model can also be obtained by a "one-step" Jackknife method. Using the maximum likelihood estimate $\hat{\boldsymbol{\theta}}$ from (4.6) as the starting value, the "one-step" estimates, $\hat{\boldsymbol{\theta}}_{-k}$ can be obtained by deleting the ith cluster, and performing one step of the Newton-Raphson algorithm,

$$\hat{\boldsymbol{\theta}}_{-k} = \hat{\boldsymbol{\theta}} + \left[\sum_{i=1, i\neq k}^{n} I_i(\hat{\boldsymbol{\theta}})\right]^{-1} \sum_{i=1, i\neq k}^{n} U_i(\hat{\boldsymbol{\theta}}).$$

Then one form of the Jackknife estimator of the variance of $\hat{\boldsymbol{\theta}}$ is given by

$$\left(\frac{n-m}{n}\right)\sum_{k=1}^{n}(\hat{\boldsymbol{\theta}}_{-k}-\hat{\boldsymbol{\theta}})(\hat{\boldsymbol{\theta}}_{-k}-\hat{\boldsymbol{\theta}})',$$

where m is the total number of parameters in $\boldsymbol{\theta}$.

A linear transformation model (3.11) can also be considered as the latency model in the marginal mixture cure model. A semiparametric estimation method under the working independence assumption is available for this model and details can be found in Chen and Lu (2012).

The parameter estimation in the marginal cure model is robust to the misspecification of the correlation structure among correlated failure times/cure statuses because the correlation is treated as a nuisance. However, it can be less efficient than the methods discussed in the next section that exploit the correlation structure.

4.2.2 Marginal Models with Specified Correlation Structures

One approach to explicitly include the correlation structure in the marginal mixture cure model is to use an adapted ES algorithm for the model (Niu and Peng, 2014). The algorithm is based on the EM algorithm for mixture cure models discussed in Section 2.3.2. Consider the marginal model (4.1), (4.2), and a PH latency submodel

$$S_u(t|\boldsymbol{x}) = S_{u0}(t;\alpha)^{\exp(\boldsymbol{\beta}'\boldsymbol{x})},$$

with $S_{u0}(t;\alpha) = \exp(-t^{\alpha})$. If we ignore the correlation within clusters and assume that the values of y_{ij}'s are all available, the complete log-likelihood function from the augmented data in the EM algorithm is

$$\begin{aligned}\ell^c(\boldsymbol{\theta}) &= \sum_{i=1}^{n}\sum_{j=1}^{n_i}\log\left(\pi(\boldsymbol{z}_{ij})^{y_{ij}}(1-\pi(\boldsymbol{z}_{ij}))^{1-y_{ij}}\right)\\ &\quad+\sum_{i=1}^{n}\sum_{j=1}^{n_i} y_{ij}t_{ij}^{\alpha}\log\left[\exp(\boldsymbol{\beta}'\boldsymbol{x}_{ij})^{\kappa_{ij}}\exp\{-\exp(\boldsymbol{\beta}'\boldsymbol{x}_{ij})\}\right]\\ &\quad+\sum_{i=1}^{n}\sum_{j=1}^{n_i}\delta_{ij}\log(\alpha t_{ij}^{\alpha-1}),\end{aligned}$$

where $\kappa_{ij} = \delta_{ij}/t_{ij}^{\alpha}$. It consists of three terms. The first term corresponds to a log-likelihood function of $\boldsymbol{\gamma}$ based on a logistic regression for y_{ij}. The second term can be viewed as a log-likelihood function for $\boldsymbol{\beta}$ based on a Poisson regression. The third term only involves α. By differentiating ℓ^c with respect to $\boldsymbol{\theta}$, we obtain the following estimating equations,

$$U_\gamma = \sum_{i=1}^{n} \left\{ \frac{\partial \pi(\boldsymbol{z}_i)}{\partial \gamma} \right\} \{\boldsymbol{A}_i^{1/2} \boldsymbol{I}_i \boldsymbol{A}_i^{1/2}\}^{-1} \{\boldsymbol{y}_i - \pi(\boldsymbol{z}_i)\} = 0, \tag{4.7}$$

$$U_\beta = \sum_{i=1}^{n} \left\{ \frac{\partial \mu(\boldsymbol{x}_i)}{\partial \gamma} \right\} \{\boldsymbol{B}_i^{1/2} \boldsymbol{I}_i \boldsymbol{B}_i^{1/2}\}^{-1} \boldsymbol{W}_i \{\boldsymbol{\kappa}_i - \mu(\boldsymbol{x}_i)\} = 0, \tag{4.8}$$

$$U_\alpha = \sum_{i=1}^{n} \sum_{j=1}^{n_i} \left[y_{ij} t_{ij}^{\alpha} \log(t_{ij}) \{\kappa_{ij} - \mu(\boldsymbol{x}_{ij})\} + \delta_{ij}/\alpha \right], \tag{4.9}$$

where

$$\begin{aligned}
\boldsymbol{y}_i &= (y_{i1}, ..., y_{in_i})', \\
\boldsymbol{\kappa}_i &= (\kappa_{i1}, ..., \kappa_{in_i})', \\
\boldsymbol{A}_i &= \text{diag}[\pi(\boldsymbol{z}_{i1})\{1 - \pi(\boldsymbol{z}_{i1})\}, ..., \pi(\boldsymbol{z}_{in_i})\{1 - \pi(\boldsymbol{z}_{in_i})\}], \\
\boldsymbol{B}_i &= \text{diag}\{\mu(\boldsymbol{x}_{i1}), ..., \mu(\boldsymbol{x}_{in_i})\}, \\
\boldsymbol{W}_i &= \text{diag}(y_{i1} t_{i1}^{\alpha}, ..., y_{in_i} t_{in_i}^{\alpha}), \\
\pi(\boldsymbol{z}_i) &= \{\pi(\boldsymbol{z}_{i1}), ..., \pi(\boldsymbol{z}_{in_i})\}', \\
\mu(\boldsymbol{x}_i) &= \{\mu(\boldsymbol{x}_{i1}), ..., \mu(\boldsymbol{x}_{in_i})\}',
\end{aligned}$$

with $\mu(\boldsymbol{x}_{ij}) = \exp(\boldsymbol{\beta}' \boldsymbol{x}_{ij})$, $\boldsymbol{I}_i$ is an $n_i \times n_i$ identity matrix, and diag($\boldsymbol{a}$) is a diagonal matrix with diagonal elements from the vector $\boldsymbol{a}$.

The E-step computes the conditional expectation of $l^c(\boldsymbol{\theta})$ with respect to y_{ij} given the observed data and the current estimates of the parameters. If the current estimates are denoted by $\boldsymbol{\theta}^{(m)} = (\gamma^{(m)}, \boldsymbol{\beta}^{(m)}, \alpha^{(m)})$, then the E-step is equivalent to computing

$$w_{ij}^{(m)} = E(y_{ij} | \boldsymbol{\theta}^{(m)}) = \delta_{ij} + \frac{(1 - \delta_{ij}) \pi(\boldsymbol{z}_{ij}) S_{u0}(t_{ij})^{\exp(\boldsymbol{\beta}' \boldsymbol{x}_{ij})}}{1 - \pi(\boldsymbol{z}_{ij}) + \pi(\boldsymbol{z}_{ij}) S_{u0}(t_{ij})^{\exp(\boldsymbol{\beta}' \boldsymbol{x}_{ij})}}. \tag{4.10}$$

The usual M-step in the EM algorithm is to solve (4.7)-(4.9) after substituting $w_{ij}^{(m)}$ for y_{ij} to update $\boldsymbol{\theta}$ and the E- and M-step iterate until the algorithm converges to obtain $\hat{\boldsymbol{\theta}}$. When the correlation within clusters is present, the above estimating equations are still unbiased if the marginal model is correctly specified. However, the estimates may not be efficient. To consider the correlation among subjects in a cluster, the identity matrix $\boldsymbol{I}_i$ in (4.7) and (4.8) can be replaced with working correlation matrices $\boldsymbol{Q}_i$ to account for the potential correlations between y_{ij}'s and between κ_{ij}'s of uncured subjects in each cluster:

$$U_{\gamma} = \sum_{i=1}^{n} \left\{ \frac{\partial \pi(\boldsymbol{z}_i)}{\partial \gamma} \right\} \{\boldsymbol{A}_i^{1/2} \boldsymbol{Q}_i(\rho_1) \boldsymbol{A}_i^{1/2}\} \{\boldsymbol{y}_i - \pi(\boldsymbol{z}_i)\} = 0, \tag{4.11}$$

$$U_{\boldsymbol{\beta}} = \sum_{i=1}^{n} \left\{ \frac{\partial \mu(\boldsymbol{x}_i)}{\partial \boldsymbol{\beta}} \right\} \{\boldsymbol{B}_i^{1/2} \boldsymbol{Q}_i(\rho_2) \boldsymbol{B}_i^{1/2}\} \boldsymbol{W}_i \{\kappa_i - \mu(\boldsymbol{x}_i)\} = 0, \tag{4.12}$$

where $\boldsymbol{Q}_i(\rho_1) = (q_{jk}(\rho_1))_{n_i \times n_i}$ and $\boldsymbol{Q}_i(\rho_2) = (q_{jk}(\rho_2))_{n_i \times n_i}$ are the working correlation matrices, and ρ_1 and ρ_2 are unknown parameters in the matrices that need to be estimated. The scale parameters ϕ_1 and ϕ_2 are incorporated in the estimating equations to accommodate potential over- or under-dispersion. The M-step with the modified estimating equations (4.11) and (4.12) is renamed as an S-step and the algorithm is called the ES algorithm (Rosen et al., 2000). The E-step and the S-step iterate until the ES algorithm converges.

Depending on the nature of the correlation structure, there are a few choices for the working correlation matrices, such as an exchangeable (equicorrelated, compound symmetric) structure with $q_{jk}(\rho) = \rho$ for $j \neq k$ and 1 otherwise, a first-order autoregressive (AR-1) structure with $q_{jk}(\rho) = \rho^{|j-k|}$ for $j \neq k$ and 1 otherwise, and an unstructured one with $q_{jk}(\rho) = \rho_{jk}$ for $j \neq k$ and 1 otherwise. If the exchangeable correlation structure for both $\boldsymbol{Q}_i(\rho_1)$ and $\boldsymbol{Q}_i(\rho_2)$ is considered, ρ_1, ρ_2, ϕ_1, and ϕ_2 can be estimated from the standardized Pearson residuals (Liang and Zeger, 1986):

$$\hat{\phi}_1 = \frac{1}{n - p_z - 1} \sum_{i=1}^{n} \sum_{j=1}^{n_i} \{\hat{r}_{ij}^{(1)}\}^2, \tag{4.13}$$

$$\hat{\rho}_1 = \frac{1}{\hat{\phi}_1 [\sum_{i=1}^{n} n_i(n_i - 1)/2 - p_z - 1]} \sum_{i=1}^{n} \sum_{j>j'} \hat{r}_{ij}^{(1)} \hat{r}_{ij'}^{(1)}, \tag{4.14}$$

$$\hat{\phi}_2 = \frac{1}{n - p_x - 1} \sum_{i=1}^{n} \sum_{j=1}^{n_i} \{\hat{r}_{ij}^{(2)}\}^2, \tag{4.15}$$

$$\hat{\rho}_2 = \frac{1}{\hat{\phi}_2 [\sum_{i=1}^{n} n_i(n_i - 1)/2 - p_x - 1]} \sum_{i=1}^{n} \sum_{j>j'} \hat{r}_{ij}^{(2)} \hat{r}_{ij'}^{(2)}, \tag{4.16}$$

where $\hat{r}_{ij}^{(1)} = \{w_{ij}^{(m)} - \pi(\boldsymbol{z}_{ij})\}/[\pi(\boldsymbol{z}_{ij})\{1 - \pi(\boldsymbol{z}_{ij})\}]^{\frac{1}{2}}$, $\hat{r}_{ij}^{(2)} = \{\kappa_{ij} - \mu(\boldsymbol{x}_{ij})\}/\{\mu(\boldsymbol{x}_{ij})\}^{\frac{1}{2}}$ and p_x and p_z are the numbers of parameters in $\boldsymbol{\beta}$ and γ respectively.

It is obvious that the ES algorithm reduces to the EM algorithm when the working correlation matrices are the identity matrix and the scale parameters ϕ_1 and ϕ_2 are set to 1. Due to the modifications in the M-step, the ES algorithm is not guaranteed to converge as the EM algorithm does. Therefore, careful checking the convergence of the algorithm is prudent, and we suggest trying different initial values if non-convergence happens. However, it is rare to see non-convergence in practice.

The baseline survival function $S_{u0}(t)$ can also be specified nonparametrically as in (4.5) and a similar estimation method is available (Niu et al., 2018a).

If the correlation is strong among observations within clusters, the marginal cure model using the working correlation matrices can improve estimation efficiency substantially compared to the models under the working independence assumption in Section 4.2.1.

4.3 Cure Models with Random Effects

4.3.1 Mixture Cure Models with Frailties

Unlike marginal models, random-effects (frailty) models account for the correlation within clusters explicitly by using shared random effects. This method has also been considered for clustered survival data with a cured fraction. Chatterjee and Shih (2001), Wienke et al. (2003), Lakhal-Chaieb and Duchesne (2017), and Su and Lin (2019) extended the mixture cure model to bivariate survival data with a cure fraction by modeling the distribution of the uncured patients with copulas, which can also be expressed as frailty models, and proposed a two-stage semiparametric estimation method. For clustered survival data, the method can be used by assuming a pairwise correlation among subjects within clusters. However, the method does not consider covariate effects in the model and it becomes infeasible when cluster size is large. In this section, we will introduce a random-effects mixture cure model (Peng and Taylor, 2011), which employs two sets of random effects to model respectively the correlation among the cure status and among the failure times for uncured subjects in the same cluster. Similar models are discussed in Yau and Ng (2001), Lai and Yau (2009) and Tawiah et al. (2019).

Let $\boldsymbol{u}' = (u_1, u_2, \dots, u_l)$ and $\boldsymbol{v}' = (v_1, v_2, \dots, v_l)$ be the random effects to model the correlation among t_{ij}^*'s and among y_{ij}'s within cluster i respectively. Given $\boldsymbol{u}$ and $\boldsymbol{v}$, t_{ij}^*'s and y_{ij}'s are assumed to be independent and follow the mixture cure model as follows

$$\begin{aligned} P(T_{ij}^* > t|\boldsymbol{u}, \boldsymbol{v}) &= S(t|\boldsymbol{u}, \boldsymbol{v}) \\ &= S_u(t|\boldsymbol{x}_{ij}\boldsymbol{\beta} + \boldsymbol{x}_{ij}^*\boldsymbol{u})\pi(\boldsymbol{z}_{ij}\boldsymbol{\gamma} + \boldsymbol{z}_{ij}^*\boldsymbol{v}) + 1 - \pi(\boldsymbol{z}_{ij}\boldsymbol{\gamma} + \boldsymbol{z}_{ij}^*\boldsymbol{v}), \end{aligned} \tag{4.17}$$

where

$$\pi(\boldsymbol{z}_{ij}\boldsymbol{\gamma} + \boldsymbol{z}_{ij}^*\boldsymbol{v}) = P(y_{ij} = 1|\boldsymbol{v}) = \frac{\exp(\boldsymbol{z}_{ij}\boldsymbol{\gamma} + \boldsymbol{z}_{ij}^*\boldsymbol{v})}{1 + \exp(\boldsymbol{z}_{ij}\boldsymbol{\gamma} + \boldsymbol{z}_{ij}^*\boldsymbol{v})},$$

$S_u(t|\boldsymbol{x}_{ij}\boldsymbol{\beta} + \boldsymbol{x}_{ij}^*\boldsymbol{u}) = P(T_{ij}^* > t|\boldsymbol{u}, y_{ij} = 1)$ can be specified using the PH model

$$S_u(t|\boldsymbol{x}_{ij}\boldsymbol{\beta} + \boldsymbol{x}_{ij}^*\boldsymbol{u}) = S_{u0}(t)^{\exp(\boldsymbol{x}_{ij}\boldsymbol{\beta} + \boldsymbol{x}_{ij}^*\boldsymbol{u})}, \tag{4.18}$$

the AFT model

$$S_u(t|\boldsymbol{x}_{ij}\boldsymbol{\beta} + \boldsymbol{x}^*_{ij}\boldsymbol{u}) = S_{u0}(t\exp(\boldsymbol{x}_{ij}\boldsymbol{\beta} + \boldsymbol{x}^*_{ij}\boldsymbol{u})),$$

or the proportional odds model

$$\text{logit}(S_u(t|\boldsymbol{x}_{ij}\boldsymbol{\beta} + \boldsymbol{x}^*_{ij}\boldsymbol{u})) = \text{logit}(S_{u0}(t)) + \boldsymbol{x}_{ij}\boldsymbol{\beta} + \boldsymbol{x}^*_{ij}\boldsymbol{u},$$

$S_{u0}(\cdot)$ is a baseline survival function for uncured individuals, and $\boldsymbol{x}^*_{ij}$ and $\boldsymbol{z}^*_{ij}$ are the coefficients for the random effect $\boldsymbol{u}$ and $\boldsymbol{v}$. The baseline survival function $S_{u0}(t)$ can be from the Weibull distribution with $S_{u0}(t) = \exp[-(t/\lambda)^p]$. To allow more flexibility in the baseline distribution, the piecewise constant hazard distribution can be considered. Let $\tau_0 = 0 < \tau_1 < \tau_2 < \cdots < \tau_K = \infty$ and $h_{u0}(t) = \exp(\alpha_j)$ if $\tau_{j-1} \leq t < t_j$, where $j = 1, \ldots, K$ and $K \geq 1$. The baseline survival function of the piecewise constant hazard distribution is

$$S_{u0}(t) = \exp\left\{ - \sum_{j:\tau_j < t} \exp(\alpha_{j+1})[\min(t, \tau_{j+1}) - \tau_j] \right\}.$$

When $K = 1$, this distribution reduces to the exponential distribution. We usually require that $\tau_1 > \min(t_{ij})$ and $\tau_{K-1} < \max(t_{ij})$. By choosing a large K, the piecewise constant hazard distribution can increase the flexibility of the parametric approach. The values $\tau_1, \ldots, \tau_{K-1}$ in this method are often chosen to make equal-spaced intervals. Since the uncensored times contribute essential information to the hazard estimation, we suggest that τ_j be the $100\frac{j}{K}$th percentile of the uncensored times so that each interval has events to estimate the hazard accurately.

For the random effects $\boldsymbol{u}$ and $\boldsymbol{v}$, we require that $E(\boldsymbol{u}) = \boldsymbol{0}$ and $E(\boldsymbol{v}) = \boldsymbol{0}$ with a joint density function $\phi[(\boldsymbol{u}', \boldsymbol{v}')', \boldsymbol{D}]$, where $\boldsymbol{D} = \boldsymbol{D}(\boldsymbol{\sigma})$ is the covariance matrix with unknown parameters $\boldsymbol{\sigma}$. The multivariate normal distribution can be considered for $\boldsymbol{u}$ and $\boldsymbol{v}$, which conveniently allow correlation within $\boldsymbol{u}$ and $\boldsymbol{v}$ as well as between $\boldsymbol{u}$ and $\boldsymbol{v}$. The correlation between $\boldsymbol{u}$ and $\boldsymbol{v}$ implies correlation between T^*_{ij} and Y_{ij} within a cluster, which, if not model properly, can cause biases in estimation. See detailed discussions on this issue in Lakhal-Chaieb and Duchesne (2017).

The marginal likelihood function for the mixture cure model with random effects above is

$$L(\boldsymbol{\theta}) = \int \prod_{i=1}^{n} \prod_{j=1}^{n_i} [\pi(\boldsymbol{z}_{ij}\boldsymbol{\gamma} + \boldsymbol{z}^*_{ij}\boldsymbol{v}) f_u(t_{ij}|\boldsymbol{x}_{ij}\boldsymbol{\beta} + \boldsymbol{x}^*_{ij}\boldsymbol{u})]^{\delta_{ij}}$$
$$\times [1 - \pi(\boldsymbol{z}_{ij}\boldsymbol{\gamma} + \boldsymbol{z}^*_{ij}\boldsymbol{v}) + \pi(\boldsymbol{z}_{ij}\boldsymbol{\gamma} + \boldsymbol{z}^*_{ij}\boldsymbol{v}) S_u(t_{ij}|\boldsymbol{x}_{ij}\boldsymbol{\beta} + \boldsymbol{x}^*_{ij}\boldsymbol{u})]^{1-\delta_{ij}}$$
$$\times \phi[(\boldsymbol{u}, \boldsymbol{v}), \boldsymbol{D}] d\boldsymbol{u} d\boldsymbol{v}, \quad (4.19)$$

where $f_u(\cdot)$ is the corresponding density function of $S_u(\cdot)$, and $\boldsymbol{\theta} = (\boldsymbol{\beta}, \boldsymbol{\gamma}, S_{u0}, \boldsymbol{\sigma})$. The integral in (4.19) is usually intractable, which makes a direct maximization of the likelihood function difficult. One can employ numerical integration methods, such as the adaptive Gaussian quadrature method, to approximate the integrals for maximization and the negative second derivative of $\log L(\boldsymbol{\theta})$ with respect to $\boldsymbol{\theta}$ to estimate the standard errors of the estimated parameters.

The EM algorithm can also be used to obtain the maximum likelihood estimate of $\boldsymbol{\theta}$ in (4.19). Given the values of $\boldsymbol{y} = (y_{11}, \ldots, y_{nn_n})$, $\boldsymbol{u}$, and $\boldsymbol{v}$, the complete log-likelihood function of the mixture cure model is

$$\ell^c(\boldsymbol{\theta}) = \sum_{i=1}^{n}\sum_{j=1}^{n_i}\{\delta_{ij}\log h_u(t_{ij}|\boldsymbol{x}_{ij}\boldsymbol{\beta} + \boldsymbol{x}_{ij}^*\boldsymbol{u}) + y_{ij}\log S_u(t_{ij}|\boldsymbol{x}_{ij}\boldsymbol{\beta} + \boldsymbol{x}_{ij}^*\boldsymbol{u})\}$$
$$+ \sum_{i=1}^{n}\sum_{j=1}^{n_i}\{y_{ij}\log \pi(\boldsymbol{z}_{ij}\boldsymbol{\gamma} + \boldsymbol{z}_{ij}^*\boldsymbol{v}) + (1-y_{ij})\log[1-\pi(\boldsymbol{z}_{ij}\boldsymbol{\gamma} + \boldsymbol{z}_{ij}^*\boldsymbol{v})]\}$$
$$+ \sum_{i=1}^{n}\log\phi[(\boldsymbol{u},\boldsymbol{v}), \boldsymbol{D}(\boldsymbol{\sigma})]. \quad (4.20)$$

The E-step of the EM algorithm computes the posterior expectation of $\ell^c(\boldsymbol{\theta})$ with respect to $\boldsymbol{y}$, $\boldsymbol{u}$, and $\boldsymbol{v}$ given the current estimates of the model parameters. Let the current estimate of $\boldsymbol{\theta}$ be $\boldsymbol{\theta}^{(r)}$. Under the PH latency model (4.18), the E-step requires evaluating the following expectations

$$E(y_{ij}|\boldsymbol{\theta}^{(r)}), \quad E\left[y_{ij}e^{\boldsymbol{x}_{ij}^*\boldsymbol{u}}|\boldsymbol{\theta}^{(r)}\right], \quad (4.21)$$
$$E\left(\log\left[1+\exp(\boldsymbol{z}_{ij}\boldsymbol{\gamma} + \boldsymbol{z}_{ij}^*\boldsymbol{v})\right]|\boldsymbol{\theta}^{(r)}\right), \quad E\left(\phi[(\boldsymbol{u},\boldsymbol{v}), \boldsymbol{D}(\boldsymbol{\sigma})]|\boldsymbol{\theta}^{(r)}\right), \quad (4.22)$$

with respect to

$$p(\boldsymbol{y},\boldsymbol{u},\boldsymbol{v}|\boldsymbol{\theta}^{(r)}) \propto \prod_{i=1}^{n}\left\{\prod_{j=1}^{n_i} e^{\delta_{ij}\boldsymbol{x}_{ij}^*\boldsymbol{u} - y_{ij}H_{u0}^{(r)}(t_{ij})\exp(\boldsymbol{x}_{ij}\boldsymbol{\beta}^{(r)} + \boldsymbol{x}_{ij}^*\boldsymbol{u})}\right.$$
$$\left.\times \prod_{j=1}^{n_i}\frac{e^{y_{ij}(\boldsymbol{z}_{ij}\boldsymbol{\gamma}^{(r)} + \boldsymbol{z}_{ij}^*\boldsymbol{v})}}{1+e^{\boldsymbol{z}_{ij}\boldsymbol{\gamma}^{(r)} + \boldsymbol{z}_{ij}^*\boldsymbol{v}}}\right\}\phi[(\boldsymbol{u},\boldsymbol{v}), \boldsymbol{D}(\boldsymbol{\sigma}^{(r)})].$$

Given $\boldsymbol{u}$ and $\boldsymbol{v}$, it is obvious that y_{ij} are independent, and $y_{ij} \equiv 1$ if $\delta_{ij} = 1$ and y_{ij} follows the binomial distribution with the following probability if $\delta_{ij} = 0$:

$$\hat{y}_{ij} = \frac{\pi(\boldsymbol{z}_{ij}\boldsymbol{\gamma}^{(r)} + \boldsymbol{z}_{ij}^*\boldsymbol{v})e^{-H_{u0}^{(r)}(t_{ij})\exp(\boldsymbol{x}_{ij}\boldsymbol{\beta}^{(r)} + \boldsymbol{x}_{ij}^*\boldsymbol{u})}}{1-\pi(\boldsymbol{z}_{ij}\boldsymbol{\gamma}^{(r)} + \boldsymbol{z}_{ij}^*\boldsymbol{v}) + \pi(\boldsymbol{z}_{ij}\boldsymbol{\gamma}^{(r)} + \boldsymbol{z}_{ij}^*\boldsymbol{v})e^{-H_{u0}^{(r)}(t_{ij})\exp(\boldsymbol{x}_{ij}\boldsymbol{\beta}^{(r)} + \boldsymbol{x}_{ij}^*\boldsymbol{u})}},$$

which is also $E(y_{ij}|\boldsymbol{\theta}^{(r)})$, and

$$E\left[y_{ij}e^{\boldsymbol{x}_{ij}^*\boldsymbol{u}}|\boldsymbol{\theta}^{(r)}\right] = \begin{cases} E\left[\hat{y}_{ij}e^{\boldsymbol{x}_{ij}^*\boldsymbol{u}}\middle|\,\boldsymbol{\theta}^{(r)}\right] & \text{if } \delta_{ij}=0, \\ E(e^{\boldsymbol{x}_{ij}^*\boldsymbol{u}}|\boldsymbol{\theta}^{(r)}) & \text{otherwise,} \end{cases}$$

where the expectations are taken with respect to the distribution of $(\boldsymbol{u}, \boldsymbol{v})$. Unfortunately, the expectations do not have closed form, and Monte Carlo methods may be used to evaluate the expectations.

The M-step maximizes the following function $Q(\boldsymbol{\theta}|\boldsymbol{\theta}^{(r)}) = Q_1(\boldsymbol{\beta}, h_{u0}|\boldsymbol{\theta}^{(r)}) + Q_2(\boldsymbol{\gamma}|\boldsymbol{\theta}^{(r)}) + Q_3(\boldsymbol{\sigma}|\boldsymbol{\theta}^{(r)})$ with respect to $\boldsymbol{\theta}$, where

$$Q_1(\boldsymbol{\beta}, h_{u0}|\boldsymbol{\theta}^{(r)}) = \sum_{i=1}^{n}\sum_{j=1}^{n_i}\left\{\delta_{ij}\left[\log h_{u0}(t_{ij}) + \boldsymbol{x}_{ij}\boldsymbol{\beta} + E(\boldsymbol{x}^*_{ij}\boldsymbol{u}|\boldsymbol{\theta}^{(r)})\right]\right.$$
$$\left. - H_{u0}(t_{ij})e^{\boldsymbol{x}_{ij}\boldsymbol{\beta}+\log E\left[y_{ij}e^{\boldsymbol{x}^*_{ij}\boldsymbol{u}}|\boldsymbol{\theta}^{(r)}\right]}\right\},$$

$$Q_2(\boldsymbol{\gamma}|\boldsymbol{\theta}^{(r)}) = \sum_{i=1}^{n}\sum_{j=1}^{n_i}\left\{E(y_{ij}|\boldsymbol{\theta}^{(r)})\boldsymbol{z}_{ij}\boldsymbol{\gamma} + E\left[y_{ij}\boldsymbol{z}^*_{ij}\boldsymbol{v}|\boldsymbol{\theta}^{(r)}\right]\right.$$
$$\left. -E\left(\log\left[1 + e^{\boldsymbol{z}_{ij}\boldsymbol{\gamma}+\boldsymbol{z}^*_{ij}\boldsymbol{v}}\right]|\boldsymbol{\theta}^{(r)}\right)\right\},$$

$$Q_3(\boldsymbol{\sigma}|\boldsymbol{\theta}^{(r)}) = \log E\{\phi[(\boldsymbol{u}, \boldsymbol{v}), \boldsymbol{D}(\boldsymbol{\sigma})]|\boldsymbol{\theta}^{(r)}\}.$$

The variances of the estimated parameters in the EM algorithm can be obtained using methods proposed in (Oakes, 1999; Meng and Rubin, 1991; Meilijson, 1989), and they closely relate to Louis' formula $-\frac{\partial^2 \log L(\boldsymbol{\theta})}{\partial\boldsymbol{\theta}\partial\boldsymbol{\theta}^T} = -E\left(\frac{\partial^2 \ell(\boldsymbol{\theta}|\mathbf{t},\boldsymbol{y},\boldsymbol{u},\boldsymbol{v})}{\partial\boldsymbol{\theta}\partial\boldsymbol{\theta}^T}\right) - Var\left(\frac{\partial \ell(\boldsymbol{\theta}|\mathbf{t},\boldsymbol{y},\boldsymbol{u},\boldsymbol{v})}{\partial\boldsymbol{\theta}}\right)$, where the expectation and the variance are taken with respect to $(\boldsymbol{y}, \boldsymbol{u}, \boldsymbol{v})$ (Louis, 1982). It is easy to see from (4.20) that both $\frac{\partial^2 \ell^c(\boldsymbol{\theta})}{\partial\boldsymbol{\theta}\partial\boldsymbol{\theta}^T}$ and $\frac{\partial \ell^c(\boldsymbol{\theta})}{\partial\boldsymbol{\theta}}$ are linear functions of $\boldsymbol{y}$. Hence the expectation and the variance can be obtained easily from the random samples obtained in the EM algorithm.

4.3.2 Non-Nixture Cure Model with Frailties

The PHC model (2.18) can be readily extended to analyze clustered survival data with a cure fraction in a similar way to how a frailty model extends the standard PH model for clustered survival data. One may assume that given a frailty ξ_i that is shared within cluster i, the conditional survival function of T_{ij} is

$$S(t|\boldsymbol{x}_{ij}, \xi_i) = \exp[-\xi_i e^{\beta_0 + \boldsymbol{x}'_{ij}\boldsymbol{\beta}} F^H(t)],$$

and ξ_i follows a prespecified frailty distribution with a fixed scale parameter. A proper cumulative distribution function is assumed for $F^H(t)$ so that $S(t|\boldsymbol{x}_{ij}, \xi_i)$ is an improper survival function and is capable to handle survival data with a cured fraction. One example of the frailty distribution is the stable distribution (Hougaard, 2000) because the resulting marginal model preserves the proportionality of the conditional model in $\boldsymbol{x}_{ij}$. Other frailty distributions, such as the gamma distribution, can also be considered.

The shared frailty model for survival data with a cure fraction can also be defined using the regular frailty model and a frailty distribution that has a probability mass at zero, similar to the discussions for (2.22) in the independent case. For example, Wienke et al. (2010) suggested the following frailty model for bivariate data conditional on ξ_{ij}:

$$S(t|\boldsymbol{x}_{ij}, \xi_i) = \exp\left[-\xi_{ij} H_0(t) e^{\boldsymbol{x}'_{ij}\boldsymbol{\beta}}\right], \quad j = 1, 2, \tag{4.23}$$

where $H_0(t)$ is a cumulative hazard function,

$$\xi_{i1} = v_{i0} + v_{i1}$$
$$\xi_{i2} = v_{i0} + v_{i2},$$

and v_{i0}, v_{i1}, and v_{i2} are independent compound Poisson-distributed random variables (Aalen, 1992). The shared v_{i0} between ξ_{i1} and ξ_{i2} induces the correlation between T^*_{i1} and T^*_{i2}. The compound Poisson distribution is a mixed type distribution with the discrete portion at 0 and the continuous portion on $(0, \infty)$ and it includes Poisson distribution as a special case. The probability mass at 0 implies that the marginal distribution of T^*_{ij} is an improper distribution and model (4.23) is suitable for correlated survival data with a cure fraction.

Another approach to extend the PHC model for clustered data is to define the frailty term ξ_i to be shared by $\tilde{T}_1, \ldots, \tilde{T}_n$'s in (2.17) from all subjects in the same clusters (Yin, 2005). The resulting frailty model is

$$S(t|\boldsymbol{x}_{ij}, \xi_i) = \exp\{-e^{\boldsymbol{\beta}_0 + \boldsymbol{z}'_{ij}\boldsymbol{\beta}}[1 - S^H(t)^{\xi_i}]\}.$$

Most of the existing methods to estimate the parameters in the models above are Bayesian methods. The promotion time distribution $F^H(t)$ can be specified parametrically or nonparametrically using a piecewise constant hazard distribution with gamma priors on the hazard segments.

The unified cure models can be adapted to model clustered survival data with a cured fraction. For example, a frailty term can be added to model (2.26) to produce a shared frailty model (Yin, 2008)

$$S(t|\boldsymbol{x}_{ij}, \boldsymbol{z}_{ij}) = \begin{cases} [1 + \lambda \xi_i e^{\boldsymbol{z}'_{ij}\boldsymbol{\beta}} F^H(t|\boldsymbol{x}_{ij})]^{-1/\lambda} & \lambda > 0 \\ \exp[-\xi_i e^{\boldsymbol{z}'_{ij}\boldsymbol{\beta}} F^H(t|\boldsymbol{x}_{ij})] & \lambda = 0, \end{cases}$$

where the frailty term ξ_i may follow a gamma distribution with a fixed scale parameter. Other distributions can also be considered for ξ_i.

4.4 Cure Models for Recurrent Event Data

For survival data with recurrent events, an individual may have multiple recurrent events or no recurrence at all. Many long-term survivors could be cured and have no recurrence, while the uncured patients could have multiple recurrences.

Suppose that there are n patients and the i-th patient has n_i episodes of recurrence. Let $(\boldsymbol{x}_{ik}, t_{ik}, \delta_{ik})$ be the covariates, survival (gap) times and censoring status for the k-th recurrence, $k = 1, ..., n_i$, and let $\boldsymbol{x}_i = (\boldsymbol{x}_{i1}, ..., \boldsymbol{x}_{in_i}), \boldsymbol{t}_i = (t_{i1}, ..., t_{in_i})$, and $\boldsymbol{\delta}_i = (\delta_{i1}, ..., \delta_{in_i})$. Let y_i be the cure status for subject i with $y_i = 1$ if the subject is not cured and 0 otherwise, and $\boldsymbol{z}_i$ be a set of covariates related to the cure status. The observed data for the i-th individual are $(\boldsymbol{z}_i, \boldsymbol{x}_i, \boldsymbol{t}_i, \boldsymbol{\delta}_i)$. Let the total number of recurrences for the i-th subject be $D_i = \sum_{k=1}^{n_i} \delta_{ik}$. When $D_i > 0$, then $y_i = 1$, as the patient experiences recurrence, hence is not cured. When $D_i = 0$, there is no recurrence, the cure status for the individual is unknown (Yu, 2008).

As discussed in previous sections, the recurrent times from an uncured subject can be correlated. We consider the multiplicative frailty model for the correlated recurrent times. The model assumes that the conditional hazard function of the recurrent time T_{ik}^* is given by $u_i h(t|\boldsymbol{x}_{ik})$ conditional on the shared common frailty $U = u_i$, where $h(t|\boldsymbol{x})$ can be specified using the PH assumption $h(t|\boldsymbol{x}) = h_0(t)\exp(\boldsymbol{\beta}'\boldsymbol{x})$ or other model assumptions discussed so far. The marginal unconditional survival function of T_{ik}^* for an uncured subject is

$$S_u(t|\boldsymbol{x}_{ik}) = E_U\big(\exp\{-UH(t|\boldsymbol{x}_{ik})\}\big) = L_U[H(t|\boldsymbol{x}_{ik})], \tag{4.24}$$

where $L_U(s) = E_U[\exp(-sU)]$ is the Laplace transformation of the frailty U (Klein and Moeschberger, 2003). Under the assumption that the recurrence times, $t_{i1}, ..., t_{in_i}$, are independent conditional on the frailty u_i if the ith individual is not cured, the joint conditional cumulative hazard function given u_i is $u_i \sum_{k=1}^{n_i} H(t_{ik}|\boldsymbol{x}_{ik})$, and the joint unconditional survival function for the uncured patient is $S_u(\boldsymbol{t}_i|\boldsymbol{x}_i) = P(T_{i1}^* > t_{i1}, \ldots, T_{in_i}^* > t_{in_i}) = L_U[\sum_{k=1}^{n_i} H(t_{ik}|\boldsymbol{x}_{ik})]$.

If the frailty U follows a gamma distribution with unit mean and variance λ, the Laplace transformation of U is $L_U(s) = (1 + \lambda s)^{-\frac{1}{\lambda}}$, and the joint unconditional survival function for the uncured patient is

$$S_u(\boldsymbol{t}_i|\boldsymbol{x}_i) = \left[1 + \lambda \sum_{k=1}^{n_i} H(t_{ik}|\boldsymbol{x}_{ik})\right]^{-\frac{1}{\lambda}}.$$

When λ goes to infinity, $L_U(s)$ degenerates to $\exp(-s)$ and this corresponds to independent recurrent times within each patient.

We assume a common frailty for all the gap times from the same uncured subject, which implies that the first gap time and the following gap times for the uncured subject have the same distribution. This assumption may not hold in practice, and it can be extended to a more general case where the frailty can vary stochastically with the indices (Yue and Chan, 1997).

For the cured patients, the frailty U is 0 as they will not experience the event of interest. The overall joint survival function is

$$S(\boldsymbol{t}_i|\boldsymbol{x}_i, \boldsymbol{z}_i) = \pi(\boldsymbol{z}_i)S_u(\boldsymbol{t}_i|\boldsymbol{x}_i) + 1 - \pi(\boldsymbol{z}_i),$$

where $\pi(\boldsymbol{z}_i)$ is specified as in (2.2). For the patient with no recurrence, i.e., $D_i = 0$, the likelihood contribution is $S(\boldsymbol{t}_i|\boldsymbol{x}_i)$. For the patient with $D_i > 0$, the likelihood contribution is $\pi(\boldsymbol{z}_i)f_u(\boldsymbol{t}_i|\boldsymbol{x}_i)$, where

$$f_u(\boldsymbol{t}_i|\boldsymbol{x}_i) = D_i \log\lambda + \log\frac{\Gamma(1/\lambda + D_i)}{\Gamma(1/\lambda)} + \sum_{k=1}^{n_i}\delta_{ik}\log[h(t_{ik}|\boldsymbol{x}_{ik})] - \left(\frac{1}{\lambda} + D_i\right)\log\left[1 + \lambda\sum_{k=1}^{n_i} H(t_{ik}|\boldsymbol{x}_{ik})\right].$$

The maximum likelihood estimates of the parameters $\boldsymbol{\theta} = (\boldsymbol{\gamma}, \boldsymbol{\beta}, h_0, \lambda)'$ can be obtained by the EM algorithm. If the cure statuses $y_i, i = 1, ..., n$, were observed, the log-likelihood function for the full data can be decomposed into two parts, $\ell^c(\boldsymbol{\theta}) = \ell_1(\boldsymbol{\gamma}) + \ell_2(\boldsymbol{\beta}, h_0, \lambda)$, where

$$\ell_1(\boldsymbol{\gamma}) = \sum_{i=1}^{n}\Big\{y_i \log\pi(\boldsymbol{z}_i) + (1 - y_i)\log(1 - \pi(\boldsymbol{z}_i))\Big\},$$

$$\ell_2(\boldsymbol{\beta}, h_0, \lambda) = \sum_{i=1}^{n} y_i\Big\{I(D_i = 0)\log S_u(\boldsymbol{t}_i|\boldsymbol{x}_i) + I(D_i > 0)\log f_u(\boldsymbol{t}_i|\boldsymbol{x}_i)\Big\}.$$

The E-step calculates the posterior expectation of y_i based on the observed data and current parameter estimates:

$$w_i = E(y_i) = I(D_i > 0) + I(D_i = 0)\frac{\pi(\boldsymbol{z}_i)S_u(\boldsymbol{t}_i|\boldsymbol{x}_i)}{\pi(\boldsymbol{z}_i)S_u(\boldsymbol{t}_i|\boldsymbol{x}_i) + 1 - \pi(\boldsymbol{z}_i)}. \tag{4.25}$$

The M-step updates the parameter estimates by maximizing $\ell_1(\boldsymbol{\gamma})$ and $\ell_2(\boldsymbol{\beta}, h_0, \lambda)$ after y_i is replaced with w_i. The estimates of $(\boldsymbol{\beta}, h_0, \lambda)$ can be obtained from $\ell_2(\boldsymbol{\beta}, h_0, \lambda)$ using the penalized likelihood method (Ripatti and Palmgren, 2000).

Estimating the variance-covariance matrix of the estimates using the methods for the EM algorithm, such as Louis (1982), requires a calculation of the complete-data variance-covariance matrix and the conditional expectation (conditional on the observed data) of the square of the complete-data score function, which can be complicated for multivariate survival data. Alternatively, the variance of the parameter estimates can be obtained by the bootstrap method (Monaco et al., 2005) or the Jackknife method (Lipsitz et al., 1994) for multivariate survival data. In the bootstrap analysis, the multiple event times for the same individual are selected simultaneously. Let $\boldsymbol{\theta}_{(b)}$ be the parameter estimate of the b-th bootstrap sample, $b = 1, ..., B$, and let $\bar{\boldsymbol{\theta}}_{(.)} = (1/B)\sum_{b=1}^{B}\hat{\boldsymbol{\theta}}_{(b)}$. The bootstrap estimate of the variance matrix is

$$\Sigma_B = \frac{1}{B-1}\sum_{b=1}^{B}(\boldsymbol{\theta}_{(b)} - \bar{\boldsymbol{\theta}}_{(.)})(\boldsymbol{\theta}_{(b)} - \bar{\boldsymbol{\theta}}_{(.)})'.$$

The confidence intervals for the regression parameters can be constructed using the normal approximation.

If there is a possibility of being cured after each event, and the probability of cure can evolve with time, the above method cannot handle this case and a random effect is also needed in the incidence submodel too. However, this case can be handled using the methods discussed in Section 4.3.1 by treating all the recurrent event times as clustered survival times. Detailed discussions can be found in Rondeau et al. (2013).

As a side note, similar cure models with a frailty in the latency submodel were also discussed in Price and Manatunga (2001); Peng and Zhang (2008a,b) for survival times without recurrences or clustering. The frailty in the models is mainly to model latent heterogeneity in data.

4.5 Cure Models for Competing-Risks Survival Data

Competing risks occur frequently in the analysis of survival data. A competing risk is an event whose occurrence precludes the occurrence of the primary event of interest. In a study examining time to death attributable to cardiovascular causes, death attributable to noncardiovascular causes is a competing risk. When estimating the crude incidence of outcomes, analysts should use the cumulative incidence function, rather than the complement of the Kaplan-Meier survival function. The use of the Kaplan-Meier survival function results in estimates of incidence that are biased upward, regardless of whether the competing events are independent of one another. When fitting regression models in the presence of competing risks, researchers can choose from two different families of models: modeling the effect of covariates on the cause-specific hazard of the outcome (Kalbfleisch and Prentice, 2002) or modeling the effect of covariates on the cumulative incidence function of the outcome (Fine and Gray, 1999, also known as the Fine-Gray model). The former allows one to estimate the effect of the covariates on the rate of occurrence of the outcome in those subjects who are currently event free and may be better suited for addressing etiologic questions. The latter allows one to estimate the effect of covariates on the absolute risk of the outcome over time and may be better suited for estimating a patient's clinical prognosis.

Survival data with cure fractions are often complicated by dependent censoring or competing risks. The analysis of this type of data typically involves untestable parametric assumptions on the dependence of the censoring mechanism and the underlying survival times. Competing risks will often hamper statistical analysis since classical methods would not be valid as ignorance of dependent censoring will typically introduce bias. Often, competing risks analysis directly works on a cumulative incidence function, for which the cause-specific hazard function has been widely used to measure the absolute risk of failure from a particular cause over time without assuming any dependence among the events. With covariates, the Fine-Gray model adapts a proportional hazards model to a cumulative incidence function and has been popularized. In the presence of a cure fraction, the proportional hazards assumption may represent a significant restriction for the analysis and the Fine-Gray model may be inappropriate for this case. In this section, we introduce two semi-parametric regression models for competing risks data with a cured fraction based on finite-mixture models.

4.5.1 Classical Approach

Suppose that during follow-up, each patient may experience one of K distinct types of failure events and $D = k$ indicates that a patient fails from the kth type of event. We use $D = 0$ for patients who are insusceptible to any type of events. Let

$$T^* = \begin{cases} T_k & D = k, \\ \infty & D = 0, \end{cases} \tag{4.26}$$

where the latent variables T_k denote the event time from cause k for uncured patients. The mixture model for T^* is given by

$$S(t) = (1 - \pi) + \sum_{k=1}^{K} \pi_k S_{ku}(t), \tag{4.27}$$

where $S_{ku}(t) = P(T^* \geq t | D = k) = P(T_k \geq t)$ is a proper sub-survival function for cause k, $\pi_k = P(D = k)$, and $\pi = \sum_{k=1}^{K} \pi_k$ is the total probability of dying from any cause (Ng and McLachlan, 2003). The mixture approach provides a unifying way to obtain estimates of the cause-specific and sub-distribution hazards as well as hazard-ratio functions for competing risks. In addition, it does not require the independence assumption between competing risks that seems questionable in most real-life situations. The mixture model also separates the long-term effect of a covariate from its short-term effect by modeling π_k and $S_{ku}(\cdot)$ separately, as we will see below.

To specify a model for $S_{ku}(t)$ to relate to covariate $\boldsymbol{x}$, a semiparametric PH model for T_k (Ng and McLachlan, 2003)

$$S_{ku}(t|\boldsymbol{x}) = S_{ku0}(t)^{\exp(-\boldsymbol{x}\boldsymbol{\beta}^{(k)})}, \tag{4.28}$$

or a semiparametric AFT model for T_k (Choi et al., 2018)

$$\log(T_k) = \boldsymbol{x}\boldsymbol{\beta}^{(k)} + \epsilon_k, \tag{4.29}$$

can be considered, where $\boldsymbol{\beta}^{(k)}$ is the set of coefficients measuring effects of $\boldsymbol{x}$ on T_k, and ϵ_k is an error term associated with T_k. Under model (4.29), we have

$$S_{ku}(t|\boldsymbol{x}) = \exp\left\{-H_k(t\exp(-\boldsymbol{x}\boldsymbol{\beta}^{(k)}))\right\},$$

where $H_k(\cdot)$ denotes the cumulative hazard function of $\exp(\epsilon_k)$ that are left unspecified. Model (4.28) and (4.29) are conditional regression models that evaluate the covariate effect on a specific event given its occurrence. Other models for $S_{ku}(t|\boldsymbol{x})$ such as linear transformation models discussed in Section 3.2.4 can also be considered (Choi and Huang, 2014; Choi et al., 2015). We further relate the probability π_k to a covariate vector $\boldsymbol{z}$ by a multinomial logistic regression model:

$$\pi_k(\boldsymbol{z}) = \frac{\exp(\boldsymbol{z}\boldsymbol{\gamma}^{(k)})}{\sum_{l=1}^{k} \exp(\boldsymbol{z}\boldsymbol{\gamma}^{(l)})}, \tag{4.30}$$

where $\boldsymbol{\gamma}^{(k)}$ is the q-vector of the parameters measuring the effects of $\boldsymbol{z}$ on the time to event of cause k. Then, the overall survival function for T^* is

$$S(t|\boldsymbol{x}, \boldsymbol{z}) = 1 - \pi(\boldsymbol{z}) + \sum_{k=1}^{K} \pi_k(\boldsymbol{z}) S_{ku}(t|\boldsymbol{x}).$$

Suppose that there are n independent subjects, and the observed data consist of observed failure time t_i, censoring indicator δ_i, cause indicator D_i, and covariates $\boldsymbol{x}_i$ and $\boldsymbol{z}_i$, $i = 1, \ldots, n$. Let $\boldsymbol{\theta}$ denote the entire set of parameters. The likelihood function for $\boldsymbol{\theta}$ based on the observed survival data is

$$L(\boldsymbol{\theta}) = \prod_{i=1}^{n} \prod_{k=1}^{K} \{\pi_k(\boldsymbol{z}_i) f_{ku}(t_i|\boldsymbol{x}_i)\}^{\delta_i I(D_i=1)} \times \left\{1 - \pi(\boldsymbol{z}_i) + \sum_{l=1}^{K} \pi_l(\boldsymbol{z}_i) S_{lu}(t_i|\boldsymbol{x}_i)\right\}^{1-\delta_i}.$$

In general, a direct maximization of the above likelihood function is difficult because of the presence of unspecified $f_{ku}(\cdot)$, $S_{ku}(\cdot)$ as well as the mixture structure. The EM algorithm can make the estimation feasible (Ng and McLachlan, 2003; Choi et al., 2018). Given the missing values of D_i's for censored times, the complete log-likelihood can be written as

$$\ell^c(\boldsymbol{\theta}) = \log \prod_{i=1}^{n} \prod_{k=1}^{K} \{\pi_k(\boldsymbol{z}_i) f_{ku}(t_i|\boldsymbol{x}_i)\}^{\delta_i I(D_i=1)} \times \left\{[1 - \pi(\boldsymbol{z}_i)]^{I(D_i=0)} \prod_{l=1}^{K} [\pi_l(\boldsymbol{z}_i) S_{lu}(t_i|\boldsymbol{x}_i)]^{I(D_i=0)}\right\}^{1-\delta_i},$$

which can be decomposed into the following components:

$$\ell_k^c = \sum_{i=1}^{n} I(D_i = k) \left[\delta_i \log h_{ku}(t_i|\boldsymbol{x}_i) - H_{ku}(t_i|\boldsymbol{x}_i)\right], \quad k = 1, \ldots, K,$$

$$\ell_\pi^c = \sum_{i=1}^{n} \sum_{k=0}^{K} I(D_i = k) \log(\pi_k(\boldsymbol{z}_i)),$$

where $\pi_0(\boldsymbol{z}_i) = 1 - \pi(\boldsymbol{z}_i)$. The E-step in the $(m+1)$th iteration of the EM algorithm computes the conditional expectation of D_i as follows given the observed data and the current estimate of $\boldsymbol{\theta}$:

$$w_{ki} = P(D_k = k) = \delta_i I(D_i = k) + (1 - \delta_i) w_k(t_i), \quad k = 0, \ldots, K,$$

where

$$w_0(t_i) = \frac{1 - \pi^{(m)}(\boldsymbol{z}_i)}{1 - \pi^{(m)}(\boldsymbol{z}_i) + \sum_{l=1}^{K} \pi_l^{(m)}(\boldsymbol{z}_i) S_{lu}^{(m)}(t_i|\boldsymbol{x}_i)},$$

$$w_k(t_i) = \frac{\pi_k^{(m)}(\boldsymbol{z}_i) S_{ku}^{(m)}(t_i|\boldsymbol{x}_i)}{1 - \pi^{(m)}(\boldsymbol{z}_i) + \sum_{l=1}^{K} \pi_l^{(m)}(\boldsymbol{z}_i) S_{lu}^{(m)}(t_i|\boldsymbol{x}_i)}, \quad k = 1, \ldots, K,$$

$\pi^{(m)}(\boldsymbol{z}_i)$ and $S_{ku}^{(m)}(t_i|\boldsymbol{x}_i)$ are respectively the values of $\pi(\boldsymbol{z}_i)$ and $S_{ku}(t_i|\boldsymbol{x}_i)$ evaluated at the parameter estimates in the mth iteration of the EM algorithm.

The M-step in the $(m+1)$th iteration of the EM algorithm maximizes the conditional expectation of the complete log-likelihood function above to update the estimates of the unknown parameters in the model after $I(D_i = k)$ is replaced with w_{ki}'s, which reduces to maximizing the following functions:

$$\sum_{i=1}^{n} \left[\Delta_{ki}\{\log h_{ku}(t_i|\boldsymbol{x}_i)\} - w_{ki} H_{ku}(t_i|\boldsymbol{x}_i)\right], \quad k = 1, \ldots, K, \tag{4.31}$$

$$\sum_{i=0}^{n} \sum_{k=0}^{K} w_{ki} \log(\pi_k(\boldsymbol{z}_i)), \tag{4.32}$$

where $\Delta_{ki} = \delta_i I(D_i = k)$ be the observed cause indicator for cause k.

The maximization of function (4.32) is relatively easy with a standard optimization algorithm or using a multinomial logistic regression program. Numerical difficulties arise when maximizing (4.31), as they involve unspecified baseline distributions. For model (4.28), a nonparametric maximum likelihood estimate of $S_{ku0}(t)$ in the $(m+1)$th iteration can be obtained in a similar way as (3.3). Let $\tau_1^{(k)} < \cdots < \tau_{n_k}^{(k)}$ be the distinct uncensored times due to cause k, $d_j^{(k)}$ be the number of uncensored times at $\tau_j^{(k)}$, and $R(t)$ be the risk set at t. Then the nonparametric estimator of the baseline survival function is

$$S_{ku0}^{(m+1)}(t) = \exp\left(-\sum_{j:\tau_j^{(k)} < t} \frac{d_j^{(k)}}{\sum_{i \in R(\tau_j^{(k)})} w_{ki} \exp(\boldsymbol{x}_i \boldsymbol{\beta}^{(k)})}\right).$$

Plug this baseline hazard estimator into (4.31) to obtain a profile log-likelihood function for $\boldsymbol{\beta}^{(k)}$, from which ${\boldsymbol{\beta}^{(k)}}^{(m+1)}$ can be obtained. An estimate of $\boldsymbol{\beta}^{(k)}$

can also be obtained from a partial log-likelihood function

$$\log \prod_{j=1}^{n_k} \frac{\exp(\boldsymbol{s}_j \boldsymbol{\beta}^{(k)})}{\left[\sum_{i \in R(\tau_j^{(k)})} w_{ki} \exp(\boldsymbol{x}_i \boldsymbol{\beta}^{(k)})\right]^{d_j^{(k)}}},$$

where $\boldsymbol{s}_j = \sum_{i:t_i=\tau_j^{(k)}, \delta_i=1, D_i=k} \boldsymbol{x}_i$.

For model (4.29), a nonparametric maximum likelihood estimate for $H_k(t)$ can be obtained as follows (Choi et al., 2015, 2018)

$$\tilde{H}_k^{(m+1)}(t; \boldsymbol{\beta}^{(k)}) = \sum_{i=1}^{n} \int_0^t \frac{dN_{ki}(ue^{-\boldsymbol{x}_i \boldsymbol{\beta}^{(k)}})}{\sum_{j=1}^{n} w_{kj} I(e^{\eta_{kj}(\boldsymbol{\beta}^{(k)})} \geq u)} du$$

$$= \sum_{i=1}^{n} \int_0^t \Delta \tilde{H}_k(u; \boldsymbol{\beta}^{(k)}) du, \quad (4.33)$$

where $N_{ki}(t) = \delta_i I(T_i \leq t, D_i = k)$ and $\eta_{ki}(\boldsymbol{\beta}^{(k)}) = \log t_i - \boldsymbol{x}_i \boldsymbol{\beta}^{(k)}$ is the residual term for cause k. Note that $\Delta \tilde{H}_k(t; \boldsymbol{\beta}^{(k)})$ represents the jump size of the discretized version of $H_k(t)$ at time t. By plugging (4.33) into (4.31) and using the martingale property that $\sum_{i=1}^{n} w_{ki} \tilde{H}_k(e^{\eta_{ki} \boldsymbol{\beta}^{(k)}}; \boldsymbol{\beta}^{(k)}) = \sum_{i=1}^{n} \Delta_{ki}$, we obtain the following profile likelihood for $\boldsymbol{\beta}^{(k)}$, ignoring the constant terms:

$$\sum_{i=1}^{n} \Delta_{ki}(-\boldsymbol{x}_i \boldsymbol{\beta}^{(k)} + \log \Delta \tilde{H}_k(e^{\eta_{ki}(\boldsymbol{\beta}^{(k)})}; \boldsymbol{\beta}^{(k)})). \quad (4.34)$$

However, maximizing (4.34) is still challenging because the estimator $\tilde{H}_k$ involves the rank of $\eta_{ki}(\boldsymbol{\beta}^{(k)})$'s only through the indicator function $I(\cdot)$ so it is very nonsmooth with respect to $\boldsymbol{\beta}^{(k)}$. Similar to the discussion in Section 3.2.2.3, a smoothed profile log-likelihood for $\boldsymbol{\beta}^{(k)}$ can be obtained following the method of Zeng and Lin (2007):

$$-\frac{1}{n}\sum_{i=1}^{n} \Delta_{ki} \boldsymbol{x}_i \boldsymbol{\beta}^{(k)} + \frac{1}{n}\sum_{i=1}^{n} \Delta_{ki} \log\left[\frac{1}{n}\sum_{j=1}^{n} \Delta_{kj} K_{h_k}(e^{\eta_{kj}(\boldsymbol{\beta}^{(k)})} - e^{\eta_{ki}(\boldsymbol{\beta}^{(k)})})\right]$$

$$-\frac{1}{n}\sum_{i=1}^{n} \Delta_{ki} \log\left[\frac{1}{n}\sum_{j=1}^{n} w_{kj} \int_{-\infty}^{e^{\eta_{kj}(\boldsymbol{\beta}^{(k)})} - e^{\eta_{ki}(\boldsymbol{\beta}^{(k)})}} K_{h_k}(u) du\right],$$

where $K_{h_k}(\cdot)$ is defined in Section 3.2.2.3 and is a symmetric kernel function with bandwidth h_k. The corresponding smoothed estimator of $H_k(t; \boldsymbol{\beta}^{(k)})$ is

$$\int_{-\infty}^{t} \frac{\sum_{i=1}^{n} \Delta_{ki} K_{h_k}(e^{\eta_{ki}(\boldsymbol{\beta}^{(k)})} - s)}{\sum_{i=1}^{n} w_{ki} \int_{-\infty}^{e^{\eta_{ki}(\boldsymbol{\beta}^{(k)})} - s} K_{h_k}(u) du} ds.$$

One advantage of the competing risks mixture model is that it is relatively easy to summarize the cumulative incidence rate for each competing cause. The cumulative incidence function corresponding to the kth event can be written as

$$F_k^*(t) = P(T \leq t, D = k) = P(T \leq t|D = k)P(D = k) = \pi_k(\boldsymbol{z})\{1 - S_{ku}(t|\boldsymbol{x})\}$$

This quantity measures the crude cumulative probability of experiencing event k over time in the presence of other causes. The implied failure time T has an improper distribution function equal to $\sum_{k=1}^{K} F_k^*(t)$ and a point mass $P(T = \infty) = 1 - \sum_{k=1}^{K} F_k^*(t)$. Therefore, the estimation of the overall survival probability is tantamount to estimation of the subdistribution for individuals who will eventually experience at least one of the failure events.

4.5.2 Vertical Approach

When modeling competing risks data, the classical approach in the last section considers factoring the subdistribution as $P(T, D|Y = 1) = P(T|D, Y = 1)P(D|Y = 1)$ and then specifying models for $P(T|D, Y = 1)$ (such as (4.28) or (4.29)) and $P(D|Y = 1)$ (such as (4.30)). In the vertical approach, the subdistribution is factored as $P(T, D|Y = 1) = P(D|T, Y = 1)P(T|Y = 1)$ and then models for $P(D|T, Y = 1)$ and $P(T|Y = 1)$ are specified (Nicolaie et al., 2019). Specifically, the Cox's PH model can be considered for $P(T|Y = 1)$ as in the non-competing risks context:

$$h_u(t) = h_{u0}(t) \exp(\boldsymbol{\beta}'\boldsymbol{x}).$$

Given $T = t$, a multinomial model can be specified for $P(D = j|T = t, Y = 1)$ as follows

$$\pi_j(t, \tilde{\boldsymbol{z}}) = \frac{\exp(\boldsymbol{b}_j' \boldsymbol{B}(t) + \tilde{\boldsymbol{z}}'\boldsymbol{\beta}^{(j)})}{\sum_{k=1}^{K} \exp(\boldsymbol{b}_k' \boldsymbol{B}(t) + \tilde{\boldsymbol{z}}'\boldsymbol{\beta}^{(k)})},$$

where $\boldsymbol{B}(t)$ is a vector of functions of t which can be in the form of polynomial or spline functions to add flexibility in the model. Due to the constraint $\sum_{j=1}^{K} \pi_j = 1$, we fix $\boldsymbol{b}_K = \boldsymbol{0}$ and $\boldsymbol{\beta}^{(K)} = \boldsymbol{0}$ and the unknown parameters are $\boldsymbol{b}_1, \ldots, \boldsymbol{b}_{K-1}$ and $\boldsymbol{\beta}^{(1)}, \ldots, \boldsymbol{\beta}^{(K-1)}$. For the latent variable Y, it's model can still be specified as in (2.2).

Given observed data $(t_i, \delta_i, D_i, \boldsymbol{x}_i, \boldsymbol{z}_i, \tilde{\boldsymbol{z}}_i)$, $i = 1, \ldots, n$, the likelihood function is

$$\log \prod_{i=1}^{n} \left[\pi(\boldsymbol{z}_i) f_u(t_i|\boldsymbol{x}_i) \prod_{j=1}^{K} \pi_j(t_i, \tilde{\boldsymbol{z}}_i)^{I(D_i=j)} \right]^{\delta_i} [1 - \pi(\boldsymbol{z}_i) + \pi(\boldsymbol{z}_i) S_u(t_i|\boldsymbol{x}_i)]^{1-\delta_i}$$

$$= \ell_1(\boldsymbol{\beta}, h_{u0}, \boldsymbol{\gamma}) + \ell_2(\boldsymbol{b}_1, \ldots, \boldsymbol{b}_{K-1}, \boldsymbol{\beta}^{(1)}, \ldots, \boldsymbol{\beta}^{(K-1)}),$$

where

$$\ell_1(\boldsymbol{\beta}, h_{u0}, \boldsymbol{\gamma}) = \log \prod_{i=1}^{n} [\pi(\boldsymbol{z}_i) f_u(t_i|\boldsymbol{x}_i)]^{\delta_i} [1 - \pi(\boldsymbol{z}_i) + \pi(\boldsymbol{z}_i) S_u(t_i|\boldsymbol{x}_i)]^{1-\delta_i},$$

$$\ell_2(\boldsymbol{b}_1, \ldots, \boldsymbol{b}_{K-1}, \boldsymbol{\beta}^{(1)}, \ldots, \boldsymbol{\beta}^{(K-1)}) = \log \prod_{i=1}^{n} \prod_{j=1}^{K} \pi_j(t_i, \tilde{\boldsymbol{z}}_i)^{\delta_i I(D_i=j)}.$$

It is easy to see that the estimates and their standard errors of $(\boldsymbol{\beta}, h_{u0}, \boldsymbol{\gamma})$ can be obtained separately from those of $(\boldsymbol{b}_1, \ldots, \boldsymbol{b}_{K-1}, \boldsymbol{\beta}^{(1)}, \ldots, \boldsymbol{\beta}^{(K-1)})$. The estimation methods discussed in previous chapters for non-competing risks data, such as the EM algorithm, can be used to estimate $\boldsymbol{\beta}$, h_{u0} and $\boldsymbol{\gamma}$ from ℓ_1 while estimation methods for multinomial logistic regression can be used to estimate $(\boldsymbol{b}_1, \ldots, \boldsymbol{b}_{K-1})$ and $(\boldsymbol{\beta}^{(1)}, \ldots, \boldsymbol{\beta}^{(K-1)})$ from ℓ_2. Thus, the vertical approach leads to a simpler estimation method than the classical approach.

4.6 Software and Applications

We show two publicly available R packages that can be used to fit some models discussed in this chapter to real-life data sets. There are few SAS macros available to fit the models. Rondeau et al. (2013) provide SAS commands to fit the models for recurrent survival times discussed in Section 4.4. The details of the SAS commands are omitted here.

4.6.1 R Package geecure

The R package `geecure` (Niu et al., 2018b) can be used to fit the marginal PH mixture cure models in Section 4.2. It allows either a parametric Weibull distribution or a nonparametric specification as the baseline distribution in the PH latency submodel.

The data we consider for the demonstration are from a tonsil cancer clinical trial study conducted by the Radiation Therapy Oncology Group in the United States (Kalbfleisch and Prentice, 2002). There are 195 patients with squamous cell carcinoma of three sites in the oropharynx between 1968 and 1972 in six participating institutions in the study. Patients in each institution were randomly assigned to one of two treatment groups: radiation therapy alone or radiation therapy together with a chemotherapeutic agent. The survival time (`time`) is defined as the time (in days) from diagnosis to death due to the cancer. Other variables include censoring indicator `cens`, `sex`, `tstage` (tumor stage with 1 for massive invasive tumor and 0 for primary tumor measuring 2 cm or less in largest diameter, the primary tumor measuring 2 to 4 cm in the largest diameter, and minimal infiltration in depth, or primary

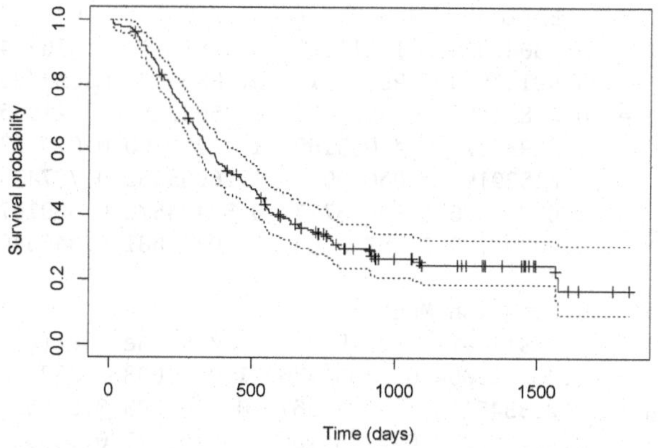

FIGURE 4.1
The Kaplan-Meier survival curve of time to death due to tonsil cancer.

tumor measuring more than 4 cm), `age`, `condition` (general condition with 0 for no disability, and 1 for cases with restricted work capability, requiring assistance with self care or bed confined), `grade` (well, moderate, and poorly differentiated respectively), and the institution code `inst`. We delete observations from patient 136, 141, and 159 due to invalid values in `grade` and `condition`. The Kaplan-Meier survival curve in Figure 4.1 levels off at about 0.18, which suggests that a cure fraction may present in this data and a cure model should be considered. The patients are clustered by institutions where the shared environment and the treatment resources may cause the correlation among the cure status and among the failure times of uncured patients in one institution. Therefore both the cure fraction and the cluster effect must be considered in a model for the data (Lai and Yau, 2008).

We first fit the parametric marginal PH mixture cure models to the tonsil data using the exchangeable correlation structure and the Weibull baseline distribution as follows. Since we are dealing with clustered survival times, the argument `id` indicates that the clusters are defined by `inst` in data.

```
> geecure(Surv(time, cens) ~ sex + grade + age + condition +
+ tstage, cureform = ~ sex + grade + age + condition + tstage, data
+ = oropharynx, id = oropharynx$inst, model = "para", corstr =
+ "exchangeable")

Call:
geecure(formula = Surv(time, cens) ~ sex + grade + age + condition +
    tstage, cureform = ~sex + grade + age + condition + tstage,
    data = oropharynx, id = oropharynx$inst, model = "para",
    corstr = "exchangeable")

Cure Probability Model:
```

```
                 Estimate  Std.Error     Z value   Pr(>|Z|)
(Intercept)    0.06087856 2.11111365  0.02883718 0.97699445
sexfemale     -0.40157588 0.98265213 -0.40866536 0.68278526
grademoderate  0.72831405 2.04364152  0.35638053 0.72155561
gradepoor     -0.71937370 0.41053169 -1.75229760 0.07972265
age            0.01529195 0.05670939  0.26965462 0.78742597
condition      1.09911676 2.09656777  0.52424576 0.60010762
tstage         0.28207183 1.45753363  0.19352681 0.84654641

Failure Time Distribution Model:
                  Estimate  Std.Error    Z value   Pr(>|Z|)
sexfemale     -0.398462004 0.37084576 -1.0744683 0.28261286
grademoderate -0.233346163 0.40609567 -0.5746088 0.56555587
gradepoor      0.252767047 0.27585106  0.9163171 0.35950059
age           -0.009463133 0.02006655 -0.4715875 0.63722128
condition      1.662646117 0.79296366  2.0967494 0.03601576
tstage         0.819346230 0.56486381  1.4505200 0.14691358

Estimated Parameters in Weibull Distribution:
            Estimate    Std.Error   Z value     Pr(>|Z|)
alpha_1 1.7491544518 2.232558e-01 7.8347543 4.662937e-15
alpha_2 0.0000214415 3.700902e-05 0.5793587 5.623472e-01

Estimated Correlation Parameters:
         Estimate
rho_1 0.014170964
rho_2 0.008035372

Number of clusters: 6       Maximum cluster size: 46
```

The semiparametric marginal PH mixture cure model with the exchangeable correlation structure is fit to the data as follows:

```
> geecure(Surv(time, cens) ~ sex + grade + age + condition +
+ tstage, cureform = ~ sex + grade + age + condition + tstage, data
+ = oropharynx, id = oropharynx$inst, model = "semi", corstr =
+ "exchangeable")

Call:
geecure(formula = Surv(time, cens) ~ sex + grade + age + condition +
    tstage, cureform = ~sex + grade + age + condition + tstage,
    data = oropharynx, id = oropharynx$inst, model = "semi",
    corstr = "exchangeable")

Cure Probability Model:
                 Estimate Std.Error     Z value   Pr(>|Z|)
(Intercept)   -0.68664791 5.6524249 -0.12147847 0.90331207
sexfemale     -0.39201499 1.6738705 -0.23419673 0.81483226
grademoderate  1.19883715 2.8942768  0.41420957 0.67872063
gradepoor     -0.78825579 0.4164993 -1.89257406 0.05841454
```

```
age              0.03654110 0.1232039  0.29659055 0.76677913
condition        0.46895261 2.5736893  0.18221026 0.85541772
tstage          -0.04874503 1.5966712 -0.03052916 0.97564504

Failure Time Distribution Model:
                  Estimate   Std.Error    Z value      Pr(>|Z|)
sexfemale       -0.4603751 0.435882517 -1.0561908 0.2908810758
grademoderate -0.2572418 0.414601417 -0.6204557 0.5349578138
gradepoor        0.1188582 0.567428059  0.2094682 0.8340827328
age             -0.0144533 0.008063506 -1.7924342 0.0730634379
condition        1.7263782 0.507008477  3.4050283 0.0006615721
tstage           0.7380744 0.595477506  1.2394665 0.2151727908

Estimated Correlation Parameters:
         Estimate
rho_1 0.005169755
rho_2 0.066172810

Number of clusters: 6       Maximum cluster size: 46
```

Both models show a weak correlation within institutions. None of the covariates has significant effects on the incidence probability of being cured. However, both the parametric and the semiparametric models show that `condition` has a significant effect on the failure time of uncured subjects, implying shortened failure times for those with disability compared to those without disability.

4.6.2 R Package intcure

The R package `intcure` can be used to fit mixture cure models with random effects discussed in Section 4.3.1. This package allows the exponential and Weibull distributions or more flexible piecewise constant hazard distribution as the baseline distribution in the mixture cure model. The random effects can be added to either part of the mixture cure model, and they are assumed to follow normal distributions. If both parts have random effects, the two random effects can be correlated.

We consider the bone marrow transplantation data set discussed in Section 3.6.5 in the demonstration. The Kaplan-Meier survival curve in Figure 3.4 suggests the existence of a cure proportion in acute leukemia patients. In addition, the patients within an institution may tend to be correlated in cure statuses and in the failure times of uncured patients due to the shared environment. Therefore, both the cure fraction and the cluster effect should be considered (Lai and Yau, 2008). The variables we consider include the disease group `g` (in three groups: acute lymphoblastic leukemia (ALL), low risk and high risk acute myelocytic leukemia (AML)), `FAB` (1 if FAB grade 4 or 5 and AML, and 0 otherwise), `inst` (institutions/hospitals: 1-The Ohio State University, 2-Alfred, 3-St. Vincent, 4-Hahnemann) and time and censoring indicator variables `time` (we divide time values by 365.25 to convert their unit from day into year) and `cens`. These variables are considered in Niu et al. (2018b) for their marginal model/generalized estimating equations approach. We consider them in the mixture cure model with random effects.

The baseline distribution we consider for the data is the Weibull distribution. The more flexible piecewise constant hazard distribution can also be considered as the baseline distribution in the random-effects mixture cure model. We start the modeling without any random effects:

```
> z = intcure(Surv(time, cens) ~ g + FAB, ~ g + FAB, data = bmt,
+ basedist = "weibull", sigma = c(NA, NA, NA), optimcfg =
+ list(method = "BFGS", hessian = T, maxit = 2000))
> summary(z)

Call:
intcure(formula = Surv(time, cens) ~ g + FAB, cureform = ~g +
    FAB, data = bmt, sigma = c(NA, NA, NA), optimcfg =
                list(method = "BFGS", hessian = T, maxit = 2000),
                basedist = "weibull", funval = F)

Mixture cure model with weibull baseline

Fixed effects in survival model:
                   Estimate    Stderr      zvalue    pvalue
gAML low risk   -0.6842093 0.5655751 -1.2097586 0.2263715
gAML high risk   0.1186363 0.5402647  0.2195891 0.8261912
FAB              0.1687005 0.4574249  0.3688048 0.7122732

Baseline parameters in survival model:
          Estimate    Stderr    zvalue       pvalue
logshape 0.3581387 0.1205748 2.9702603 0.002975475
lograte  0.2926832 0.3261439 0.8974051 0.369502792

Fixed effects in logistic model:
                   Estimate    Stderr    zvalue       pvalue
(Intercept)     -0.4219126 0.3880971 -1.087131 0.276978742
gAML low risk   -1.7954045 0.6565482 -2.734612 0.006245384
gAML high risk  -0.1696658 0.6217394 -0.272889 0.784938552
FAB              1.7755283 0.5689114  3.120922 0.001802856

Random effects:
NULL

Maximum log-likelihood: -84.17185
```

The result shows that only `FAB` has a significant effect in the incidence model. We then add a random institution effect in the latency part as follows:

```
> summary(intcure(Surv(time, cens) ~ g + FAB + cluster(inst), ~ g +
+ FAB, data = bmt, basedist = "weibull", bt = z$bt, gm  =z$gm,
```

```
+ basepara = z$basepara, sigma = c(-2, NA, NA), optimcfg =
+ list(method = "BFGS", hessian = T, maxit = 2000)))

Call:
intcure(formula = Surv(time, cens) ~ g + FAB + cluster(inst),
    cureform = ~g + FAB, data = bmt, bt = z$bt, gm = z$gm,
               basepara = z$basepara, sigma = c(-2, NA, NA),
               optimcfg = list(method = "BFGS", hessian = T,
    maxit = 2000), basedist = "weibull", funval = F)

Mixture cure model with weibull baseline

Fixed effects in survival model:
                   Estimate    Stderr      zvalue    pvalue
gAML low risk  -0.7793680 0.5902657 -1.3203682 0.1867121
gAML high risk  0.1283226 0.5282317  0.2429286 0.8080607
FAB             0.1621599 0.4554964  0.3560070 0.7218353

Baseline parameters in survival model:
          Estimate    Stderr   zvalue      pvalue
logshape 0.3960895 0.1274036 3.108936 0.001877626
lograte  0.4995367 0.4255788 1.173782 0.240482466

Fixed effects in logistic model:
                   Estimate    Stderr      zvalue      pvalue
(Intercept)    -0.4340039 0.3848586 -1.1276971 0.259447864
gAML low risk  -1.7656216 0.6563998 -2.6898569 0.007148267
gAML high risk -0.1718087 0.6186691 -0.2777069 0.781237356
FAB             1.7844899 0.5697220  3.1322115 0.001734948

Random effects:
          Estimate    Stderr
lsigmau -0.9801852 0.9376209

Maximum log-likelihood: -83.80412
```

The maximum log-likelihood increases slightly and the fixed effects do not change substantially in the model. The estimated variance of the random effect is $\exp(2 \times -0.9801852) = 0.14$ and a 95% confidence interval is (0.003, 5.558).

If we instead add the random institution effect in the incidence part as follows, the impact of the random effect is even smaller:

```
> summary(intcure(Surv(time, cens) ~ g + FAB, ~ g + FAB +
+ cluster(inst), data = bmt, basedist = "weibull", bt = z$bt, gm
+ =z$gm, basepara = z$basepara, sigma = c(NA, -2, NA), optimcfg =
+ list(method = "BFGS", hessian = T, maxit = 2000)))

Call:
intcure(formula = Surv(time, cens) ~ g + FAB, cureform = ~g +
```

```
    FAB + cluster(inst), data = bmt, bt = z$bt, gm = z$gm,
                basepara = z$basepara, sigma = c(NA, -2, NA),
                optimcfg = list(method = "BFGS", hessian = T,
    maxit = 2000), basedist = "weibull", funval = F)

Mixture cure model with weibull baseline

Fixed effects in survival model:
                  Estimate    Stderr     zvalue    pvalue
gAML low risk  -0.6842530 0.5654734 -1.2100534 0.2262584
gAML high risk  0.1192150 0.5400794  0.2207361 0.8252979
FAB             0.1692987 0.4572134  0.3702838 0.7111710

Baseline parameters in survival model:
          Estimate    Stderr    zvalue      pvalue
logshape 0.3580047 0.1205544 2.9696530 0.002981363
lograte  0.2931282 0.3260803 0.8989449 0.368681986

Fixed effects in logistic model:
                  Estimate    Stderr     zvalue      pvalue
(Intercept)    -0.4233170 0.3963146 -1.0681337 0.285460215
gAML low risk  -1.7964643 0.6958665 -2.5816221 0.009833719
gAML high risk -0.1691668 0.6241080 -0.2710537 0.786349731
FAB             1.7759149 0.6196306  2.8660866 0.004155806

Random effects:
         Estimate   Stderr
lsigmav -2.000062 19.10945

Maximum log-likelihood: -84.17244
```

The maximum log-likelihood is literally unchanged compared to the value from the model without any random effects. The estimated variance is even smaller and the 95% confidence interval is even wider, suggesting that it is unnecessary to include a random institution effect in the incidence part. For the information purpose, we show the command below to further fit the data with institution random effects in both parts and correlated and the result does not change substantially from we got above.

```
> intcure(Surv(time, cens) ~ g + FAB + cluster(inst), ~ g + FAB +
+ cluster(inst), data = bmt, basedist = "weibull", bt = z$bt, gm
+ =z$gm, basepara = z$basepara, sigma = c(-2, -2, 0), optimcfg =
+ list(method = "BFGS", hessian = T, maxit = 2000)
```

If one doubts the suitability of the Weibull distribution as the baseline distribution in the model, one can use `basedist = "piecewise"` to fit the model with a piecewise constant hazard distribution. If a 3-piecewise constant hazard distribution is considered with the interior cutpoints set to `piececut = c(0.13, 1.6)`, the model does provide a better fit to the data than using the Weibull baseline distribution. However, the fixed effects do not change substantially and the random effects behave similarly as observed in the model with the Weibull baseline distribution. The detailed R results are omitted.

4.7 Summary

This chapter presented cure models for correlated survival data and competing risks data with a cured fraction. One type of correlated survival data is clustered survival times or multivariate survival data. We discussed two classes of models for this type of data. One class is the marginal models, which only assume marginal distributions for individual survival times. The correlation among survival times is either ignored or replaced with a working correlation structure, and a set of generalized estimating equations can be used to estimate the parameters in the marginal models. The second class is frailty/random-effects models. A joint distribution for the correlated survival times is usually specified under these models. Compared to the marginal models, the frailty/random-effects models are usually estimated with likelihood-based approaches and are easier to apply the likelihood-based inferential methods to the models. But their estimation methods tend to be more time consuming. The frailty models were also introduced for the recurrent survival time data, another type of correlated survival times.

Another type of data considered in this chapter is competing-risks data. The correlation between competing risks times cannot be identified because of the competing nature, and thus the models developed for correlated survival times are not appropriate. We introduced two approaches to model competing risks data with a cured fraction: One is a classical approach that models the unconditional probability of the cause of risks and the conditional survival time distribution given the cause of risks. Another newer approach is so-called vertical approach, which models the unconditional distribution of time and the conditional probability of cause of risks given the time.

There are not many software packages available for models discussed in this chapter. We reviewed two R packages that are available to fit marginal and frailty/random-effects models to clustered survival times with a cured fraction.

A related topic to competing risks data is multistate data, where the states for uncured patients can be either recurrent or dead while for cured patients, the only state is dead. For uncured patients, the recurrence and death are two semi-competing risks states because a death prevents recurrence from being observed but a recurrence does not prevent death from being observed. Multistate Markov cure models have been proposed for such data, and we refer readers to Conlon et al. (2014) and Beesley and Taylor (2019) for details.

5

Joint Modeling of Longitudinal and Survival Data with a Cure Fraction

5.1 Introduction

Longitudinal data consist of repeated outcome measurements from the same subjects over time and are frequently collected in medical and social science studies along with time to event data from the subjects. Even though longitudinal data and time to event data can be analyzed separately by existing statistical models, a joint analysis of the longitudinal and survival data becomes very popular in recent years because it may provide more efficient estimation than the separate analyses when longitudinal data and survival data are highly correlated (Ibrahim et al., 2010; Rizopoulos, 2012; Gould et al., 2015). In this chapter, we will introduce some methods for a joint analysis of longitudinal data and survival data when some subjects are cured and thus a cured fraction has to be properly taken into account in the joint analysis. The chapter is organized as follows: Section 5.2 introduces examples of longitudinal data and survival data from the same group of study subjects and notations that will be used in this chapter. Section 5.3 and 5.4 discuss a shared random effects approach to jointly model longitudinal continuous and proportional data and survival data with a cured fraction. Section 5.5 presents another approach for the joint model by including the trajectory of the longitudinal model in the cure model for survival data. Finally, applications of some joint models to data from in a breast cancer clinical trial are given in Section 5.6.

5.2 Longitudinal and Survival Data with a Cured Fraction

As an illustration, we consider the longitudinal quality of life (QoL) and survival data from the MA.5 trial conducted by the Canadian Cancer Trials Group, which compared two chemotherapy regimens for early breast cancer patients: a new and intensive treatment of cyclophosphamide, epirubicin, and fluorouracil (CEF) and the standard treatment of cyclophosphamide,

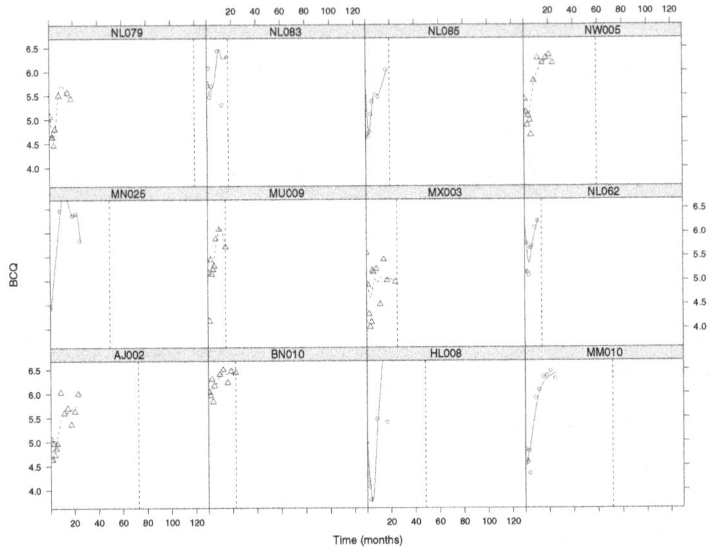

FIGURE 5.1
Trajectories of average BCQ from 12 randomly selected patients from the CEF (red circles with red lines as the fitted lowess curves) and CMF (blue triangles with blue dashed lines as the fitted lowess curves). Dashed vertical line indicates the recurrent-free survival time.

methotrexate, and fluorouracil (CMF) (Levine et al., 1998, 2005). The trial randomized 716 pre-menopausal women with early-stage breast cancer to two chemotherapy treatments, among them 356 patients were randomly assigned to CEF arm and 360 patients to the CMF arm. Both CEF and CMF were administered monthly for six months. The primary endpoint of this trial was the time to relapse or recurrence-free survival (RFS) time. The median follow-up time of all patients is 59 months, and there are 169 and 132 uncensored RFS times from patients randomized to CEF and CMF respectively in the data set.

The QoL of patients in the trial was assessed by the self-answered Breast Cancer Questionnaire (BCQ), which consists of 30 questions measuring different dimensions of QoL and was administered at each of the clinical visits (every one during the treatment and then every 3 months after the completion of the treatment) until the end of the second year or until recurrence or death, whichever came first. The specific QoL scale of interest is the global QoL of patients defined as the means of the answers to all 30 questions. There are 7769 QoL measurements from both arms. Figure 5.1 shows the trajectories of the longitudinal data from 12 randomly selected patients along with their RFS times.

The longitudinal QoL measurements can be analyzed by standard statistical methods for repeated measurements, such as linear mixed models (Fairclough, 2010), and the survival data can be analyzed by standard survival models (Kalbfleisch and Prentice, 2002). These models provide valid statistical inference when longitudinal measurements are complete in all patients. In cancer clinical trials where the QoL is measured, however, some seriously ill patients may drop out of the study because of worse QoL, disease recurrence or death, and their QoL measurements are incomplete. In this case, the missing of QoL measurements caused by the dropout of the patients is informative and may not be assumed as missing at random. Patients' poor QoL can also lead to censoring in survival time. Using standard longitudinal models for the data without taking into account of informative dropout in this context will lead to biased results, and failure to consider the correlation between the longitudinal and survival data can reduce the efficiency of the modeling. A joint modeling framework for longitudinal QoL measurements and survival data allows modeling both longitudinal measurements and survival times jointly to accommodate the association between them. As pointed out by Ibrahim et al. (2010), Diggle et al. (2008), Zeng and Cai (2005), Tsiatis and Davidian (2004), and Wulfsohn and Tsiatis (1997), joint analysis of longitudinal QoL data together with survival data, such as disease-free or overall survival times, would reduce bias and improve efficiency in the estimation of treatment effects on both QoL and time to event endpoints.

Another feature of such data is that a fraction of patients may be immune to the event of interest. With advances in cancer treatments, some patients may become cured and their cancer will not recur after a long-term follow-up. As discussed in early chapters, this is usually evidenced by a plateau in Kaplan-Meier survival curves based on survival times from a study with a sufficient follow-up. The Kaplan-Meier RFS estimate based on the data in the MA.5 trial for early-stage breast cancer is shown in Figure 5.2. The plateau in the curves demonstrates that there is a substantial fraction of early-stage breast patients who may be deemed as cured, particularly with the long follow-up of about 12 years. The standard survival models, such as Cox's PH model, may not be suitable to model censored survival times when some patients are cured.

Moreover, the longitudinal trajectory of cured patients may be different from uncured patients. Law et al. (2002) considered a case from a prostate cancer study where the longitudinal prostate-specific antigen (PSA) values of cured patients became stable after an initial decline, while those uncured patients increased steadily. Thus, it is important to take the cured patients into account when jointly analyzing the longitudinal and survival data.

In this chapter, we denote the longitudinal data by $\tilde{\boldsymbol{y}}_i = (\tilde{y}_{i1}, \ldots, \tilde{y}_{in_i})'$ and $\tilde{\boldsymbol{t}}_i = (\tilde{t}_{i1}, \ldots, \tilde{t}_{in_i})'$, where $\tilde{y}_{ij}$ is a longitudinal measurement from subject i at time $\tilde{t}_{ij}$, $j = 1, \ldots, n_i$, $i = 1, \ldots, n$. The observed data from subject i are $(\tilde{\boldsymbol{y}}_i, t_i, \delta_i, \dot{\boldsymbol{X}}_i, \tilde{\boldsymbol{X}}_i, \boldsymbol{x}_i, \boldsymbol{z}_i)$, where $\dot{\boldsymbol{X}}_i$ and $\tilde{\boldsymbol{X}}_i$ are matrices of values of some covariates ($\tilde{t}_{ij}$ may be included in the matrices, and the two matrices may or

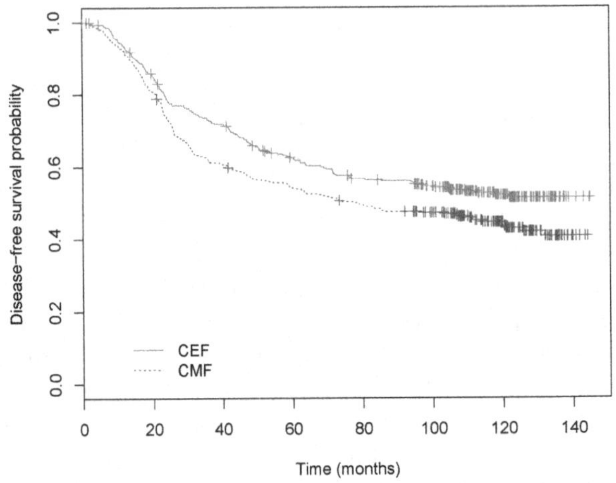

FIGURE 5.2
Kaplan-Meier recurrent-free survival curves for early breast cancer patients in the two treatments (CMF vs CEF).

may not be equal) from longitudinal data, and $\boldsymbol{x}_i$ and $\boldsymbol{z}_i$ are two vectors of covariates at the subject level.

5.3 Joint Modeling Longitudinal and Survival Data with Shared Random Effects

Random effects models are often used to analyze longitudinal data (Verbeke and Molenberghs, 2009). A simple approach to jointly analyze longitudinal and survival data is to allow the random effects in the model for longitudinal data to be shared in the model for the survival data so that the correlation between the two types of data can be accounted for. For example, a linear mixed-effects model can be considered for longitudinal QoL data as follows (Song, 2007):

$$\tilde{\boldsymbol{y}}_i = \dot{\boldsymbol{X}}_i\boldsymbol{\theta} + \tilde{\boldsymbol{X}}_i\boldsymbol{\alpha}_i + \boldsymbol{e}_i, \tag{5.1}$$

where $\boldsymbol{\theta}$ is a vector of fixed effects, $\boldsymbol{\alpha}_i$ is a $q \times 1$ vector of random effects, and $\boldsymbol{e}_i$ is the random error. The survival data can be modeled by a mixture cure model such as (2.1) or a non-mixture cure model such as (2.18) to take a cure fraction of subjects into account. A joint model can be defined by using a shared latent variate ξ_i to connect the longitudinal model and the cure model in the following way. Assume ξ_i follows a gamma distribution with the density function $\psi(\cdot|\eta,\eta)$ so that $E[\xi_i]=1$ and $var[\xi_i]=1/\eta$. Given ξ_i, $\boldsymbol{\alpha}_i$ and $\boldsymbol{e}_i$ are assumed to be independent and both are normal random variates with $\boldsymbol{\alpha}_i|\xi_i \sim N(\mathbf{0}, \boldsymbol{\Sigma}_\alpha/\xi_i)$ and $\boldsymbol{e}_i|\xi_i \sim N(\mathbf{0}, \boldsymbol{I}_{n_i \times n_i}\sigma_e^2/\xi_i)$. For survival data, if the PHC model (2.18) is considered, the survival time T_i in the joint model is assumed to follow a conditional distribution with the following survival function

$$S(t|\boldsymbol{x}_i,\xi_i)=\exp[-\xi_i e^{\boldsymbol{x}_i'\boldsymbol{\beta}}F^H(t)], \tag{5.2}$$

given ξ_i (to simplify our notation, the intercept term in (2.18) is absorbed into $\boldsymbol{\beta}$).

It can be shown that the marginal distributions of $\boldsymbol{\alpha}_i$ and $\boldsymbol{e}_i$ are respectively $t_q(\mathbf{0},\boldsymbol{\Sigma}_\alpha,2\eta)$ and $t_{n_i}(\mathbf{0},\sigma_e^2\boldsymbol{I}_{n_i\times n_i},2\eta)$, where $t_n(\mathbf{0},\boldsymbol{\Sigma}_{n\times n},2\eta)$ is an n-dimensional t distribution with mean 0, a positive definite scale matrix $\boldsymbol{\Sigma}_{n\times n}$ and a degree of freedom 2η (Pinheiro et al., 2001). Since the marginal variances of $\boldsymbol{\alpha}_i$ and $\boldsymbol{e}_i$ are respectively $var[\boldsymbol{\alpha}_i]=\frac{\eta}{\eta-1}\boldsymbol{\Sigma}_\alpha$ and $var[\boldsymbol{e}_i]=\frac{\eta}{\eta-1}\sigma_e^2\boldsymbol{I}_{n_i\times n_i}$, a condition $\eta>1$ in the joint model is required to guarantee the existence of the variances. The unconditional cure probability for a subject with $\boldsymbol{x}_i$ under this model is $\lim_{t\to\infty}\int_0^\infty S(t|\boldsymbol{x}_i,\xi_i)\psi(\xi_i|\eta,\eta)d\xi_i=\left(\frac{1}{\eta}e^{\boldsymbol{x}_i'\boldsymbol{\beta}}+1\right)^{-\eta}$ (Song et al., 2016b).

To estimate the unknown parameters, a maximum likelihood approach can be used (Song et al., 2012). For the sake of simplicity, we only consider $q=1$ with $\tilde{\boldsymbol{X}}_i=1$ and $\alpha_i|\xi_i\sim N(0,\sigma_\alpha^2/\xi_i)$. Conditional on α_i,ξ_i, the contribution of $\tilde{\boldsymbol{y}}_i$ to the likelihood under (5.1) is

$$L_{li}(\alpha_i,\xi_i)=\frac{1}{(\sqrt{2\pi\sigma_e^2/\xi_i})^{n_i}} \times \exp\left[-\frac{1}{2\sigma_e^2/\xi_i}(\tilde{\boldsymbol{y}}_i-\dot{\boldsymbol{X}}_i\boldsymbol{\theta}-\alpha_i)'(\tilde{\boldsymbol{y}}_i-\dot{\boldsymbol{X}}_i\boldsymbol{\theta}-\alpha_i)\right]$$

and the contribution of (t_i,δ_i) to the likelihood under (5.2) and independent censoring is

$$L_{si}(\alpha_i,\xi_i)=[\xi_i e^{\boldsymbol{x}_i'\boldsymbol{\beta}}f^H(t_i)]^{\delta_i}\exp[-\xi_i e^{\boldsymbol{x}_i'\boldsymbol{\beta}}F^H(t_i)]$$

where $f^H(\cdot)$ is the density function corresponding to $F^H(\cdot)$. The observed likelihood of the unknown parameters $\Theta=(\boldsymbol{\beta},\ \boldsymbol{\theta},\ \eta,\ \sigma_\alpha,\ \sigma_e,\ F^H(t))$ for the proposed joint model based on all observed data is

$$L(\Theta)=\prod_{i=1}^n\iint L_{li}(\alpha_i,\xi_i)L_{si}(\alpha_i,\xi_i)\varphi(\alpha_i|0,\sigma_\alpha^2/\xi_i)\psi(\xi_i|\eta,\eta)d\alpha_i d\xi_i,$$

where $\varphi(\cdot|0,\sigma_\alpha^2/\xi_i)$ is the density function of the normal distribution with mean 0 and variance σ_α^2/ξ_i. The unknown parameters in this likelihood function can be obtained using the EM algorithm. If α_i and ξ_i are observed, the complete log-likelihood from the joint model is $l^c = l_l + l_s + l_\alpha + l_\xi$, where

$$l_l = \sum_{i=1}^{n} \left[\frac{n_i}{2}(\log \xi_i - \log \sigma_e^2) - \frac{\xi_i}{2\sigma_e^2}(\tilde{\boldsymbol{y}}_i - \dot{\boldsymbol{X}}_i\boldsymbol{\theta} - \alpha_i)^T(\tilde{\boldsymbol{y}}_i - \dot{\boldsymbol{X}}_i\boldsymbol{\theta} - \alpha_i) \right],$$

$$l_s = \sum_{i=1}^{n} \left[\delta_i(\log f^H(t_i) + \log \xi_i + \boldsymbol{x}_i'\boldsymbol{\beta}) - \xi_i \exp(\boldsymbol{x}_i'\boldsymbol{\beta}) F^H(t_i) \right],$$

$$l_\alpha = \sum_{i=1}^{n} \left[\frac{1}{2}(\log \xi_i - \log \sigma_\alpha^2) - \frac{\xi_i \alpha_i^2}{2\sigma_\alpha^2} \right],$$

$$l_\xi = \sum_{i=1}^{n} [\eta \log \eta - \log \Gamma(\eta) + (\eta - 1)\log \xi_i - \eta \xi_i].$$

Let Θ_k be the estimate of Θ in the kth iteration. The E-step in the $(k+1)$th iteration of the EM algorithm computes the conditional expectation of l^c with respect to α_i and ξ_i, which is equivalent to evaluating the following four conditional expectations: $E[l_l|\Theta_k]$, $E[l_s|\Theta_k]$, $E[l_\alpha|\Theta_k]$, $E[l_\xi|\Theta_k]$. A closed-form of the expectations can be obtained and details can be found in Song et al. (2016b). The M-step in the $(k+1)$th iteration of the EM algorithm maximizes $E[l_l|\Theta_k]$, $E[l_\alpha|\Theta_k]$, and $E[l_\xi|\Theta_k]$, which can be accomplished using the Newton-Raphson method. To update the parameters $(\boldsymbol{\beta}, F^H(t))$ in $E[l_s|\Theta_k]$, the semiparametric method of Tsodikov et al. (2003) can be used to maximize $E[l_s|\Theta_k]$. The maximum likelihood estimates of the parameters are obtained after iterating the E-step and M-step until convergence. The variance of the parameter estimates can be obtained using the method of Louis (1982).

5.4 Modeling Longitudinal Proportional Data in Joint Modeling

The joint model discussed in Section 5.3 is suitable for continuous longitudinal data that can be approximated by a symmetric distribution, such as the normal distribution or t distribution. However, some longitudinal data in joint modeling may not satisfy this requirement. One particular case is QoL measurements from clinical trials, which are usually answers from patients to many questions on an ordinal Likert scale. The questions on a QoL questionnaire are usually divided into a few domains or items, which assess some specific aspects of QoL. For a given patient, his/her score on a specific QoL domain or item is obtained by the sum of the answers to all questions which define this domain or item. The values of the score are restricted in an interval with the minimum and maximum as respectively the score when answers to all questions are at the lowest and highest end of the ordinal scale for each question. Because of many potential values for these scores, they are usually considered as continuous and transformed linearly to a scale from 0 to 100 or from 0 to 1 for analysis. For example, the score on overall BCQ domain (or BCQ for short) for a patient in the study of Levine et al. (1998) is defined as the sum of her answers to all 30 questions in the questionnaire, each on a Likert scale from 0 to 7 with the best outcome marked as 7. The minimum and maximum of the BCQ score are respectively 0 and 210. It is difficult to treat these scores as ordinal data because of many potential values. For the analysis, they are usually assumed to be continuous and the raw scores are transformed to the unit interval $(0, 1)$. Such longitudinal data confined to (0, 1) are known as longitudinal proportional data (Song and Tan, 2000) or bounded data (Lesaffre et al., 2007).

In practice, the longitudinal proportional data are often treated as continuous data, or even further as normally distributed data. Song and Tan (2000) pointed out that ignoring the (0, 1) constraint may result in misleading conclusions. A more intuitive approach to analyze proportional data would be to transform the proportional data first using a logit function and then to assume a normal distribution for the logit-transformed proportional data, as suggested by Lesaffre et al. (2007), although, as pointed by Song and Tan (2000) and Qiu et al. (2008), it may be difficult to interpret the results obtained from this approach.

The simplex distribution (Barndorff-Nielsen and Jørgensen, 1991) provides an alternative way to directly model the marginal means of the longitudinal proportional responses, and it has been used in a generalized linear mixed model for longitudinal proportional data (Qiu et al., 2008). This approach can be used in the joint modeling for the longitudinal data. Specifically, we assume the following generalized linear mixed-effect model (GLMM) for the longitudinal proportional measurement $\tilde{y}_{ij}$:

$$\eta_{ij} = g(\mu_{ij}) = \dot{\boldsymbol{x}}_{ij}'\boldsymbol{\theta} + \alpha_i, \tag{5.3}$$

where α_i is a random effect with $\alpha_1, \ldots, \alpha_n \overset{\text{i.i.d.}}{\sim} \varphi(\alpha|0, \sigma_\alpha^2)$, $\boldsymbol{\theta}$ is a column vector of fixed effects, μ_{ij} is the mean of $\tilde{y}_{ij}$, and g is a link function. Given the random effect α_i, the longitudinal proportional measurement $\tilde{y}_{ij}|\alpha_i$ follows a simplex distribution with the density function

$$f(y|\mu_{ij}, \sigma^2) = a(y; \sigma^2) \exp\left[-\frac{d(y; \mu_{ij})}{2\sigma^2}\right], \ y \in (0, 1), \tag{5.4}$$

where

$$d(y; \mu_{ij}) = \frac{(y - \mu_{ij})^2}{y(1 - y)\mu_{ij}^2(1 - \mu_{ij})^2}, \ 0 < \mu_{ij} < 1,$$
$$a(y; \sigma^2) = [2\pi\sigma^2(y(1 - y))^3]^{-1/2}, \ \sigma^2 > 0.$$

The unit deviance function $d(y; \mu_{ij})$ is a nonlinear function measuring the discrepancy between the observed y and the expected μ_{ij} and the normalizing factor $a(y; \sigma^2)$ depends on the dispersion parameter σ^2 only. When the deviance d takes the squared Euclidean distance $(y - \mu_{ij})^2$, the density function implies the normal distribution. When the dispersion parameter σ^2 is small, the simplex density is similar to the normal distribution with the same mean and variance, due to the small-dispersion asymptotics (Song, 2007); when the dispersion parameter is large, the simplex density provides a more flexible distribution accommodating various features of data. For the link function in (5.3), we choose the logit link $g(\mu_{ij}) = \log \frac{\mu_{ij}}{1-\mu_{ij}}$. This simplex distribution model for $\tilde{y}_{ij}$ allows a directly modeling effects of $\dot{\boldsymbol{x}}_{ij}$ on the mean of $\tilde{y}_{ij}$. The effect of $\dot{\boldsymbol{x}}_{ij}$ on the mean, measured by $\boldsymbol{\theta}$, can be easily interpreted similarly as the log odds ratio in the logistic regression.

For survival data with a cure fraction, we still consider the PHC with a random effect similar to (5.2). Given the random effect α_i, this model specifies a conditional survival function as

$$S(t|\boldsymbol{x}_i, \alpha_i) = \exp[-F^H(t) e^{\boldsymbol{x}_i'\boldsymbol{\beta} + \nu\alpha_i}], \tag{5.5}$$

where ν is the coefficient of the random effect α_i (similarly, the intercept term in (2.18) is absorbed into $\boldsymbol{\beta}$ in this expression).

Model (5.3) and (5.5) together define a joint model for the longitudinal proportional data and survival data with a cure fraction. It is easy to see that similar to the joint model in the last section, this joint model also connects the models for longitudinal data and survival data via shared random effects, but in a slightly different way. The random effect α_i in the joint model reflects the unobserved heterogeneity in the mean of the longitudinal data and the hazard of survival time for different subjects, and ν characterizes the correlation between the longitudinal proportional measurements and survival times, which can be seen from the joint density function of T_i^* and $\tilde{Y}_{ij}$

$$f(t, y) = f^H(t)[2\pi\sigma^2(y(1-y))^3]^{-1/2} e^{\boldsymbol{x}_i'\boldsymbol{\beta}}$$
$$\times \int_{-\infty}^{+\infty} e^{\nu\alpha - F^H(t) e^{\dot{\boldsymbol{x}}_i'\boldsymbol{\beta} + \nu\alpha}} \exp\left[- \frac{\left(y - \frac{e^{\dot{\boldsymbol{x}}_{ij}'\boldsymbol{\theta}+\alpha}}{1+e^{\dot{\boldsymbol{x}}_{ij}'\boldsymbol{\theta}+\alpha}}\right)^2}{2\sigma^2 y(1-y) \frac{e^{2(\dot{\boldsymbol{x}}_{ij}'\boldsymbol{\theta}+\alpha)}}{(1+e^{\dot{\boldsymbol{x}}_{ij}'\boldsymbol{\theta}+\alpha})^4}} \right] \varphi(\alpha) d\alpha.$$

When $\nu = 0$, the survival times and longitudinal measurements will be independent conditional on the observed covariates because $f(t, y) = f(t) \int_{-\infty}^{+\infty} f(y|\alpha)\varphi(\alpha)d\alpha = f(t)f(y)$.

To estimate the parameters in the model, denoted as $\Theta = (\boldsymbol{\theta}, \nu, \boldsymbol{\beta}, f^H(t), \sigma^2, \sigma_\alpha^2)'$, consider the marginal log-likelihood of the proposed joint model based on the observed data:

$$l(\Theta) = \log \prod_{i=1}^{n} \int \left[\prod_{j=1}^{n_i} f(\tilde{y}_{ij}|\mu_{ij}, \sigma^2) \right] \times [f^H(t_i) e^{\boldsymbol{x}_i'\boldsymbol{\beta}_i + \nu\alpha_i}]^{\delta_i} e^{-F^H(t_i)e^{\boldsymbol{x}_i'\boldsymbol{\beta}_i + \nu\alpha_i}} \varphi(\alpha_i|0, \sigma_\alpha^2) d\alpha_i. \quad (5.6)$$

Since the marginal log-likelihood (5.6) involves an integration that does not have a closed-form, it is difficult to maximize it directly. A Laplace approximation to the marginal likelihood function can be used to obtain the estimates of the unknown parameters (Ripatti and Palmgren, 2000; Song et al., 2016a). The first-order and second-order Laplace approximation to the log-likelihood (5.6) are, respectively,

$$\tilde{l}(\Theta) = -\frac{\sum_{i=1}^n n_i}{2} \log \sigma^2 - \frac{n}{2} \log \sigma_\alpha^2 + \sum_{i=1}^n \lambda_c(\hat{\alpha}_i),$$

$$\tilde{\tilde{l}}(\Theta) = -\frac{\sum_{i=1}^n n_i}{2} \log \sigma^2 - \frac{n}{2} \log \sigma_\alpha^2 + \sum_{i=1}^n \lambda_c(\hat{\alpha}_i) - \frac{1}{2} \sum_{i=1}^n \log |\lambda_c^{(2)}(\hat{\alpha}_i)|,$$

where

$$\lambda_c(\alpha_i) = -\frac{1}{2\sigma^2} \sum_{j=1}^{n_i} d(\tilde{y}_{ij}; \mu_{ij}) + \delta_i(\log f^H(t_i) + \boldsymbol{x}_i'\boldsymbol{\beta} + \nu\alpha_i) - F^H(t_i)e^{\boldsymbol{\beta}'\boldsymbol{x}_i + \nu\alpha_i} - \frac{\alpha_i^2}{2\sigma_\alpha^2},$$

$$\lambda_c^{(2)}(\alpha_i) = -\frac{1}{2\sigma^2} \sum_{j=1}^{n_i} \frac{\partial^2 d(\tilde{y}_{ij}; \mu_{ij})}{\partial {\alpha_i}^2} - F^H(t_i)e^{\boldsymbol{\beta}'\boldsymbol{x}_i + \nu\alpha_i}\nu^2 - \frac{1}{\sigma_\alpha^2},$$

and $\hat{\alpha}_i = \text{argmax}_{\alpha_i} \lambda_c(\alpha)$. Noted that $\lambda_c(\alpha_i)$ can be viewed as a penalized joint log-likelihood for subject i with $-\frac{\alpha_i^2}{2\sigma_\alpha^2}$ as the penalty term if σ_α^2 is known and α_i is considered as a fixed effect, we can replace the two middle terms in $\lambda_c(\alpha_i)$, which correspond to the log-likelihood function for the survival times, by the corresponding partial likelihood and obtain the following first-order and the second-order penalized joint cure partial log-likelihoods:

$$\tilde{l}^p(\Theta^*) = -\frac{\sum_{i=1}^n n_i}{2} \log \sigma^2 - \frac{n}{2} \log \sigma_\alpha^2 + \sum_{i=1}^n \tilde{\lambda}_c(\hat{\alpha}_i),$$

$$\tilde{\tilde{l}}^p(\Theta^*) = -\frac{\sum_{i=1}^n n_i}{2} \log \sigma^2 - \frac{n}{2} \log \sigma_\alpha^2 + \sum_{i=1}^n \tilde{\lambda}_c(\hat{\alpha}_i) - \frac{1}{2} \sum_{i=1}^n \log |\tilde{\lambda}_c^{(2)}(\hat{\alpha}_i)|,$$

where $\Theta^* = (\boldsymbol{\theta}, \nu, \boldsymbol{\beta}, \sigma^2, \sigma_\alpha^2)$,

$$
\begin{aligned}
\tilde{\lambda}_c(\alpha_i) &= -\frac{1}{2\sigma^2}\sum_{j=1}^{n_i} d(\tilde{y}_{ij}; \mu_{ij}) \\
&\quad + \delta_i \left[\boldsymbol{\beta}'\boldsymbol{x}_i + \nu\alpha_i - \log \sum_{k \in R(t_i)} e^{\boldsymbol{\beta}'\boldsymbol{x}_k + \nu\alpha_k}\right] - \frac{\alpha_i^2}{2\sigma_\alpha^2}, \\
\tilde{\lambda}_c^{(2)}(\alpha_i) &= -\frac{1}{2\sigma^2}\sum_{j=1}^{n_i} \frac{\partial^2 d(\tilde{y}_{ij}; \mu_{ij})}{\partial {\alpha_i}^2} \\
&\quad - \delta_i \frac{e^{\boldsymbol{\beta}'\boldsymbol{x}_i + \nu\alpha_i}\nu^2}{\sum_{k \in R(t_i)} e^{\boldsymbol{\beta}'\boldsymbol{x}_k + \nu\alpha_k}} \left(1 - \frac{e^{\boldsymbol{\beta}'\boldsymbol{x}_i + \nu\alpha_i}}{\sum_{k \in R(t_i)} e^{\boldsymbol{\beta}'\boldsymbol{x}_k + \nu\alpha_k}}\right) - \frac{1}{\sigma_\alpha^2},
\end{aligned}
$$

$R(t)$ is the set of subjects who are at risk at time t and $\hat{\alpha}_i = \text{argmax}_{\alpha_i} \tilde{\lambda}_c(\alpha)$. To estimate Θ^*, we first fix $\sigma^2, \sigma_\alpha^2, \nu$ at some initial values. Since omitting the complicated term $\log|\lambda_c^{(2)}(\hat{\alpha}_i)|$ would have a negligible effect on the parameter estimation but could make the computation fast (Ripatti and Palmgren, 2000; Ye et al., 2008), we update $\boldsymbol{\theta}, \boldsymbol{\beta}$ by maximizing $\tilde{l}^p(\Theta^*)$. With updated estimates of $\boldsymbol{\theta}$ and $\boldsymbol{\beta}$, we maximize the second-order $\tilde{\tilde{l}}^p(\Theta^*)$ with respect to σ^2, σ_α^2 and ν. The maximization can be carried out with the Newton-Raphson method.

To estimate baseline $f^H(t)$, we maximize the marginal likelihood $\tilde{l}(\Theta)$ at $(\hat{\boldsymbol{\theta}}, \hat{\boldsymbol{\beta}}, \hat{\sigma}^2, \hat{\sigma}_\alpha^2, \hat{\nu}, \hat{\alpha}_i)$. This is equivalent to maximizing

$$
\sum_{i=1}^{n}[\delta_i(\log f^H(t_i) + \hat{\boldsymbol{\beta}}'\boldsymbol{x}_i + \hat{\nu}\hat{\alpha}_i) - F^H(t_i)e^{\hat{\boldsymbol{\beta}}'\boldsymbol{x}_i + \hat{\nu}\hat{\alpha}_i}] \tag{5.7}
$$

with respect to $f^H(t)$. It is easy to see that this is the log-likelihood of the PHC model. Therefore, the estimation can be carried out by assuming that $F^H(t)$ is nonparametric and using the semiparametric method of Tsodikov et al. (2003) and Song et al. (2012) through EM algorithm.

The variances of these parameter estimates can be approximated by inverting the information matrices of $\tilde{l}^p$ for parameters $(\boldsymbol{\theta}, \boldsymbol{\beta})$ and of $\tilde{\tilde{l}}^p$ for parameters $(\sigma^2, \sigma_\alpha^2, \nu)$, and of (5.7) for $F^H(t)$. The details of these matrices can be found in Song et al. (2016a).

5.5 Joint Modeling by Including Longitudinal Effects in Cure Model

Another approach to jointly model longitudinal and survival data is to directly incorporate the effects of longitudinal data into the cure model, often by viewing the longitudinal measurement as a time-dependent covariate in the latency part of the cure model (Law et al., 2002; Yu et al., 2004b, 2008). Consider longitudinal PSA data and survival data with a cure fraction from prostate cancer patients as an example. The longitudinal data are modeled by nonlinear random effects exponential decay and exponential growth model $\tilde{y}_{ij} = g(\tilde{t}_{ij}) + e_{ij}$, where

$$g(t|\boldsymbol{\alpha}_i) = \exp(\alpha_{i1} - e^{\alpha_{i2}}t) + \exp(\alpha_{i3} + e^{\alpha_{i4}}t),$$

$\boldsymbol{\alpha}_i' = (\alpha_{i1}, \alpha_{i2}, \alpha_{i3}, \alpha_{i4})$ are random effects, and e_{ij} is the error term following $N(0, \sigma_e^2)$ (a t distribution with degree of freedom 2η, mean 0 and scale σ_e similar to the one discussed in Section 5.3 may be considered to allow a larger variation in error). The random effects $\boldsymbol{\alpha}_i$ follows a normal distribution:

$$\begin{aligned}
\boldsymbol{\alpha}_i &\sim N(\boldsymbol{\theta}_1'\dot{\boldsymbol{X}}_i^{(1)}, \boldsymbol{\Sigma}_1) && \text{if } y_i = 1,\\
\boldsymbol{\alpha}_{i(-4)} &\sim N(\boldsymbol{\theta}_2'\dot{\boldsymbol{X}}_i^{(2)}, \boldsymbol{\Sigma}_2) && \text{if } y_i = 0,\\
\alpha_{i4} &\sim N(-6, \sigma_{44}) && \text{if } y_i = 0,
\end{aligned}$$

where $\dot{\boldsymbol{X}}_i^{(1)} = I_4 \otimes \dot{\boldsymbol{x}}_i$, $\dot{\boldsymbol{X}}_i^{(2)} = I_3 \otimes \dot{\boldsymbol{x}}_i$ and $\otimes$ is the Kronecker product, which basically allows the longitudinal PSA values to behavior differently between cured and uncured subjects.

For the survival data, a PH mixture cure model (2.2) and (2.5) with time-dependent longitudinal effects is considered. That is, given the random effects $\boldsymbol{\alpha}_i$,

$$h_u(t) = h_{u0}(t) \exp\left[\boldsymbol{\beta}'\boldsymbol{x}_i + \beta^{(1)} \log(g(t|\boldsymbol{\alpha}_i) + 1) + \beta^{(2)}|g^{(1)}(t|\boldsymbol{\alpha}_i)|\right],$$

where $g^{(1)}(t|\boldsymbol{\alpha}_i) = \partial g(t|\boldsymbol{\alpha}_i)/\partial t$.

Given observed longitudinal and survival data, the observed likelihood function for the unknown parameters $\Theta = (\boldsymbol{\theta}_1, \boldsymbol{\theta}_2, \boldsymbol{\Sigma}_1, \boldsymbol{\Sigma}_2, \sigma_{44}, \boldsymbol{\beta}, \beta^{(1)}, \beta^{(2)}, h_{u0}(t), \sigma_e, \boldsymbol{\gamma})'$ is

$$\begin{aligned}
\prod_{i=1}^{n} \Bigg\{ \pi(\boldsymbol{z}_i) \int f_u(t_i|\boldsymbol{x}_i, \boldsymbol{\alpha}_i)\phi\left[(\tilde{\boldsymbol{y}}_i - g(\tilde{\boldsymbol{t}}_i|\boldsymbol{\alpha}_i))\sigma_e^{-1}\right] \\
\times \phi\left[(\boldsymbol{\alpha}_i - \boldsymbol{\theta}_1'\dot{\boldsymbol{X}}_i^{(1)})\boldsymbol{\Sigma}_1^{-1/2}\right] d\boldsymbol{\alpha}_i \Bigg\}^{\delta_i} \\
\times \Bigg\{ \pi(\boldsymbol{z}_i) \int S_u(t_i|\boldsymbol{x}_i, \boldsymbol{\alpha}_i)\phi\left[(\tilde{\boldsymbol{y}}_i - g(\tilde{\boldsymbol{t}}_i|\boldsymbol{\alpha}_i))\sigma_e^{-1}\right] \phi\left[(\boldsymbol{\alpha}_i - \boldsymbol{\theta}_1'\dot{\boldsymbol{X}}_i^{(1)})\boldsymbol{\Sigma}_1^{-1/2}\right] d\boldsymbol{\alpha}_i \\
+ [1 - \pi(\boldsymbol{z}_i)] \int \phi\left[(\tilde{\boldsymbol{y}}_i - g(\tilde{\boldsymbol{t}}_i|\boldsymbol{\alpha}_i))\sigma_e^{-1}\right] \phi\left[(\boldsymbol{\alpha}_{i(-4)} - \boldsymbol{\theta}_2'\dot{\boldsymbol{X}}_i^{(2)})\boldsymbol{\Sigma}_2^{-1/2}\right] \\
\times \phi((\alpha_{i4} + 6)/\sigma_{44}) d\boldsymbol{\alpha}_i \Bigg\}^{1-\delta_i}.
\end{aligned}$$

Directly maximizing this observed likelihood function can be challenging, and the EM algorithm is preferred to estimate the parameters in the model. Given the values of cure status y_i's and the random effects $\boldsymbol{\alpha}_i$'s, the complete likelihood function for Θ is $L(\Theta) = \prod_{i=1}^n L_i(\Theta)$, where

$$\begin{aligned} L_i(\Theta) = \Bigg\{ & \pi(\boldsymbol{z}_i) f_u(t_i|\boldsymbol{x}_i, \boldsymbol{\alpha}_i) \phi\left[(\tilde{\boldsymbol{y}}_i - g(\tilde{\boldsymbol{t}}_i|\boldsymbol{\alpha}_i))\sigma_e^{-1}\right] \\ & \qquad \times \phi\left[(\boldsymbol{\alpha}_i - \boldsymbol{\theta}_1' \dot{\boldsymbol{X}}_i^{(1)})\boldsymbol{\Sigma}_1^{-1/2}\right] \Bigg\}^{y_i\delta_i} \\ & \times \Bigg\{ \pi(\boldsymbol{z}_i) S_u(t_i|\boldsymbol{x}_i, \boldsymbol{\alpha}_i) \phi\left[(\tilde{\boldsymbol{y}}_i - g(\tilde{\boldsymbol{t}}_i|\boldsymbol{\alpha}_i))\sigma_e^{-1}\right] \\ & \qquad \times \phi\left[(\boldsymbol{\alpha}_i - \boldsymbol{\theta}_1' \dot{\boldsymbol{X}}_i^{(1)})\boldsymbol{\Sigma}_1^{-1/2}\right] \Bigg\}^{y_i(1-\delta_i)} \\ & \times \Bigg\{ [1 - \pi(\boldsymbol{z}_i)] \phi\left[(\tilde{\boldsymbol{y}}_i - g(\tilde{\boldsymbol{t}}_i|\boldsymbol{\alpha}_i))\sigma_e^{-1}\right] \phi\left[(\boldsymbol{\alpha}_{i(-4)} - \boldsymbol{\theta}_2' \dot{\boldsymbol{X}}_i^{(2)})\boldsymbol{\Sigma}_2^{-1/2}\right] \\ & \qquad \times \phi((\alpha_{i4} + 6)/\sigma_{44}) \Bigg\}^{(1-y_i)(1-\delta_i)}. \end{aligned}$$

The E-step in the mth step calculates $E[\log L_i(\Theta|\Theta^{(m)})]$ concerning y_i and $\boldsymbol{\alpha}_i$. For uncensored subjects, $y_i \equiv 1$ and the posterior density function of $\boldsymbol{\alpha}_i$ is

$$p(\boldsymbol{\alpha}_i|\Theta^{(m)}) = \frac{f_u^{(m)} \phi_{\tilde{\boldsymbol{y}}}^{(m)} \phi_{\boldsymbol{\alpha}1}^{(m)}}{\int f_u^{(m)} \phi_{\tilde{\boldsymbol{y}}}^{(m)} \phi_{\boldsymbol{\alpha}1}^{(m)} d\boldsymbol{\alpha}_i},$$

where

$$\begin{aligned} f_u^{(m)} &= f_u(t_i|\boldsymbol{x}_i, \boldsymbol{\alpha}_i)|_{\boldsymbol{\beta}=\boldsymbol{\beta}^{(m)}, \beta^{(1)(m)}, \beta^{(2)(m)}, h_{u0}(t)=h_{u0}(t)^{(m)}}, \\ \phi_{\tilde{\boldsymbol{y}}}^{(m)} &= \phi\left[(\tilde{\boldsymbol{y}}_i - g(\tilde{\boldsymbol{t}}_i|\boldsymbol{\alpha}_i))\sigma_e^{-1}\right]\Big|_{\sigma_e=\sigma_e^{(m)}}, \\ \phi_{\boldsymbol{\alpha}1}^{(m)} &= \phi\left[(\boldsymbol{\alpha}_i - \boldsymbol{\theta}_1' \dot{\boldsymbol{X}}_i^{(1)})\boldsymbol{\Sigma}_1^{-1/2}\right]\Big|_{\boldsymbol{\theta}_1=\boldsymbol{\theta}_1^{(m)}, \boldsymbol{\Sigma}_1=\boldsymbol{\Sigma}_1^{(m)}}. \end{aligned}$$

Thus $E[\log L_i(\Theta|\Theta^{(m)})] = \int L_i(\Theta|\Theta^{(m)}) p(\boldsymbol{\alpha}_i|\Theta^{(m)}) d\boldsymbol{\alpha}_i$.

For censored subjects,

$$\begin{aligned} E[\log L_i(\Theta|\Theta^{(m)})] = & \int L_i(\Theta|\Theta^{(m)}) p(\boldsymbol{\alpha}_i|\Theta^{(m)}, y_i = 1) p(y_i = 1|\Theta^{(m)}) d\boldsymbol{\alpha}_i \\ & + \int L_i(\Theta|\Theta^{(m)}) p(\boldsymbol{\alpha}_i|\Theta^{(m)}, y_i = 0) p(y_i = 0|\Theta^{(m)}) d\boldsymbol{\alpha}_i, \end{aligned}$$

where

$$
\begin{aligned}
p(\boldsymbol{\alpha}_i|\Theta^{(m)}, y_i = 1) =& \frac{S_u^{(m)}\phi_{\tilde{\boldsymbol{y}}}^{(m)}\phi_{\boldsymbol{\alpha}1}^{(m)}}{\int S_u^{(m)}\phi_{\tilde{\boldsymbol{y}}}^{(m)}\phi_{\boldsymbol{\alpha}1}^{(m)}d\boldsymbol{\alpha}_i},\\
p(\boldsymbol{\alpha}_i|\Theta^{(m)}, y_i = 0) =& \frac{\phi_{\tilde{\boldsymbol{y}}}^{(m)}\phi_{\boldsymbol{\alpha}2}^{(m)}}{\int \phi_{\tilde{\boldsymbol{y}}}^{(m)}\phi_{\boldsymbol{\alpha}2}^{(m)}d\boldsymbol{\alpha}_i},\\
p(y_i = 1|\Theta^{(m)}) =& \frac{\int \pi^{(m)} S_u^{(m)}\phi_{\tilde{\boldsymbol{y}}}^{(m)}\phi_{\boldsymbol{\alpha}1}^{(m)}d\boldsymbol{\alpha}_i}{\int \pi^{(m)} S_u^{(m)}\phi_{\tilde{\boldsymbol{y}}}^{(m)}\phi_{\boldsymbol{\alpha}1}^{(m)}d\boldsymbol{\alpha}_i + \int [1-\pi^{(m)}] S_u^{(m)}\phi_{\tilde{\boldsymbol{y}}}^{(m)}\phi_{\boldsymbol{\alpha}2}^{(m)}d\boldsymbol{\alpha}_i},\\
p(y_i = 0|\Theta^{(m)}) =& 1 - p(y_i = 1|\Theta^{(m)}),\\
\pi^{(m)} =& \pi(\boldsymbol{z}_i)|_{\boldsymbol{\gamma}=\boldsymbol{\gamma}^{(m)}},\\
S_u^{(m)} =& S_u(t_i|\boldsymbol{x}_i, \boldsymbol{\alpha}_i)|_{\boldsymbol{\beta}=\boldsymbol{\beta}^{(m)}, \boldsymbol{\beta}^{(1)(m)}, \boldsymbol{\beta}^{(2)(m)}, h_{u0}(t)=h_{u0}(t)^{(m)}},\\
\phi_{\boldsymbol{\alpha}2}^{(m)} =& \phi\left[(\boldsymbol{\alpha}_{i(-4)} - \boldsymbol{\theta}_2'\dot{\boldsymbol{X}}_i^{(2)})\boldsymbol{\Sigma}_2^{-1/2}\right]\\
& \times \phi((\alpha_{i4} + 6)/\sigma_{44})\Big|_{\boldsymbol{\theta}_2=\boldsymbol{\theta}_2^{(m)}, \boldsymbol{\Sigma}_2=\boldsymbol{\Sigma}_2^{(m)}, \sigma_{44}=\sigma_{44}^{(m)}}.
\end{aligned}
$$

The M-step in the mth iteration maximizes $\sum_{i=1}^{n} E[\log L_i(\Theta|\Theta^{(m)})]$ with respect to Θ via the Newton-Raphson method. When update $h_{u0}(t)$, a non-parametric estimate by assuming a discrete baseline distribution at the observed uncensored times can be obtained.

The standard errors of the estimates can be obtained using the method Louis (1982). The details can be found in Law et al. (2002) and Yu et al. (2004b).

In addition to the maximum likelihood estimation method, the Bayesian method based on Markov chain Monte Carlo (MCMC) is also employed to estimate the parameters in joint models (Brown and Ibrahim, 2003; Chen et al., 2004; Yu et al., 2008). However, due to the complexity of the joint models, MCMC usually takes a long time to converge than the likelihood methods (Yu et al., 2008).

5.6 Applications

We consider an application of some joint models discussed in previous sections to the data described in Section 5.2. A preliminary examination of QoL data revealed that patterns of change in the QoL scores are different in different periods and different treatment groups (Figure 5.3). The nature of the QoL data leads us to consider the joint model in Section 5.4 with the following piecewise polynomial linear predictors in the longitudinal part of the joint

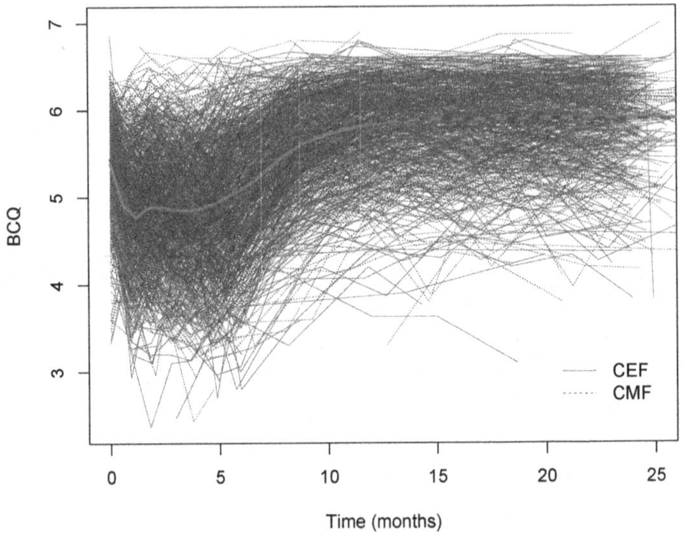

FIGURE 5.3
Trajectories of QoL BCQ scores for patients in CEF (red solid thin lines) and CMF (blue dashed thin lines) groups and the fitted lowess curves (thick lines).

model:

$$\begin{aligned}\eta_{ij} = \dot{\boldsymbol{x}}_{ij}'\boldsymbol{\theta} + \alpha_i = [\theta_0 + \theta_1 x_i + \theta_2 \tilde{t}_{ij} + \theta_3 x_i \tilde{t}_{ij} + \theta_4 \tilde{t}_{ij}^2 + \theta_5 x_i \tilde{t}_{ij}^2] I_{\tilde{t}_{ij} \in [0,2)} \\ + [\theta_6 + \theta_7 x_i + \theta_8 \tilde{t}_{ij} + \theta_9 x_i \tilde{t}_{ij} + \theta_{10} \tilde{t}_{ij}^2 + \theta_{11} x_i \tilde{t}_{ij}^2] I_{\tilde{t}_{ij} \in [2,9)} \\ + [\theta_{12} + \theta_{13} x_i + \theta_{14} \tilde{t}_{ij} + \theta_{15} x_i \tilde{t}_{ij}] I_{\tilde{t}_{ij} \in [9,\infty)} + \alpha_i,\end{aligned}$$

where x_i is the binary treatment indicator (1 for CEF and 0 for CMF) and $I_{t \in A}$ is an indicator function with value 1 if t is in A and 0 otherwise. The survival part of the joint model includes x_i as the only covariate in the cure model.

Table 5.1 summarizes the estimates of the parameters and their standard errors in the joint model. First of all, the significance of the difference of $\hat{\nu}$ from 0 indicates a strong dependence between the longitudinal QoL and RFS in the data. The hazard of the RFS times is significantly lower for patients randomized to CEF than those to CMF (p-value 0.017). The marginal cure rate is 52% for the CEF group and 42% for the CMF group, and the difference is statistically significant. For QoL, the two treatment groups do not have a statistically significant difference at any given time in the treatment. However, the two treatment groups do have significantly different QoL change rates in the early period of treatment. For example, the QoL of patients

TABLE 5.1
Estimates (Est) and their standard errors (SE) from the joint model for the data from MA.5 trial (the estimates with statistical significance are in bold).

Random effects in joint model						
Effect	Est	SE				
σ_α^2	**0.178**	0.010				
ν	**0.344**	0.143				
Fixed effects in cure model part						
Effect	Est	SE				
Intercept	-0.146	0.057				
CEF	**-0.268**	0.112				
Fixed effects in longitudinal model part						
	Time interval (months)					
	$[0, 2)$		$[2, 9)$		$[9, \infty)$	
Effect	Est	SE	Est	SE	Est	SE
Intercept	1.052	0.032	0.743	0.079	1.436	0.040
CEF	0.035	0.045	-0.015	0.112	0.011	0.057
Time	**-0.217**	0.062	-0.031	0.032	**0.007**	0.002
Time^2	0.039	0.033	**0.010**	0.003	-	-
CEF × Time	**-0.435**	0.090	-0.011	0.045	0.001	0.003
CEF × Time^2	**0.190**	0.045	**0.002**	< 0.001	-	-

deteriorates faster in the CEF than in CMF in the first two months and slightly recovers faster between two and nine months. The fitted trajectory curves and their confidence bands of the longitudinal QoL for CEF and CMF are given in Figure 5.4. Both curves show a similar trend. The mean BCQ score in the CMF group decreases to a nadir after randomization and then increases steadily over the next 7 months. In contrast, the mean BCQ score in the CEF group decreases more quickly to a nadir and gradually increases in the remaining months of chemotherapy treatment. After 6-month of the chemotherapy treatments, the scores of both arms tend to be stable. This implies that patients treated by CEF had worse QoL than those treated by CMF at the very beginning but gradually recovered to a slightly better level than those treated by CMF.

5.7 Summary

Joint models are useful tools to analyze longitudinal and survival data efficiently. There are extensive studies on joint models for longitudinal and survival data without a cure fraction. However, when there is a cure fraction in

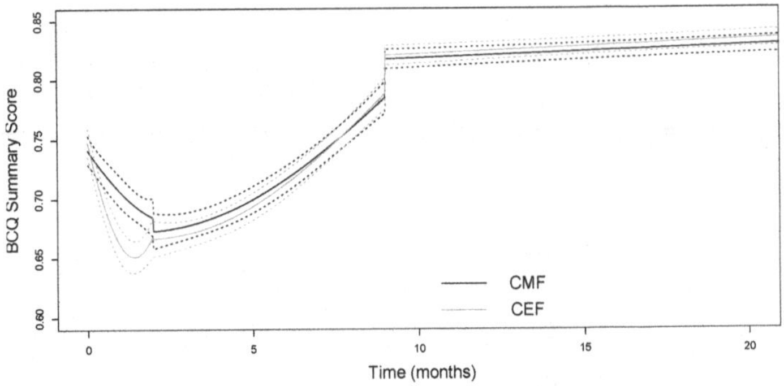

FIGURE 5.4
Estimated η as functions of time for the two treatment groups and their confidence bands in the longitudinal part of the joint model.

the data, there are only a handful models that can take the cured fraction into account. This chapter first introduced clinical trials for breast cancer and prostate cancer where both longitudinal data and survival data with a cure fraction are observed from each patient. Then two classes of the joint models were discussed in detail. One is the class of joint models where the longitudinal submodel and the survival submodel are connected by shared random effects. The other is the class of joint models where the longitudinal submodel enters the survival submodel as a time-dependent variable. The longitudinal outcomes can be continuous data with or without a boundary.

The computation methods for joint models tend to be complicated and time consuming due to complexity of the joint models. This chapter focused on the likelihood estimation methods based on the EM algorithm and approximations only. Bayesian methods are also employed in joint models in the literature. They are conceptually easier to develop but time-consuming to complete because of the numerical MCMC used in the methods, while the likelihood methods tend to be difficult to develop but usually require less time to complete.

6

Testing the Existence of Cured Subjects and Sufficient Follow-up

6.1 Introduction

As indicated in previous chapters, cure models are useful for survival data from a population where a subset of subjects are immune to the event of interest and can be considered as cured. However, in the presence of censored observations, the cured subjects usually are not explicitly identified. If τ, the upper bound of the uncured survival time as defined in Section 2.2, is finite, subjects with survival times greater than τ are considered cured. Otherwise, cured subjects are usually inferred from long-term censored times, but not directly observable. Uncensored observations can only be from uncured subjects while censored observations may be from either cured or uncured patients. Therefore, it is not obvious to tell whether cured subjects exist or not from data directly. Even when there is a substantial fraction of cured subjects in data, as demonstrated in Peng and Taylor (2014), a cure model can still overestimate the cure probability if the follow-up in the study is not long enough to cover the domain of the distribution of the failure time of an uncured subject (i.e., the follow-up duration is less than τ). Thus, it is important to have a priori judgement on the existence of cured subjects and sufficient follow-up before applying a cure model in an analysis. Such a priori judgement may be from experts in the subject area, clinical experience with the disease, biological evidence, or the study design. If the judgement cannot be obtained, statistical methods may be considered to help an investigator to decide whether the conditions for using cure models are met or not, and this will be the focus of this chapter. We will discuss some statistical methods for testing the existence of cured subjects in Section 6.2. Section 6.3 will provide some methods to address the sufficient follow-up condition.

6.2 Tests for Existence of Cured Subjects

We consider tests for testing the existence of cured subjects in a study when sufficient follow-up is available in this section. There are two approaches to define cured subjects, depending on the type of a study. In the first approach, a subject is deemed as cured if the event of interest, such as relapse due to cancer, will not happen with a long follow-up. This approach is often used in clinical trial data analyses. The other approach is to define a subject as cured if the subject has similar survival experience as the general disease-free population. This approach is often used in population-based studies because the event of interest is often death in these studies and death always happens whether or not a subject is cured or not. In this case, cured subjects are those with death rate at the same level of the general disease-free population. In this section, we will focus on the first approach only. Readers interested in the second approach can find details in Chapter 8.

6.2.1 Without Covariates

We first consider statistical tests for the existence of cured subjects based on data. If we consider the mixture cure model (2.1) for survival data, testing the existence of cured subjects is equivalent to testing hypotheses

$$H_0\colon \pi = 1 \text{ vs } H_1\colon \pi < 1. \tag{6.1}$$

If a test produces a small p-value, say less than 0.05, it implies that the data show significant evidence of existence of cured subjects. Otherwise, the data do not provide strong evidence for the existence of cured subjects.

Knowing that the parameter space for π is $(0, 1]$ and H_0 is at the boundary of the parameter space of π, this hypothesis testing problem is a so-called non-standard problem (Self and Liang, 1987; Everitt, 1988) as the standard statistical tests and their asymptotic null distribution (the distribution of the tests under H_0) are developed when H_0 is an interior point of the parameter space. Thus the asymptotic null distribution of the standard tests for testing (6.1) can be different from the usual distribution used under standard conditions.

6.2.1.1 Likelihood Ratio Test

Consider the LRT for (6.1). If the log likelihood for a mixture cure model $\ell(\boldsymbol{\theta})$ is given in (2.12), then the LRT for (6.1) is

$$d_n = -2[\ell(\hat{\boldsymbol{\theta}}_0) - \ell(\hat{\boldsymbol{\theta}}_1)]$$

where $\hat{\boldsymbol{\theta}}_1 = \arg\max_{\boldsymbol{\theta}} \ell(\boldsymbol{\theta})$ and $\hat{\boldsymbol{\theta}}_0 = \arg\max_{\boldsymbol{\theta}/\pi=1} \ell(\boldsymbol{\theta})$ ($\max_{\boldsymbol{\theta}/\pi=1}$ means maximization over $\boldsymbol{\theta}$ with π fixed at 1). Under the exponential and gamma mixture cure model without any covariates, it has been shown under mild conditions (Zhou and Maller, 1995; Maller and Zhou, 1995; Vu et al., 1998) that the asymptotic null distribution of the LRT statistic d_n for H_0 follows a 50-50 mixture of a chi-squared distribution and the probability mass at zero

$$P(d_n < t) \to \frac{1}{2} + \frac{1}{2}P(\chi_1^2 < t). \tag{6.2}$$

This result was further examined numerically under other distributions for the latency part (Peng et al., 2001), and it generally holds. However, the asymptotic null distribution of the LRT can deviate substantially from the suggested distribution under moderate sample sizes when the censoring rate is small or the hazard rate is large. That is, the percentiles of the observed null distribution of the LRT can be substantially smaller than the percentiles from the suggested distribution, which makes the test reject H_0 less often than anticipated. Consequently, caution is needed in this case to determine the presence of cured patients, and other computational intensive methods, such as the bootstrap method, may be considered to simulate the null distribution of the LRT.

Consider the leukemia data in Table 2.1. The existence of cured subjects in the data is supported by the plateau at the right tails of the Kaplan-Meier survival curves in Figure 2.4 and by clinical evidence for leukemia. If we are interested in statistical evidence to support the existence of cured subjects in the two treatment groups, we can consider the LRT test to generate the evidence. For the allogeneic group, it has been shown that the exponential distribution fits the data well (Maller and Zhou, 1995). Therefore, we conduct the test under the exponential distribution assumption for the latency part and obtain $\ell(\hat{\boldsymbol{\theta}}_0) = -90.35$ and $\ell(\hat{\boldsymbol{\theta}}_1) = -78.86$. It is easy to see that the p-value of the LRT under the distribution (6.2) is < 0.001. We have strong statistical evidence for the existence of cured subjects in this group.

For the autologous group, however, the exponential distribution does not fit the data well. As demonstrated in Section 2.6, the lognormal distribution for the latency part provides an acceptable fit to the data. We can proceed with the LRT for the existence of cured patients in the autologous group under the lognormal mixture model. The maximum log-likelihoods are $\ell(\hat{\boldsymbol{\theta}}_0) = -58.79$ and $\ell(\hat{\boldsymbol{\theta}}_1) = -73.88$. Thus $d_n = -2 \times (-73.88 + 58.79) = 30.18$, and the p-value from the distribution (6.2) is < 0.001. We reject H_0 and consider that there is strong evidence in the data for the presence of cured patents in the autologous group.

6.2.1.2 Score Test

The score test can also be considered as an alternative to the likelihoods ratio test for testing (6.1) (Zhao et al., 2009). Let $\boldsymbol{\theta}$ be partitioned into (π, $\boldsymbol{\theta}^{(2)}$), where $\boldsymbol{\theta}^{(2)}$ includes all parameters in $\boldsymbol{\theta}$ except π, and $\boldsymbol{U}(\boldsymbol{\theta})$ and $\boldsymbol{I}(\boldsymbol{\theta})$ be the first and the second derivatives of the log-likelihood function $\ell(\boldsymbol{\theta})$ and

$\boldsymbol{U}(\boldsymbol{\theta})' = (\boldsymbol{U}_1(\boldsymbol{\theta})', \boldsymbol{U}_2(\boldsymbol{\theta})')$ corresponding to the partition of $\boldsymbol{\theta}$. The score test for (6.1) can be written as follows:

$$s_n = (\mathbf{0}', \boldsymbol{U}_2(\hat{\boldsymbol{\theta}}_0)')\boldsymbol{I}^{-1}(\hat{\boldsymbol{\theta}}_0)\begin{pmatrix}\mathbf{0}\\ \boldsymbol{U}_2(\hat{\boldsymbol{\theta}}_0)\end{pmatrix}$$

where $\boldsymbol{U}_2(\hat{\boldsymbol{\theta}}_0) = \boldsymbol{U}_2(\boldsymbol{\theta})|_{\boldsymbol{\theta}=\hat{\boldsymbol{\theta}}_0}$ and $\boldsymbol{I}(\hat{\boldsymbol{\theta}}_0) = \boldsymbol{I}(\boldsymbol{\theta})|_{\boldsymbol{\theta}=\hat{\boldsymbol{\theta}}_0}$. Due to the asymptotic equivalence between the likelihood ratio test and the score test, it has been suggested that the score test for (6.1) also follows the 50-50 mixture of a chi-squared distribution and the probability mass at zero

$$P(s_n < t) \to \frac{1}{2} + \frac{1}{2}P(\chi_1^2 < t).$$

The performance of this test is similar to the likelihood ratio test.

This test can also be used for clustered survival data under the random-effects model discussed in Section 4.3.1. See details in Zhao et al. (2009).

6.2.2 With Covariates

When the cure rate is potentially dependent on a covariate $\boldsymbol{z}$, testing the existence of cure fraction becomes even more complicated and elusive (Hsu et al., 2016). If a cured fraction exists, it may exist for some values of $\boldsymbol{z}$. Thus the hypotheses becomes

$$H_0\text{: } \pi(\boldsymbol{z}) = 1 \text{ for all } \boldsymbol{z} \text{ vs } H_1\text{: } \pi(\boldsymbol{z}) < 1 \text{ for some } \boldsymbol{z}. \tag{6.3}$$

Consider the logistic model (2.2) in $\pi(\boldsymbol{z})$ and suppose that $\boldsymbol{\gamma}' = (\gamma_0, \boldsymbol{\gamma}^{*\prime})$ and $\boldsymbol{z}' = (1, \boldsymbol{z}^{*\prime})$ (we separate the intercept from other parameters in the logistic model, and $\boldsymbol{z}^*$ includes all covariates but 1). If we confines $\boldsymbol{\gamma}^*$ to a compact set, i.e., $\sup_{\boldsymbol{\gamma}^* \in \boldsymbol{\Gamma}^*} \|\boldsymbol{\gamma}^*\| \leq M$ for some $M < \infty$ ($\boldsymbol{\Gamma}^*$ is the parameter space for $\boldsymbol{\gamma}^*$), it is easy to see that H_0 above corresponds to $\gamma_0 = \infty$, or $\psi = 0$ if $\psi = \exp(-\gamma_0)$. Given $\pi(\boldsymbol{z}) = [1 + \psi \exp(-\boldsymbol{\gamma}^{*\prime}\boldsymbol{z}^*)]^{-1}$, it implies that $\boldsymbol{\gamma}^*$ is not identifiable under H_0.

Given $\boldsymbol{\gamma}^*$, a score test can be considered for H_0. Let $\boldsymbol{\lambda} = (\boldsymbol{\beta}', \boldsymbol{\alpha}')'$ and $\boldsymbol{\theta} = (\psi, \boldsymbol{\gamma}^{*\prime}, \boldsymbol{\lambda}')$, the test is given as follows

$$\hat{s}_n(\boldsymbol{\gamma}^*) = \frac{1}{n}\hat{u}_n(\boldsymbol{\gamma}^*)^2 \hat{\imath}(\boldsymbol{\gamma}^*) I(\hat{u}_n(\boldsymbol{\gamma}^*) \geq 0)$$

where

$$\hat{u}_n(\boldsymbol{\gamma}^*) = \left.\frac{\partial \ell(\boldsymbol{\theta})}{\partial \psi}\right|_{\psi=0, \boldsymbol{\lambda}=\hat{\boldsymbol{\lambda}}}$$

$$\hat{\imath}(\boldsymbol{\gamma}^*) = \left[-E\left\{\frac{\partial^2 \ell(\boldsymbol{\theta})}{\partial \psi^2}\right\} \right.$$
$$\left.\left. -E\left\{\frac{\partial^2 \ell(\boldsymbol{\theta})}{\partial \psi \partial \boldsymbol{\lambda}}\right\}' \left(-E\left\{\frac{\partial^2 \ell(\boldsymbol{\theta})}{\partial \boldsymbol{\lambda} \partial \boldsymbol{\lambda}'}\right\}\right)^{-1} E\left\{\frac{\partial^2 \ell(\boldsymbol{\theta})}{\partial \psi \partial \boldsymbol{\lambda}}\right\}\right]^{-1}\right|_{\psi=0, \boldsymbol{\lambda}=\hat{\boldsymbol{\lambda}}}$$

$\ell(\boldsymbol{\theta})$ is the observed log-likelihood function (2.12) for the mixture cure model, $\hat{\boldsymbol{\lambda}}$ is the estimate of $\boldsymbol{\lambda}$ under H_0. To remove the dependence of the test on γ^*, a supremum score test of the following can be used:

$$\mathcal{T}_n = \sup_{\gamma^* \in \boldsymbol{\Gamma}^*} \hat{s}_n(\gamma^*).$$

Similar to the likelihood ratio test (6.2), for each γ^*, $\hat{s}_n(\gamma^*)$ follows a 50-50 mixture of a chi-squared distribution and the probability mass at zero. Unfortunately, the asymptotic distribution of $\mathcal{T}_n$ is difficult to obtain and a resampling based method is required to approximate the null distribution of the test.

A numerical study (Hsu et al., 2016) shows that the supremum score test tends to be slightly conservative for light censoring in that it rejects the H_0 less often than anticipated, similar to the observation for the LRT in the last section. A heuristic explanation for this phenomenon is that when censoring is light, few subjects have censored failure times, leading to a smaller chance for the test to reject H_0. To the extreme, if there is no censoring, then cure is practically improbable, and the test is unlikely to commit a type I error.

6.3 Testing for Sufficient Follow-up

A sufficient follow-up in a study is important when considering a cure model for survival data from the study. It was briefly discussed in Section 3.3.1 and mentioned in other sections and chapters. However, there are very few studies on formal statistical tests for sufficient follow-up. This section will introduce the existing statistical methods to address sufficient follow-up for cure models.

Following the notations of (3.3.1), let $t_{(n)} = \max\{t_i\colon i = 1, \ldots, n\}$, $t^1_{(n)} = \max_{i:\delta_i=1}(t_i)$, $\tau_u = \sup\{t\colon S_u(t) > 0\}$ and $\tau_G = \sup\{t\colon G(t) > 0\}$, where $G(t)$ is the survival function of the censoring time distribution function. A study from which data were drawn has a sufficient follow-up if $\tau_u \leq \tau_G$. Testing a sufficient follow-up is equivalent to testing in the following hypotheses:

$$H_0\colon \tau_u \leq \tau_G \text{ vs } H_1\colon \tau_u > \tau_G \tag{6.4}$$

If H_0 is rejected, failures may occur after the maximum follow-up period and then it is not possible to determine which proportion of the late censored data has been generated by cured subjects. Thus, it is important to have sufficient follow-up to avoid overestimation of a cure rate.

The first approach to test the hypotheses is based on the number uncensored survival times in the interval $(2t^1_{(n)} - t_{(n)}, t^1_{(n)}]$, denoted as N_n, and the

p-value of the test is approximated by (Maller and Zhou, 1994)

$$\alpha_n = \left(1 - \frac{N_n}{n}\right)^n.$$

This test suggests that H_0 be rejected whenever $\alpha_n < 0.05$. However, a numerical study shows that this test is too conservative. A modified version of this test is (Maller and Zhou, 1996)

$$q_n = \frac{N_n}{n}.$$

Unfortunately, the null distribution of this test is not available. Simulation methods may be used to obtain the null distribution of q_n if parametrical assumptions are made for $S_u(t)$, which may limit the use of this test in general.

Klebanov and Yakovlev (2007) later argued that the above approach cannot be improved because it deals with observations close to the end of an observation period where the Kaplan-Meier survival estimator and related statistics are extremely unstable in the presence of censoring. They suggested to test whether there is sufficient follow-up to detect the presence of cured subject in data. That is, instead of testing general sufficient follow-up H_0 in (6.4) for any cure rate estimation, they suggested to test whether or not there is sufficient follow-up to detect H_0 in (6.1), which can also be written as H_0: $S(t) = S_u(t)$. Let $\tilde{\tau}$ be the length of follow-up. For any $t_0 < \tilde{\tau}$, under mild assumption on $S_u(t)$ such as non-decreasing hazard rate, a lower bound of π can be obtained from

$$\pi_n^* = \max\left\{1 - \frac{1 - \hat{S}^{KM}(\tilde{\tau})}{1 - \hat{S}^{KM}(t_0)^{\tilde{\tau}/t_0}}, 0\right\},$$

where $\hat{S}^{KM}(\cdot)$ is defined in Section 3.3.1. Then the hypothesis H_0 in (6.1) will be rejected if $\pi_n^* > 0$. The value of t_0 can be chosen initially between $(0, \tilde{\tau}/2)$ and then optimized by maximizing π_n^*. They suggest that $\tilde{\tau}$ is set to different values between 0 and $t_{(n)}$ to examine how π_n^* changes.

Even though this method does not test sufficient follow-up directly, it does have a monotonic behaviour: the longer the follow-up, the more likely it is sufficient for making inferences about existence of cured subjects. The method based on N_n above does not have this behaviour.

6.4 Summary

This chapter first introduced statistical tests for the existence of cured subjects in data. Cure models should only be considered for data with a fraction of cured subjects. Unfortunately, cured subjects are usually not self-identified as cured in many studies and they are usually inferred based on later censored times. Without subject knowledge, it is not easy to differentiate later censoring from uncured subjects and censoring from cured subjects. Without covariates, we introduced a likelihood ratio test and a score test for testing the existence of cured subjects and their asymptotic distributions under the null hypothesis. With covariate, a supremum score test can be employed to test the existence of cured subjects. Unfortunately, the null distribution of the supremum score test is not available and a resampling method has to be used to determine the significance of the test for a given data.

Sufficient follow-up is another important issue in cure models. Unlike some standard survival models, such as Cox's PH model, where the length of follow-up is usually not an issue and a shorter follow-up may only affect estimation of certain quantiles, insufficient follow-up can lead to biased estimates in cure models. We introduced some heuristic approaches to determine whether a given data set provides substantial evidence for sufficient follow-up. The sufficient follow-up is also required for the validity of the tail-restriction methods discussed in Section 3.2.1.1 to enhance the identifiability of the semiparametric estimation method for mixture cure models.

A related issue to the topics in this chapter is the identifiability of cure models. This is different from the above identifiability issue. The former is usually caused by the estimation method of a cure model, particularly for a semiparametric estimation method, while the latter is about the uniqueness of the parameters in the cure models, which is independent of censoring, follow-up and estimation methods. Compared to the standard survival models, cure models tend to be more complicated with more components and parameters. For a given cure model, one has to ensure that the parameters in the model can be uniquely determined or identified before they are estimated under the sufficient follow-up condition and confirmation of the existence of cured subjects. There are a few existing papers to address this issue, including Li et al. (2001) for mixture cure models, Peng and Zhang (2008b) for mixture cure models with frailty, and more recently Hanin and Huang (2014) for both mixture cure models and PHC models. They showed that cure models are generally identifiable if the latency distribution is a proper distribution, covariates are present in cure models and not shared in different components of cure models, and the design space of covariates are not degenerate. See these papers for the detailed conditions for cure model identifiability.

We only considered tests for existence of cured subjects in this chapter. There are other tests that extend the log-rank test to compare treatment effects among different treatments with the presence of cured subjects. Some early work can be found in Gray and Tsiatis (1989), Broët et al. (2001), Broët et al. (2003), Broët et al. (2004), and Li and Feng (2005). Chapter 9 provides details of tests for comparing treatments in cancer clinical trials in the presence of cured subjects and delayed effects.

7

Bayesian Cure Model

7.1 Introduction

In additional to the likelihood and frequentist approaches to cure modeling, Bayesian methods have also been applied to survival data with a cure fraction. Ibrahim et al. (2001) provided a comprehensive review of the Bayesian analysis for survival data, and some of the discussions in the review focus on cure rate models, particularly the non-mixture cure model described in Section 2.4.1. The advantage of this type of non-mixture cure model is that the hazard functions are proportional when covariates are used in the analysis. Ibrahim et al. (2001) considered the Bayesian inference for parametric and semiparametric cure models as well as multivariate cure models. The readers are referred to Ibrahim et al. (2001) for detailed discussions of the non-mixture Bayesian cure models. In this chapters, we describe the Bayesian inference including the prior specification, computational methods, posterior distribution, and the model comparison criteria for several alternative parametric and semiparametric cure models. The flexible cure model with latent activation schemes is described in Section 7.2 and the Bayesian cure model with generalized modified Weibull distribution is described in Section 7.3. Section 7.4 presents a Bayesian cure models with spatial random effects. For the three sections, the statistical methods are followed by illustrative examples with BUGS code (Lunn et al., 2009). In Section 7.5, we discuss the general implementation of Bayesian analysis using BUGS language.

7.2 Flexible Cure Model with Latent Activation Schemes

The non-mixture models proposed by Yakovlev et al. (1994b) and Wang et al. (2012a) are motivated by the mechanisms of cancer metastasis. These models assume that an individual is at the risk of failure if a certain number of latent risk factors are activated. Cooner et al. (2007) proposed a unifying class of cure models by accounting for uncertainty in the underlying mechanisms leading to disease manifestation. They called this class of hierarchical models as the flexible cure model under latent activation schemes.

7.2.1 Model Formulation and Inference

Under the latent activation schemes, the observed failure time T is generated by the N latent event times $\tilde{T}_1, \ldots, \tilde{T}_N$. If $N = 0$, then the individual is not exposed to any of the latent events and is considered cured. For a given N, the latent event times $\tilde{T}_1, \ldots, \tilde{T}_N$ are independently identically distributed with a survival function, $P(\tilde{T} > t) = S^H(t) = 1 - F^H(t)$, which is independent of N. A popular choice of parametric distribution is the Weibull distribution, where

$$S^H(t) = \exp\left(-\exp(\mu)t^{\sigma}\right), \tag{7.1}$$

where μ is the scale parameter and σ is the shape parameter. Let $\tilde{T}_{(1)}, \ldots, \tilde{T}_{(N)}$ be the ordered failure times of $\tilde{T}_1, \ldots, \tilde{T}_N$. Under the general latent activation schemes, r out of N latent factors need to activate for the subject to fail, then $T = \tilde{T}_{(r)}$ for $1 \leq r \leq N$. The rank of the order statistics for the activation of failure r may be a fixed constant, a function of N, or be specified as a random variable conditional on N.

The conditional survival function of $T = \tilde{T}_{(r)}$ given N and r can be written as

$$\begin{aligned} S(t|N,r) &= P(T \geq t|N,r) \\ &= I(N=0) + IB(S^H(t); N-r+1, r)I(1 \leq r \leq N), \end{aligned} \tag{7.2}$$

where $I(\cdot)$ is the indicator function and

$$IB(S^H(t); N-r+1, r) = N \begin{pmatrix} N-1 \\ r-1 \end{pmatrix} \int_0^{S^H(t)} u^{N-r}(1-u)^{r-1}du$$

is the incomplete beta function (Cooner et al., 2007). The unconditional survival function $S(t)$ is a mixture of cure ($N = 0$) and the latency distribution for uncured individuals

$$\begin{aligned} S(t) &= E[P(T \geq t|N,r)] \\ &= P(N=0) + E_{N,r}[IB(S^H(t); N-r+1, r)I(1 \leq r \leq N)] \end{aligned} \tag{7.3}$$

where the expectation $E_{N,r}$ is taken over the joint distribution of (N, r). Note that the latency distribution $0 \leq S^H(t) \leq 1$ for any valid distribution of (N, r) with restriction $1 \leq r \leq N$. The cure probability $1 - \pi = P(N = 0)$ only depends on the distribution of N. Usually, the variable N is not observed and parametric distribution may be used. For example, one may assume that $N \sim \text{Poisson}(\lambda)$ with probability density function

$$P(N = k) = \frac{\lambda^k \exp(-\lambda)}{k!}. \tag{7.4}$$

The corresponding cure rate is $P(N = 0) = \exp(-\lambda)$. Other possible distributions for N include Bernoulli, binomial and geometric distributions, and each has its own biological motivations. See Section 2.4 for more discussions.

The marginal distribution of $S(t)$ can be obtained by specifying the joint distribution of r and N through a marginal specification for N and a conditional distribution for r given N. Cooner et al. (2007) considered various latent activation schemes. For example, the first activation scheme is generated by setting $r = 1$. This implies that the event occurs by activating any one of the N latent events, i.e.,

$$T = \tilde{T}_{(1)} = \min\{\tilde{T}_1, \ldots, \tilde{T}_N\}.$$

The last activation scheme is generated by setting $r = N$, where

$$T = \tilde{T}_{(N)} = \max\{\tilde{T}_1, \ldots, \tilde{T}_N\}.$$

Both the first-activation and last-activation schemes may be generated from certain mechanisms of carcinogenics. For certain types of cancer, the first-activation scheme involves metastasis-competent mutation of the tissue mass that generates the first primary cancer. During the short interval of this mutation, the subject's immune response may be activated to initiate N immune responses to this mutation. When there is no mutation, then $N = 0$ and the subject is not susceptible to the cancer. Each immune response is a latent factor capable of resisting disease manifestation or death until its promotion time. Failure occurs after all of the N factors have been activated, so the observed failure time is $T = \max\{\tilde{T}_1, \ldots, \tilde{T}_N\}$, resulting in the last-activation scheme. More generally, a mixture scheme can be generated by a mixture distribution of r given N, where

$$P(r = 1|N) = p \text{ and } P(r = N|N) = 1 - p \tag{7.5}$$

for $0 < p < 1$. The resulting survival function is a mixture of survival functions for the first-activation and last-activation schemes.

In the presence of covariates, one may assume that the parameters μ in equation (7.1) and λ in equation (7.4) are related to covariates. Suppose there are n subjects. For the ith subject, the observed data consist of $(t_i, \delta_i, \boldsymbol{x}_i)$, $i = 1, \ldots, n$, where t_i is the observed failure time, δ_i is the failure indicator, and $\boldsymbol{x}_i$ is a set of covariates. Let μ_i and λ_i be the scale and cure parameters for the ith subject, $i = 1, \ldots, n$. When the covariates are related to the latent event times, one may assume that $\mu_i = \boldsymbol{x}_i'\boldsymbol{\beta}$. When the covariates are related to the cure rate and the complementary log-log link function $\log(\lambda_i) = \boldsymbol{x}_i'\gamma$ is used, the cure rate is given by

$$1 - \pi(\boldsymbol{x}_i) = \log(-\log(\boldsymbol{x}_i'\gamma)). \tag{7.6}$$

The logit link function can also be considered for the cure rate model. In the situation that covariates are related to both latent survival times and cure, the regression models for the marginal survival function $S(t)$ may not identifiable. For the issue of identifiability, see further discussions in Cooner et al. (2007).

Let $\boldsymbol{\theta} = (\boldsymbol{\beta}, \boldsymbol{\gamma}, \sigma, \psi)$ denote collection of all parameters to be estimated, where $\boldsymbol{\beta}$ and $\boldsymbol{\gamma}$ are the regression coefficients for μ_i and λ_i and ψ denotes set of other hyperparameters that may arise in specific models. The contribution of the ith subject to the likelihood is

$$L(\boldsymbol{\theta}, N_i, r_i) = S(t_i|N_i, r_i)^{1-\delta_i} f(t_i|N_i, r_i)^{\delta_i},$$

where $f(t_i|N_i, r_i) = -\frac{dS(t_i|N_i,r_i)}{dt_i}$ is the corresponding density function of $S(t_i|N_i, r_i)$ in Equation (7.2). The posterior distribution of $\boldsymbol{\theta}$ by marginalizing over N_i and r_i can be written as

$$P(\boldsymbol{\theta}) \propto \prod_{i=1}^{n} \sum_{N_i, r_i} P(\boldsymbol{\theta}, N_i, r_i) \times L(\boldsymbol{\theta}, N_i, r_i), \tag{7.7}$$

where $P(\boldsymbol{\theta}, N_i, r_i)$ are the joint prior probabilities. In general, marginalization in (7.7) is analytically intractable and may be obtained using a MCMC algorithm (Gilks et al., 1995; Carlin and Louis, 2010).

7.2.2 Bayesian Cure Model with Negative Binomial Distribution

As the validity of Poisson distribution for N is questionable (Tucker and Taylor, 1996), de Castro et al. (2009) and Cancho et al. (2011) proposed to use the negative binomial (NB) distribution for N with the probability density function

$$P(N = k|\alpha, \lambda) = \frac{\Gamma(\alpha^{-1} + k)}{\Gamma(\alpha^{-1})k!} \left(\frac{\alpha\lambda}{1 + \alpha\lambda}\right)^k (1 + \alpha\lambda)^{-\frac{1}{\alpha}},$$

where $\lambda > 0, \alpha \geq -1$ and $\alpha > -1/\lambda$.

Under the first-activation scheme, the probability generating function for the NB distribution is $G(s) = \{1 + \alpha\lambda(1 - s)\}^{-1/\alpha}, 0 \leq s \leq 1$. The corresponding marginal survival and density functions are given by

$$\begin{aligned} S(t) &= G(S^H(t)) = \{1 + \alpha\lambda F^H(t)\}^{-1/\alpha}, \\ f(t) &= \{1 + \alpha\lambda F^H(t)\}^{-1/\alpha}\lambda f^H(t). \end{aligned} \tag{7.8}$$

The cure fraction is $1 - \pi = \lim_{t\to\infty} S(t) = (1 + \alpha\lambda)^{-1/\alpha}$. Both the complementary log-log link function and the logit link function can be used in the regression model for the cure rate. Note that the parameter λ is a function of α and cure rate $1 - \pi$, i.e.,

$$\lambda = \begin{cases} [(1 - \pi)^{-\alpha} - 1]/\alpha & \text{if } \alpha \neq 0 \text{ and } \alpha > -1 \\ -\log(1 - \pi) & \text{if } \alpha = 0 \end{cases}.$$

The parameters related to cure rate in model (7.8) are α and γ, which have intuitive biological interpretations. The parameter λ is the mean number of competing causes and α accounts for the inter-individual variance of the number of causes. For the count data with over-dispersion, the parameter α control the dispersion. As $\alpha \to 0$, we obtain the Poisson distribution for N and the PHC model or the promotion time cure model (Chen et al., 1999). Under the first-activation scheme, $r = 1$ for all subjects and the likelihood contribution for the ith subject is

$$L(\boldsymbol{\theta}, N_i) = S(t_i|N_i)^{1-\delta_i} f(t_i|N_i)^{\delta_i},$$

where $S(t|N) = S(t|N, r = 1)$ is defined as equation (7.2). A Weibull distribution or a piecewise exponential distribution (Chen et al., 1999) may be used for the latent survival function $S^H(t)$. The piecewise exponential distribution results a semiparametric alternative to the Weibull distribution. Let the time axis be partitioned into L intervals $(0, \tau_1], (\tau_1, \tau_2], \ldots, (\tau_{L-1}, \tau_L]$. If a constant baseline hazard rate λ_j is assumed at the jth interval $(\tau_{j-1}, \tau_j], j = 1, \ldots, L$, the latent survival function can be written as

$$S^H(t) = \exp\left(-\sum_{l=1}^{j-1} \lambda_l(\tau_l - \tau_{l-1}) - \lambda_j(t - \tau_{j-1})\right) \tag{7.9}$$

for $\tau_{j-1} < t \leq \tau_j$. The overall survival function can be written as

$$S(t) = \begin{cases} \{1 + [(1-\pi)^{-\alpha} - 1]F^H(t))\}^{-1/\alpha} & \text{if } \alpha \neq 0 \\ (1-\pi)^{F^H(t)} & \text{if } \alpha = 0 \end{cases}$$

and the density function is

$$f(t) = \begin{cases} \frac{(1-\pi)^{-\alpha}-1}{\alpha} f^H(t)\{1 + [(1-\pi)^{-\alpha} - 1]F^H(t)\}^{-\frac{1}{\alpha}-1} & \text{if } \alpha \neq 0 \\ -\log(1-\pi)(1-\pi)^{F^H(t)} f^H(t) & \text{if } \alpha = 0 \end{cases}.$$

In the presence of covariates $\boldsymbol{x}_i$, the corresponding survival and density functions can be written as $S(t|\boldsymbol{x}_i)$ and $f(t|\boldsymbol{x}_i)$. For the observed survival data $(t_i, \delta_i, \boldsymbol{x}_i), i = 1, \ldots, n$, the loglikelihood function can be written as

$$L(\boldsymbol{\theta}) \propto \prod_{i=1}^{n} f(t_i|\boldsymbol{x}_i, \boldsymbol{\theta})^{\delta_i} S(t_i|\boldsymbol{x}_i, \boldsymbol{\theta})^{1-\delta_i},$$

where $\boldsymbol{\theta} = (\alpha, \boldsymbol{\lambda}, \gamma)$, α is the dispersion parameter of the NB distribution, γ is the regression coefficients related to cure rate and $\boldsymbol{\lambda} = (\lambda_1, \ldots, \lambda_L)$ are the constant hazard rates for the piecewise exponential distribution. For Bayesian inference, one may assume that α, γ and $\boldsymbol{\lambda}$ are independent a priori, i.e.,

$$p(\boldsymbol{\theta}) = p(\alpha)p(\gamma)p(\boldsymbol{\lambda}),$$

where $p(\cdot)$ is the prior density functions for the parameters. A discrete uniform prior for α may be used, i.e., $\alpha \in \Omega_\alpha = \{\alpha_1, \ldots, \alpha_A\}$ with probability $1/A$, $A \geq 1$. Yin and Ibrahim (2005a) emphasized that in most real applications there is weak evidence about the specific value of α. If a possible range of α

TABLE 7.1
Specifications of the Bayesian cure models for melanoma survival data

Model	μ	$1-\pi=\exp(-\lambda_i)$	N
1	$\mu_i=\boldsymbol{\beta}'\boldsymbol{x}_i$	$\lambda_i=\lambda$	Poisson(λ)
2	$\mu_i=\mu$	$\log(\lambda_i)=\boldsymbol{\beta}'\boldsymbol{x}_i$	Poisson(λ_i)
3	$\mu_i=\mu$	$\log(\lambda_i)=\boldsymbol{\beta}'\boldsymbol{x}_i$	NB(α,λ_i)

values are used, the final model can be seen as an average of models among the grid Ω_α. The prior distribution for the regression coefficients γ may be multivariate normal, i.e., $\gamma \sim MVN(\boldsymbol{\mu}_\gamma, \Sigma_\gamma)$. For the piecewise exponential distribution (7.9), let $\xi_j = \log(\lambda_j), j = 1, \ldots, L$. The prior distributions for $\xi_1, \ldots, \xi_L$ can be specified as

$$\xi_j|\xi_{j-1}, \sigma_j^2 \sim N(\xi_{j-1}, \sigma_\xi^2), j = 1, \ldots, L,$$

and $\sigma_\xi^2 \sim IG(a, b)$ with $\xi_0 = 0$, where $IG(a, b)$ denotes a inverse-gamma distribution with shape parameter a and scale parameter b. Again, the joint posterior density is analytically intractable because the integration of the joint posterior density is not easy to perform. The Bayesian inference based on the MCMC method is described in de Castro et al. (2009).

7.2.3 Application

The melanoma data from the Eastern Cooperative Oncology Group (ECOG) phase III clinical trial E1684 which is used for modeling semiparametric PH mixture cure model (Kirkwood et al., 1996). The survival endpoint is the time to cancer relapse. The covariates include binary variable of sex (0=male, 1=female), binary treatment variable (0=control, 1=IFN treatment) and centered continuous variable for age. In the data set, there are 171 males and 113 females and 140 are in the control group and 144 receive the IFN treatment. The Kaplan-Meier survival curves of the two treatment groups are shown in Figure 7.1. The survival curves of cancer relapse time reach plateaus after six months of treatment, indicating a possibility of cure among the patients.

We apply the Bayesian cure models with different latent activation schemes, the NB distribution for the number of latent events, and the Weibull distribution for the latent distribution. We consider three models and the model specifications are shown in Table 7.1. The three covariates are used in the scale parameter of the Weibull distribution in Model 1 and in the cure probability in Models 2 and 3. Model 1 and 2 consider a mixture of the first-activation and last-activation schemes with the mixing probability p. As recommended by Cooner et al. (2007), we consider a mixture model (7.5) for last-activation and first-activation schemes and use the prior $p \sim U(0, 1)$. For Model 1, all patients have the same number of latent events from a Poisson distribution $N \sim$ Poisson(λ), thus the same cure rate $1 - \pi = \exp(-\lambda)$ for

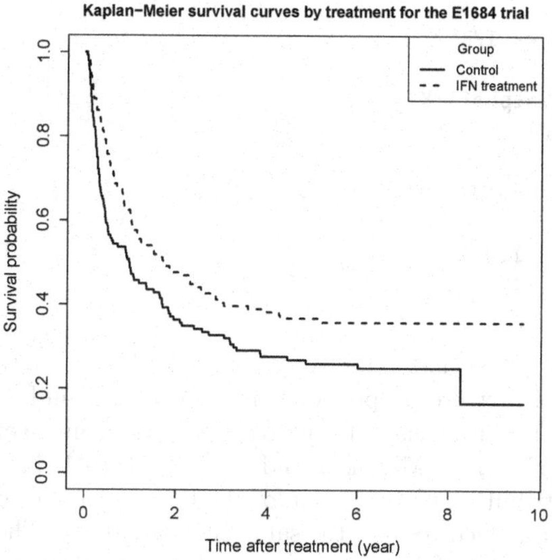

FIGURE 7.1
Kaplan-Meier curves of cancer relapse time for melanoma patients in the E1684 trial.

all subjects. For Model 2, the number of latent events for the ith patient is N_i = Poisson(λ_i) and the cure rates are dependent on the covariates of the subjects. Model 3 considers a last-activation scheme but introduces an extra parameter α in the NB distribution for the number of latent events. For each analysis, we run two initially dispersed parallel MCMC chains for 10,000 iterations each as burn-in, then 25,000 addition runs with thinning factor of 2 to yield 2×25,000 = 50,000 samples for posterior analysis. The sample OpenBUGS code for fitting Model 3 is as follows:

```
model {
for (i in 1:n) {
  # CDF and pdf
  F[i] <- 1 - exp(-exp(eta)*pow(t[i],gamma))
  f[i] <- exp(eta) * gamma * pow(t[i],gamma-1)) * (1-F[i])

  # Cure rate
  p.cure[i]<-exp(-exp(inprod(beta[1:L],x[i,1:L])))

  # Log-likelihood
  loglik[i]<-(delta[i]*log((pow(p.cure[i],-alpha)-1)/alpha*f[i])
       -(delta[i]+1/alpha)*log(1+(pow(p.cure[i],-alpha)-1)*F[i]))
  zeros[i] ~ dloglik(loglik[i])
}

# Prior distributions
```

```
for (j in 1:K) {
  pi.alpha[j] <- 1/K
}
ind ~ dcat(pi.alpha[1:K])
alpha <- A[ind]
for (j in 1:L) {
  beta[j] ~ dnorm(0,0.01)
}
gamma~dgamma(0.1,0.1)
eta~dnorm(0,0.01)
}
```

The parameter estimates for the three models are shown in Table 7.2. The estimates of mixture proportion p from Models 1 and 2 are above 0.83, indicating that the data is more likely to arise from the first-activation scheme. The estimates of σ from Models 1 and 2 are close to 1, indicating that the exponential distribution may be used for the latent distribution. For Model 1, all patients are assumed to have the same cure rate 0.284. The IFN treatment group has a lower latent hazard rate than the control group with a hazard ratio $\exp(-0.184) = 0.831$ and 95% confidence interval (0.582, 1.192), which is not statistically significant. For Model 2, the covariates are assumed to be related to the cure rate as $1 - \pi(\boldsymbol{x}) = \exp(-\exp(\boldsymbol{x}^{'}\boldsymbol{\beta}))$, and thus a negative coefficient means a higher cure rate for a larger value of a covariate in $\boldsymbol{x}$. For example, the parameter estimate for IFN treatment is -0.393 with 95% confidence interval (-0.697, -0.107), which implies that the patients in the IFN treatment group have statistically significantly higher cure rate than the patients in the control group. The three covariates are assumed to be related to cure fraction in Model 3 in the same way as in Model 2. The parameter estimate of IFN treatment is -0.155 with 95% confidence interval (-0.295, -0.041). Age and sex are not statistically significantly associated with the cure rate in Model 2 and 3.

To evaluate the goodness-of-fit of the three models, we show the estimated survival curves by treatment and sex. We assume that the age for prediction is the average age in the group defined by treatment and sex. For comparison, we also show the Kaplan-Meier curves for cancer relapse by treatment and sex. The plots of the survival curves are shown in Figure 7.2. The dashed, dotted and dash-dotted lines are the predictions from Models 1, 2 and 3, respectively. Model 1 assumes that the cure rates are the same for all patients and Models 2 and 3 assume that the cure rates are associated with treatment and sex. Overall, we see that Models 2 and 3 provide a better fit to the long-term survival rate than Model 1. The estimated survival from Model 3 is between the estimates from Models 1 and 2. Model 3 appears to have a better fit to the early survival than Models 1 and 2. As Cooner et al. (2007) recommended, scientific consideration should guide the final model selection when several models fit the data adequately well. In the E1684 study, treatment, age and

TABLE 7.2
Parameter estimates from the Bayesian cure models with a mixture latent activation scheme

	Model 1				Model 2				Model 3			
Parameter	Mean	SD	95% CI		Mean	SD	95% CI		Mean	SD	95% CI	
Intercept	-0.349	0.155	-0.656	-0.054	0.427	0.125	0.180	0.670	0.319	0.113	0.124	0.581
Treatment	-0.184	0.186	-0.542	0.176	-0.393	0.151	-0.697	-0.107	-0.155	0.064	-0.295	-0.041
Sex	0.146	0.183	-0.206	0.505	-0.048	0.153	-0.353	0.243	0.008	0.057	-0.110	0.116
Age	-0.007	0.006	-0.020	0.005	0.006	0.006	-0.005	0.018	0.001	0.002	-0.003	0.006
Cure $1-\pi$	0.284	0.028	0.234	0.342								
μ					-0.357	0.126	-0.597	-0.100	-4.350	1.490	-8.524	-2.425
p (α)	0.861	0.108	0.599	0.995	0.838	0.108	0.584	0.990	6.398	1.411	4.000	9.000
σ	1.009	0.060	0.892	1.127	1.014	0.057	0.901	1.124	2.244	0.336	1.651	2.964

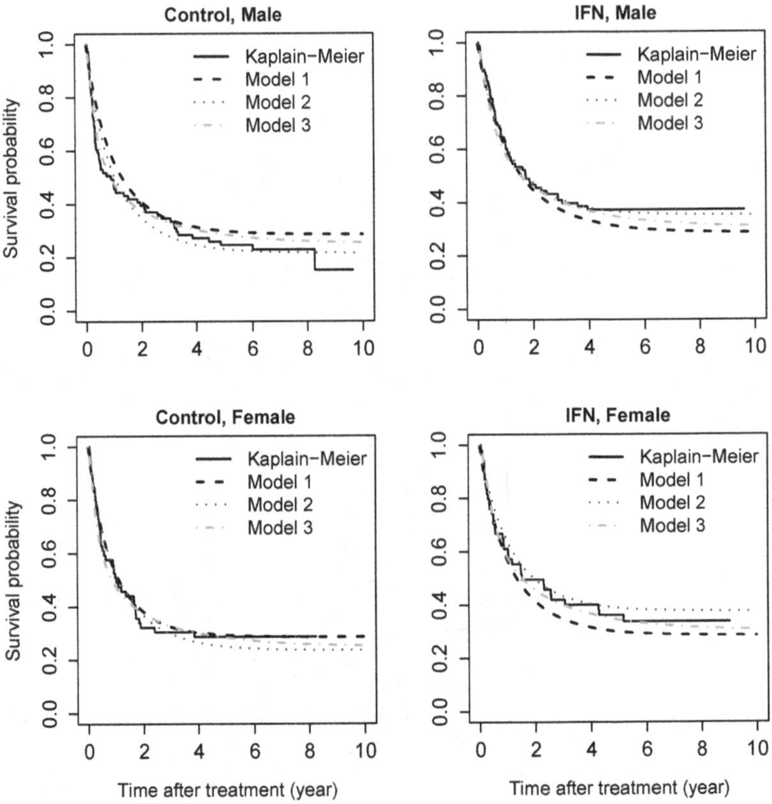

FIGURE 7.2
Comparison of the predicted survival from the three models for the E1684 study.

sex are significant prognostic factor of cure, therefore Models 2 and 3 that assume a covariate-dependent cure rate are more scientifically appropriate.

7.3 Bayesian Cure Models with Generalized Modified Weibull Distribution

7.3.1 Model Formulation and Inference

We introduce here a Bayesian analysis for the cure models based on the generalized modified Weibull (GMW) distribution, which is a very general class of

TABLE 7.3
Parametric distributions as special cases of the GMW distribution

Distribution	Parameter restrictions
Weibull	$\delta = 0, \beta = 1$
Exponential	$\delta = 0, \beta = 1, \eta = 1$
Rayleigh	$\delta = 0, \beta = 1, \eta = 2$
Type I Extreme value	$\beta = 1, \eta = 0$
Exponentiated Weibull	$\delta = 0$
Exponentiated Exponential	$\delta = 0, \eta = 1$
Generalized Rayleigh	$\delta = 0, \eta = 2$
Modified Weibull	$\beta = 1$

distributions and easy to implement (Martinez et al., 2013). The mixture cure model is given by (2.1) with the GMW distribution as the latency distribution with the following survival and density functions:

$$S_u(t) = 1 - \{1 - \exp[-\alpha t^\eta \exp(\delta t)]\}^\beta,$$
$$f_u(t) = \frac{\alpha\beta t^{\eta-1}(\eta + \delta t)\exp[\delta t - \alpha t^\eta \exp(\delta t)]}{1 - \exp[-\alpha t^\eta \exp(\delta t)]^{1-\beta}},$$

where $\alpha > 0, \beta > 0, \eta \geq 0$ and $\delta \geq 0$, but η and δ cannot be 0 simultaneously. The GMW distribution is denoted by $GMW(\alpha, \beta, \eta, \delta)$. The parameter α is a scale parameter and β and η are shape parameters. The four-parameter distribution was introduced by Carrasco et al. (2008) and it is flexible to accommodate many forms of the hazard rate function, including bathtub-shaped hazard rate function. Table 7.3 shows several standard parametric distributions as the special cases of the four-parameter GMW distribution. The corresponding density function of the GMW distribution is given by

Assume that $\pi_c(\boldsymbol{x}) = 1 - \pi(\boldsymbol{x})$ and

$$\pi_c(\boldsymbol{x}) = \frac{\exp(\boldsymbol{x}'\gamma)}{1 + \exp(\boldsymbol{x}'\gamma)}, \tag{7.10}$$

The overall survival function of the mixture cure model is

$$S(t|\boldsymbol{x}) = \pi_c(\boldsymbol{x}) + (1 - \pi_c(\boldsymbol{x}))S_u(t),$$

For observed survival data $(t_i, \delta_i, \boldsymbol{x}_i), i = 1, \ldots, n$, the likelihood function for the mixture cure model is given by

$$L(\boldsymbol{\theta}) = \prod_{i=1}^{n} [(1 - \pi_c(\boldsymbol{x}_i))f_u(t_i)]^{\delta_i} [\pi_c(\boldsymbol{x}) + (1 - \pi_c(\boldsymbol{x}))S_u(t)]^{1-\delta_i}. \tag{7.11}$$

For the non-mixture cure model, the survival function is given by

$$S(t|\boldsymbol{x}) = \{\pi_c(\boldsymbol{x})\}^{F_u(t)} = \exp\{\log(\pi_c(\boldsymbol{x})F_u(t))\},$$

where $F_u(t) = 1 - S_u(t)$ is a proper cumulative distribution function. Unlike the mixture cure model, $F_u(t)$ cannot be interpreted as the cumulative distribution function for the uncured patients. The likelihood function for the non-mixture cure model is given as

$$L(\boldsymbol{\theta}) = \prod_{i=1}^{n} \{-\log(\pi_c(\boldsymbol{x})F_u(t))\}^{\delta_i} \exp\{\log(\pi_c(\boldsymbol{x})F_u(t))\}. \tag{7.12}$$

For a Bayesian analysis of the both types of cure models, we assume gamma and half-normal (HN) prior distributions for the parameters α, β, η and δ considering the fact that these parameters are real and positive numbers:

$$\alpha \sim \text{Gamma}(a_\alpha, b_\alpha), \quad \beta \sim \text{Gamma}(a_\beta, b_\beta),$$
$$\eta \sim \text{HN}(a_\eta, b_\eta), \quad \delta \sim \text{HN}(a_\delta, b_\delta),$$

where a_α, b_α, a_β, b_β, a_η, b_η, a_δ and b_δ are known hyperparameters and Gamma(a, b) denotes a Gamma distribution with mean a/b and and variance a/b^2.

It is important to note that one or more of these parameters may be fixed with constant values when considering the special cases of the GMW distribution. For example, if considering the exponentiated exponential distribution, $\eta = 1$ and $\delta = 0$. For the regression coefficients $\boldsymbol{\gamma}$ for cure rate, we assume a multivariate normal distribution where $\boldsymbol{\gamma} \sim MNV(0, \Sigma_\gamma)$.

7.3.2 Application

As an illustration, we apply the Bayesian mixture and non-mixture cure models with the GMW distribution to survival data from an International Bone Marrow Transplant Registry study of alternative donor bone marrow transplants (BMT) reported in Szydlo et al. (1997). As in many BMT studies, there are two competing risks of treatment failure in this study; relapse (n=311/1715 cases), i.e., recurrence of the primary disease, and death in complete remission (n=557/1715), also known as treatment-related mortality. This study consisted of patients with acute lymphoblastic leukemia (ALL) (n=537), acute myelogenous leukemia (AML) (n=340), or chronic myelogenous leukemia (CML) (n=838). Patients were transplanted with their disease in an early (n=1026), intermediate (n=410), or advanced (n=279) stage based on remission status. The initial Karnofsky performance score was greater than or equal to 90 in 1382 cases. Of primary interest is the comparison of relapse and treatment-related mortality between patients with different donor types. There were 1224 with a human leukocyte antigen (HLA)-identical sibling donor, 383 with an HLA-matched unrelated donor, and 108 cases with an HLA-mismatched unrelated donor. The data were analyzed as an example of competing-risk analysis in Klein and Andersen (2005).

We restricted the analysis to the patients with CML and considered the event as relapse or treatment-related mortality. Therefore, the cured patients

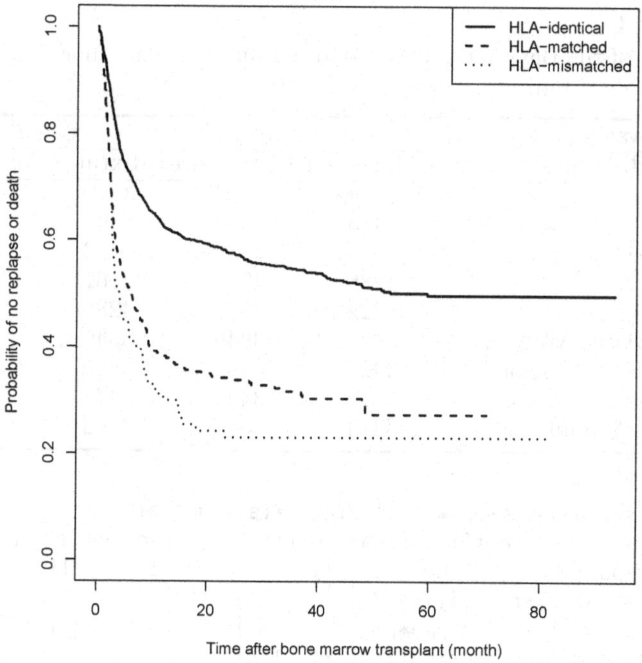

FIGURE 7.3
Kaplan-Meier survival curves for the CML patients with 3 donor types.

are those who did not have either event. The Kaplan-Meier survival curves for the 3 donor groups are shown in Figure 7.3. The survival curves clearly reach a plateau in 60 months after bone marrow transplant. The patients with HLA-identically matched donors have the highest long-term survival rates.

We fit the Bayesian cure models with the GMW distribution and its special cases listed in Table 7.3 to the BMT data. Figure 7.3 shows that the HLA donor type is a strong predictor of long-term survival rates. Thus, we use it as a categorical covariate in the incidence model (7.10) for the cure rate. We also consider covariates in the scale parameter α as $\alpha(\boldsymbol{x}) = \exp(\beta_\alpha \boldsymbol{x})$. Following Carrasco et al. (2008), we use the Deviance Information Criterion (DIC) for model selection. Models with smaller DIC values are better supported by the data. The DIC values for the various cure models are shown in Table 7.4. The model with the smallest DIC 3340 is the mixture cure model with exponentiated Weibull distribution and the covariate donor type is only used for the cure rate in this model. The WinBUGS code for fitting this model is as follows:

```
model {
for (i in 1:N) {
```

TABLE 7.4
DIC values of the Bayesian mixture and non-mixture cure models with different latency distributions

Use of covariate	π_c only		π_c and α	
Latency distribution	Mixture	Non-mixture	Mixture	Non-mixture
GMW	3364	3343	3370	3344
Weibull	3413	3384	3390	3380
Exponential	3435	3386	3402	3379
Rayleigh	4288	4081	4161	4001
Type I Extreme Value	4322	4276	4288	4268
Exponentiated Weibull	3361	3340	3349	3341
Exponentiated Exponential	3428	3387	3400	3381
Generalized Rayleigh	3510	3449	3475	3437
Modified Weibull	3414	3386	3392	3381

```
  f0A1[i]<-alpha*beta*pow(t[i],eta-1)*(eta+delta*t[i])
  f0A2[i]<-exp(delta*t[i]-alpha*pow(t[i],eta)*exp(delta*t[i]))
  f0B[i]<-pow(1-exp(-alpha*pow(t[i],eta)*exp(delta*t[i])),1-beta)
  f0[i]<-(f0A1[i]*f0A2[i])/f0B[i]
  S0[i]<-1-pow(1-exp(-alpha*pow(t[i],eta)*exp(delta*t[i])),beta)
  logit(p[i])<-inprod(gamma[1:K],x[i,1:K])
  F0[i] <- 1-S0[i]
  h[i] <- -(log(p[i]))*f0[i]
  L[i] <- pow(h[i],d[i])*exp(F0[i]*log(p[i]))
  logL[i] <- log(L[i])
  zeros[i] ~ dloglik(logL[i])
}

for (i in 1:K) {
  gamma[i]~dnorm(0,0.01)
}

alpha ~ dgamma(1,1)
beta ~ dgamma(1,1)
eta ~ dnorm(0,0.01)I(0,)
delta<-0
}
```

We present the model fit for this model in Figure 7.4. We see the model fits the data well and the cure rates are 57.2%, 24.8% and 17.2% for the patients with identical, matched and mismatched donors, respectively.

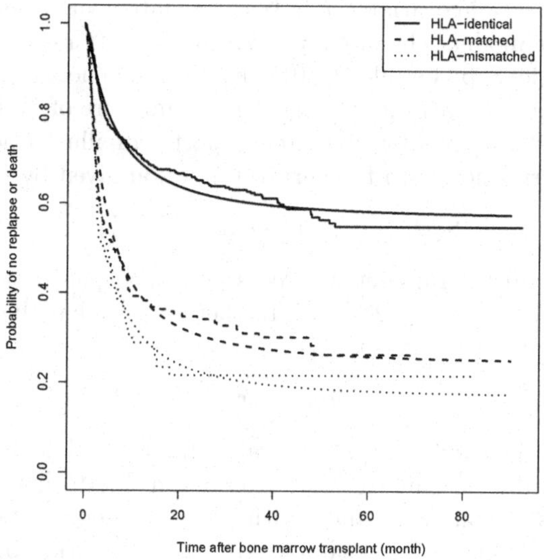

FIGURE 7.4
Estimated survival curves from the Bayesian cure model for the BMT data.

7.4 Bayesian Mixture Cure Model with Spatially Correlated Frailties

7.4.1 Spatial Mixture Cure Model

Bayesian methods have been used to fit the cure model with random effects (frailty). For example, de Souza et al. (2017) used a discrete probability distribution including zero for the frailty in the mixture cure model. Rahimzadeh et al. (2010) used two different types of frailty with the bivariate log-normal distribution instead of the gamma distribution in the non-mixture cure models. Cooner et al. (2006) proposed a non-mixture cure model with spatial frailties for geographically referenced survival data and Banerjee and Carlin (2004) developed a parametric spatial cure rate models for interval-censored survival data from smoking cessation trials. Seppa et al. (2010) and Yu and Tiwari (2012) proposed similar mixture cure models with spatial frailties for population-based cancer survival data. In this section, we briefly describe the mixture cure model with spatially correlated frailties for population-based cancer survival data.

The survival function of the mixture cure model is specified as

$$S(t|\boldsymbol{x}) = \pi_c(\boldsymbol{x}) + (1 - \pi_c(\boldsymbol{x}))S_u(t|\boldsymbol{x}), \tag{7.13}$$

where the cure fraction $\pi_c(\boldsymbol{x})$ is modeled as in (7.10). For the sake of simplicity, we use the same set of covariates $\boldsymbol{x}$ in both the latency and incidence parts of the mixture cure model. The latency distribution $S_u(t|\boldsymbol{x})$ may be parametric or semiparametric. Seppa et al. (2010) considered a generalized gamma distribution and Yu and Tiwari (2012) considered a mixture of Weibull, lognormal and loglostic distributions for the latency part. For illustration, we consider the Weibull distribution with the survival function given by

$$S_u(t|\boldsymbol{x}) = \exp\{-\exp[\mu(\boldsymbol{x})]\, t^{\sigma}\},$$

where μ is the rate parameter and σ is the scale parameter. The median survival time is $[\exp(-\mu)\log(2)]^{\frac{1}{\sigma}}$. We further assume that the rate or location parameter is related to covariates as

$$\mu(\boldsymbol{x}) = \boldsymbol{x}'\boldsymbol{\beta}. \tag{7.14}$$

For population-based cancer survival data, we will focus on the cause-specific survival due to cancer, where the death due to cancer is treated as event while loss to follow-up and death due to other causes are treated as censoring. Because of the large sample size, the population-based cancer survival data may be stratified by variables like age, calendar year and cancer stages at diagnosis. In addition, the survival times after diagnosis are grouped into monthly or annual intervals $I_j = [t_{j-1}, t_j), j = 1, 2, \ldots, J$, where t_J is the study cutoff time. For the stratum with covariates $\boldsymbol{x}$, let n_{xj} be the number of people alive at the beginning of interval I_j. For cause-specific cancer survival analysis, we consider d_{xj} as the number of patients dying from cancer of interest and l_{xj} as the number of patients lost to follow-up or dying from other causes in interval I_j. Using the actuarial assumption, the adjusted number of person-years at risk is $r_{xj} = n_{xj} - 0.5l_{xj}$. The probability of dying from cancer during the interval I_j given that a subject is alive at the beginning of the interval is given by

$$p_j(\boldsymbol{x}) = P(T < t_j | T \geq t_{j-1}; \boldsymbol{x}) = 1 - \frac{S(t_j|\boldsymbol{x})}{S(t_{j-1}|\boldsymbol{x})}, \tag{7.15}$$

where $S(t|\boldsymbol{x})$ is the survival function defined in (7.13).

The number of deaths due to cancer in an interval is usually assumed to follow a binomial distribution, i.e., $d_{xj} \sim \text{Binomial}(r_{xj}, p_j(\boldsymbol{x}))$. When the cancer has a good prognosis or curable, the number of deaths due to cancer may be sparse or even zero in late intervals, especially for small geographical regions in spatial analysis. In this situation, the binomial distribution may not be appropriate and a Poisson distribution may be used, i.e.,

$$d_{xj} \sim \text{Poisson}(r_{xj} p_j(\boldsymbol{x})).$$

Let $\boldsymbol{\theta} = (\boldsymbol{\beta}, \boldsymbol{\gamma}, \sigma)$ be the vector of all parameters to be estimated. The corresponding likelihood function is written as

$$L(\boldsymbol{\theta}) = \prod_{\boldsymbol{x}} \prod_{j=1}^{J} (r_{xj} p_j(\boldsymbol{x}))^{d_{xj}} \exp(-r_{xj} \times p_j(\boldsymbol{x})). \tag{7.16}$$

The results from the two distributional assumptions for the number of deaths are usually very similar since the log-likelihoods are similar for survival data with moderate or low annual death rates (Dickman et al., 2004).

The spatial pattern and the temporal trends of cancer survival are gaining more interest recently, and health policy makers and public health researchers started to investigate the spatial association and patterns of health outcomes. Suppose that there are I geographical regions and let $\boldsymbol{r}_i = (r_{i1}, r_{i2})$ be the bivariate random effects (frailties), where r_{i1} denotes the frailty for the cure fraction and r_{i1} denotes the frailty for the survival for the uncured patients. Similar to the models discussed in Section 4.3.1, the cure fraction and the location parameter for the uncured patients for the ith geographic region can be written as

$$\pi_{ci}(\boldsymbol{x}) = \frac{\exp(\boldsymbol{x}'\gamma + r_{i1})}{1 + \exp(\boldsymbol{x}'\gamma + r_{i1})} \tag{7.17}$$

and

$$\mu_i(\boldsymbol{x}) = \boldsymbol{x}'\boldsymbol{\beta} + r_{i2}, \tag{7.18}$$

respectively. The multivariate conditionally autoregressive (CAR) distributions can be used for the spatial random effects in the baseline hazard rate and the spatial frailties. Most CAR models are members of the family developed by Mardia (1988). Specifically, the multivariate CAR of Gamerman et al. (2003) generalizes the univariate pairwise difference joint prior as

$$\pi(\boldsymbol{r}_1, \ldots, \boldsymbol{r}_I|\Omega_r) \propto |\Omega_r|^{-I/2} \exp\left\{\sum_{i \neq j}^{I} c_{ij}(\boldsymbol{r}_i - \boldsymbol{r}_j)'\Omega_r^{-1}(\boldsymbol{r}_i - \boldsymbol{r}_j)\right\},$$

where $\boldsymbol{r}_i = (r_{i1}, \ldots, r_{ip})', i = 1, \ldots, I$, be the multivariate p-dimensional ($p \geq 2$, $p = 2$ in the mixture cure model above) vector of spatially correlated Gaussian random effects in the I areas, Ω_r is the dispersion matrix and $c_{ij} = 1$ if area i and j are adjacent and 0 otherwise (Congdon, 2007). The intrinsic multivariate CAR prior with 0-1 adjacency weights (Besag et al., 1991) gives the conditional distribution

$$\boldsymbol{r}_i|\boldsymbol{r}_{(-i)} \sim \text{MVN}_p(\bar{\boldsymbol{r}}_i, V/n_i),$$

where $\boldsymbol{r}_{(-i)}$ denotes the elements of the $2 \times I$ matrix excluding the ith area (column), $\bar{\boldsymbol{r}}_i = (\bar{r}_{i1}, \bar{r}_{i2})$ with $\bar{r}_{ip} = \sum_{j \in \delta_i} r_{jp}/n_i$, δ_i and n_i denote the set of labels of the neighbors of area i and the number of neighbors, respectively, and V is a 2×2 dispersion matrix. The intrinsic multivariate CAR is currently implemented in GeoBUGS, a module of WinBUGS (Lunn et al., 2009). The syntax for a CAR distribution is

```
R[1:p,1:J] ~ mv.car(adj[], weights[], num[], omega[,])
```

where `adj[]` is a vector that represents the adjacency matrix for the study region, `weights[]` gives unnormalized weights associated with each pair of areas, `num[]` gives the number of neighbors for each area and `omega[,]` is the precision matrix.

Let $p(\boldsymbol{\theta})$ be the joint prior distribution of $\boldsymbol{\theta}$ and let $L(\boldsymbol{\theta})$ be the likelihood function for the grouped cause-specific survival data given by (7.16). The joint posterior distribution of $\boldsymbol{\theta}$ is

$$p(\boldsymbol{\theta}) \propto L(\boldsymbol{\theta})p(\boldsymbol{\theta}).$$

We assume that the prior distributions for the parameters are mutually independent, i.e.,

$$p(\boldsymbol{\theta}) = p(\boldsymbol{\beta})p(\boldsymbol{\gamma})p(\sigma)p(\boldsymbol{r}),$$

where $p(\boldsymbol{\beta})$ and $p(\boldsymbol{\gamma})$ are the priors for regression coefficients, $p(\sigma)$ is the prior for the scale parameter and $p(\boldsymbol{r}) = p(\boldsymbol{r}_1, \ldots, \boldsymbol{r}_I|\Omega_r)$ is the prior for the spatial random effects. In particular, we assume conjugate prior for the model parameters: $p(\boldsymbol{\beta}) \sim MVN(\mu_{\boldsymbol{\beta}}, \Sigma_{\boldsymbol{\beta}}), p(\boldsymbol{\gamma}) \sim MVN(\mu_{\boldsymbol{\gamma}}, \Sigma_{\boldsymbol{\gamma}})$, $p(\sigma^2) \sim IG(a, b)$, where $IG(a, b)$ denotes an inverse gamma distribution with shape parameter a and scale parameter b. In addition, we also assume that the hyperprior for Ω_r is an inverse Wishart distribution with scale matrix C_γ and ν_γ degrees of freedom.

We use the MCMC algorithm for parameter estimation and inferences. The proposed method can be implemented in the freely available software WinBUGS or OpenBUGS (Lunn et al., 2009). After a sufficient number of burn-in iterations, we use the remaining samples from the MCMC simulations to estimate any function of the parameters of interest. In order to see how stable the final estimates are, multiple MCMC runs are conducted with different initial values and starting points. The convergence of the MCMC samples of the parameters after excluding the initial burn-in samples are monitored using the R package `CODA` (Best et al., 1995). For example, Gelman and Rubin (1992) used a 'potential scale reduction factor' for each parameter in $\boldsymbol{\theta}$, together with upper and lower confidence limits.

7.4.2 Application

We apply the spatial mixture cure model to estimate the survival and cure rate for patients diagnosed with lung and bronchus cancer from 1992 to 2013 in Iowa. The survival data was extracted from the Surveillance, Epidemiology, and End Results (SEER) 13 registries and the cutoff date for survival analysis is the end of 2013. The relative survival data are stratified by SEER historical stage and 99 counties in Iowa. The SEER historical stage is a summary stage that categorize how far a cancer has spread from its point of origin. It is a combination of the most precise clinical and pathological documentation of the extent of disease. The SEER Program classifies the historical stages into Localized, Regional and Distant stages consistently for all cancer sites for the appropriate years. The maximum follow-up time is 21 years, with sufficient time to observing the possible plateau of survival curve if there is a cure. The survival times are grouped into annual intervals. The survival data include the number of subjects being alive in the beginning of the interval, the number of subjects dying from lung and bronchus cancer and the number of loss of follow-up during each of the intervals. The WinBUGS code for fitting the Bayesian spatial cure model is as follows:

```
model {
for (i in 1:Nx) {
  # probability and mean number of deaths in each intervals
  logit(p.cure[i])<-inprod(alpha[1:3],x[i,1:3])+R[1,G[i]]
  mu[i]<-inprod(beta[1:3],x[i,1:3])+R[2,G[i]]
  for (j in 1:maxT) {
    S[i,j]<-p.cure[i]+(1-p.cure[i])*exp(-exp(mu[i])*pow(j,sigma))
  }
  p[i,1]<-(1-S[i,1])*n[i,1]
  for (j in 2:nFup[i]) {
        p[i,j]<-(1-S[i,j]/S[i,j-1])*n[i,j]
  }

  # poisson model for number of deaths
  for (j in 1:nFup[i]) {
        d[i,j]~dpois(p[i,j])
  }
}

# priors for alpha, beta and sigma
alpha[1]~dnorm(0,0.01)
beta[1]~dnorm(0,0.01)
for (i in 2:3) {
  alpha[i]~dnorm(0,0.01)I(,0)
  beta[i]~dnorm(0,0.01)I(0,)
}
sigma~dexp(1)

# priors for spatial random effect
for (i in 1:nsum) {
  weights[i]<-1
}
R[1:2,1:M] ~ mv.car(adj[], weights[], num[], tau[,])
tau[1:2,1:2] ~ dwish(A.tau[,],2)
}
```

In the analysis, the total number of patients diagnosed with lung and bronchus cancer is 212,619. The historical stage is used as a categorical covariates in both cure fraction and latency distribution as specified in (7.10) and (7.14). The posterior mean, standard deviation (SD) and 95% confidence interval (CI) of the parameters are shown in Table 7.5. The reference group is the patients with localized cancer, the cure rate estimate is 62.7% with 95% CI (58.5%, 69.8%). Compared to the patients with localized cancer, the patients

TABLE 7.5
Parameter estimates for the spatial mixture cure model for lung and bronchus cancer survival data

	Latency distribution			Cure		
Variable	Mean	SD	(95% CI)	Mean	SD	(95% CI)
Intercept	-2.133	0.067	(-2.264,-2.002)	0.520	0.091	(0.343, 0.698)
Localized						
Regional	1.101	0.068	(0.968, 1.235)	-0.679	0.086	(-0.848, -0.510)
Distant	2.060	0.069	(1.924, 2.196)	-2.449	0.091	(-2.626, -2.271)
σ	0.639	0.005	(0.628, 0.649)			

TABLE 7.6
Mean, minimum and maximum cure fraction and median survival time for the uncured patients.

Stage	Median survival for uncured			Cure fraction (%)		
	Minimum	Mean	Maximum	Minimum	Mean	Maximum
Localized	12.7	15.9	19.6	56.2	62.7	68.9
Regional	2.3	2.8	3.5	39.4	46.1	52.9
Distant	0.5	0.6	0.8	10.0	12.7	16.1

with regional and distant cancers have significantly higher hazard of dying from lung and bronchus cancer and significantly lower cure rates. Therefore, the cancer stage is a significant prognostic factor for cancer survival. This also implies the importance of early diagnosis for survival. Table 7.6 shows the mean, minimum and maximum of the cure fractions and median survival times for the uncured patients for the 99 counties by SEER historic stage.

The mean cure rate for the distant lung and bronchus cancer for the 99 counties is 12.7% with a range of 10.0%–16.1%. The cure rates for the localized cancer have a wider range of 56.2%–68.9% and mean 62.7%. We show the map of the county-level cure rates for localized lung and bonchus cancer in Figure 7.5. From this map, we see that the northern Iowa counties tend to have slightly higher cure rates than the southern counties. This is probably due to the differences in patient characteristics or health care quality in this area. It provides useful information to health care planners for allocating limited resources for cancer control.

7.5 Implementation

We consider the example of the Bayesian cure model with latent activation schemes, discussed in Section 7.2. The survival data include cancer relapse

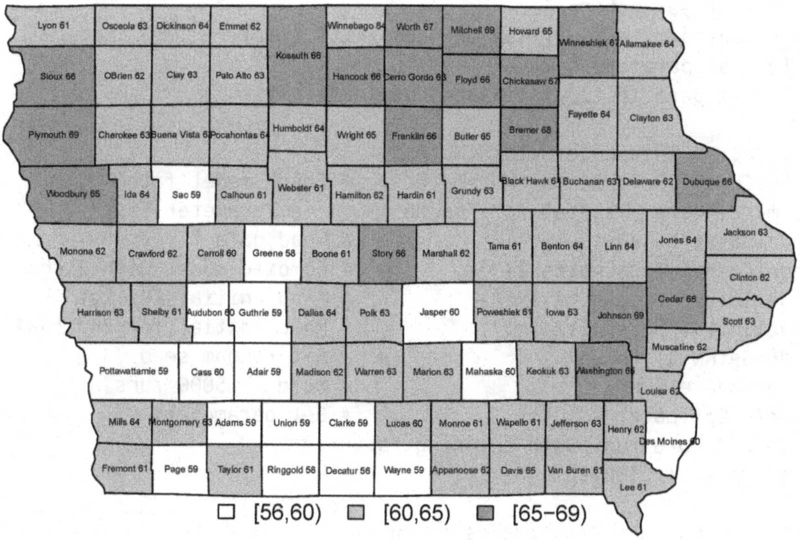

FIGURE 7.5
Map of cure rate (%) for localized lung and bronchus cancer in Iowa.

time `y` and event indicator `d` for n patients, and the data matrix `x` include `K` columns for $K-1$ covariates and one column of constant 1. The parameters to be estimated are $\boldsymbol{\beta}, \theta, \sigma$ and p. The BUGS syntax code for the Bayesian cure model is specified in Section 7.4.2.

Bayesian cure model has been implemented using the OpenBUGS, which can be called within R using BRugs (Thomas et al., 2006). BRugs is a collection of R functions that allow users to analyze graphical models using MCMC techniques. BRugs uses the same model specification language as WinBUGS or OpenBUGS and the same format for data and initial values. The BRugs functions can be split into two groups: those associated with setting up and simulating the graphical model and those associated with making statistical inference. In general, the R functions in BRugs correspond to the command buttons and text entry fields in the menus of WinBUGS. The example syntax of using BRugs is shown below:

```
library("BRugs")
# Setting up the data list and initial parmaters
data.list<-list(n=n,y=y,x=x,d=d,K=K)
parm.init1<-list(beta = rep(0,4), theta = 0.5, sigma = 1.0, p=0.5)
parm.init2<-list(beta = rnorm(4), theta = 0.4, sigma = 1.0, p=0.2)

# Create files for data, initial parameters
# Create data file
bugsData(data.list, fileName="bugsData.txt")
```

```
# Initial parameters 1
bugsData(parm.init1, fileName="bugsInit1.txt")
# Initial parameters 2
bugsData(parm.init2, fileName="bugsInit2.txt")

# Bayesian inference with MCMC
modelCheck("BayesianCureModel.txt")  # Check model file
parm<-c("beta","theta","p","sigma")     # Parameter list
modelData("bugsData.txt")            # Read data file
modelCompile(numChains=2)            # Compile model with 2 chains
modelInits("bugsInit1.txt")          # Read initial for 1st chain
modelInits("bugsInit2.txt")          # Read initial for 2nd chain
modelSetRN(1)                        # Set random seed
modelUpdate(5000)                    # Burn in 5000 runs
samplesSet(parm)                     # Set parameters
# 10,000 more runs with thinning factor 2
modelUpdate(10000,thin=2)

# output parameter estimates and plots
# Output estimates to a data frame
parm.estimate=samplesStats("*")
# plot the sample history
samplesHistory("*",mfrow=c(2,4),ask=FALSE)
# plot the sample density
samplesDensity("*",mfrow=c(2,4),ask=FALSE)
# Auto-correlation of beta in 1st chain
samplesAutoC("beta",chain=1)
```

In the set-up stage, the analysis data file is generated from a data list `data.list` and two files for initial parameters are generated from two data lists. After the MCMC simulations, the parameter estimates can be saved into a data frame `parm.estimate`. An alternative way to call WinBUGS/OpenBUGS is to use the R package `R2WinBUGS`:

```
library("R2WinBUGS")
data.list<-list(n=n, y=y, x=x, d=d,K=K)
inits<-list(parm.init1, parm.init2)
parm<-c("beta","theta","sigma","p")

BayesianCureModel<-bugs(
 data.list,
 inits,
 model.file="BayesianCureModel.txt",
 parameters.to.save=parm,
 n.chains=2,
 n.iter=20000,
 n.burnin=10000,
 n.thin=2,
 bugs.directory="C:/WinBUGS/winbugs14_full_patched/WinBUGS14",
 working.directory="C:/Cure Model Book/chapter7",
```

```
  codaPkg=TRUE,
  debug=TRUE
)
```

The input data set `data.list` is either a named list with names corresponding to variable names in the model file or a list of the names of the data objects used by the model. The initial value `inits` is a list with `n.chains` elements; each element of the list is itself a list of starting values for the model, or a function creating possibly random initial values. Alternatively, if `inits=NULL`, initial values are generated by WinBUGS. If `inits` is a character vector with `n.chains` elements, it is assumed that `inits` have already been written to the working directory. The vector of parameters `parm` includes the parameters to be monitored. The arguments `n.chain`, `n.iter`, `n.burnin` and `n.thin` are the number of chains, number of MCMC iterations, burn-ins and thinning factors, respectively. Readers are referred to Sturtz et al. (2005) for details.

7.6 Summary

Bayesian analysis of cure models is increasingly used because of the convenience of the MCMC method. In this chapter, we described several extensions and implementation of the mixture and non-mixture cure models. Non-informative or weakly informative priors are used to reduce the impact of priors. We consider using DIC as the goodness-of-fit measure for model selection. For the cure model with latent activation schemes, Cooner et al. (2007) mentioned that the DIC may not be appropriate because that the likelihood function is not log-concave and suggested using the L-measure. Furthermore, it is challenging to determine how to use the covariates in the regression for the parameters in the cure models. In practice, the goodness-of-fit from different models may be very close, and scientific knowledge should be used to guide how to pick the covariates and select the final models.

The Bayesian framework is easy to implement and can be extended to more general situations, e.g., the Bayesian cure model with frailty (de Souza et al., 2017) and Bayesian cure model that accommodates both multiplicative and additive covariates (Nieto-Barajas and Yin, 2009). Bremhorst and Lambert (2016) proposed a flexible estimation method using Bayesian P-splines for cure models.

Recently, the Bayesian methods are increasingly used in clinical trials. For example, informative priors that incorporate historical data or expert opinions are necessary because of limited data. Bayesian design that use historical data may be used for clinical trials for pediatric populations or rare indications with cure rate (Psioda and Ibrahim, 2018). It is of interest to explore how to use power prior to utilize historical data to reduce the number of patients in the control group (Chen et al., 2002).

8

Analysis of Population-Based Cancer Survival Data

8.1 Introduction

Cancer is the second leading cause of death around the globe. The World Health Organization (WHO) estimates that cancer is responsible for approximately 9.8 million deaths in 2018 worldwide and about 1 in 6 deaths are due to cancer. The American Cancer Society (ACS) predicts that there are 1,735,350 new cancer cases diagnosed and 609,640 death due to cancer in the United States in 2018 (Siegel et al., 2018). As the global population age, it is expected that the number of cancer incidences and cancer patients being treated will keep increasing in the coming decades. Over the years, progress in cancer research has led to substantial improvement in cancer prevention, screening and treatment. More cancer patients are living longer and if diagnosed early, some are even cured of cancer.

Cancer data are important resources for public health and medical research. For patients and health care providers, data from a patient's diagnosis and treatment history may provide valuable insight for determining the most effective treatment and survival prognosis. For government agencies and decision-makers, the cancer data and statistics may be used to understand the burden and trends of various cancers, to assess the quality of cancer care, and to measure progress of cancer control and prevention efforts. Cancer registry is an information system designed for the collection, management, and analysis of cancer data for patients who are diagnosed with a malignant or neoplastic cancer. The main missions of a cancer registry include (a) establishing and maintaining of a reporting system for new cancer incidences, (b) serving as an information resource for the investigation of cancer and its causes and (c) providing data for the planning and evaluation of cancer prevention and control efforts.

Several key statistics have been used to measure the impact of cancer on the society. The popular metrics for cancer burden include incidence, mortality, prevalence and survival (Ellis et al., 2014; Kamangar et al., 2006). A cancer incidence is defined as the newly diagnosed cancer case during a specific time period and the incidence rate is usually expressed as the number of cancer incidence cases per 100,000 population at risk. Cancer mortality rate is defined as the number of deaths with cancer as the underlying cause of death during a specific time period, which is also expressed as the number of cancer death per 100,000 population. Cancer prevalence (rate) is defined as the number (proportion) of people alive on a specific date but previously having diagnosis of a certain type of cancer. The prevalent cases include both newly diagnosed cases and pre-existing cases. Cancer survival is typically expressed as the proportion of patients alive at certain time point after the diagnosis of cancer. These cancer statistical metrics are inter-related but distinct measures of cancer burden and progress of cancer treatment. Cancer incidence is the main measure of cancer burden in a population and cancer mortality rates is usually regarded as the best indicator of progress against cancer. Cancer survival is a primary endpoint for evaluating cancer treatment efficacy and an important metric for monitoring and evaluating the progress of cancer control and treatment.

In this chapter, we discuss the analysis of population-based cancer survival data with cure models. In Section 8.2, we describe the population-based cancer registry and survival data, which has different structures and features from the survival data in clinical trials. In Section 8.3, we discuss the popular parametric cure models for analyzing the population-based cancer survival data and describe the implementation of several R packages. In Section 8.4, we present a log-rank test for the existence of statistical cure from the population-based perspective. An example of colorectal cancer survival data is used to estimate the cure rate by gender and cancer stages in Section 8.5.

8.2 Population-Based Cancer Registry and Survival Data

Population-based cancer registries are an essential part of an effective program of cancer control and treatment (Brewster et al., 2005). In comparison to the hospital-based cancer registry, the data collected by the population-based registry serves a wider range of purposes. Data from population-based registries can be used for monitoring the distribution of cancer cases with late diagnosis for which early diagnosis is crucial for better survival and prognosis. Many countries and regions have established population-based cancer registry programs to collect continuous, robust and unbiased cancer data at population level (Bouchardy et al., 2014; Parkin, 2006). For example, SEER Program is supported by the National Cancer Institute in the United States (James and Smith, 2009) and the European Network of Cancer Registries (ENCR) is established within the framework of the Europe Against Cancer Programme of the European Commission, has been in operation since 1990 (Forsea, 2016). At a regional level, the Ontario Cancer Registry (OCR) is a passive, population-based cancer registry that captures diagnostic and demographic information of all incident cases of cancer diagnosed in the province of Ontario, Canada (Hall et al., 2006).

Population-based cancer survival is a key measure of cancer patient care and cancer treatment progress. The optimal method for monitoring and evaluating the effectiveness of cancer treatment and diagnosis can only be achieved by the population-based study of cancer survival. The most commonly used concept in population-based cancer survival studies is the net cancer-specific survival, which is defined as the probability of surviving cancer in the absence of other competing causes of death, e.g., cardiovascular diseases or Alzheimer's disease. The measure of net survival is not influenced by changes in mortality from other causes and, therefore, provides a useful measure for cancer survival trends across time, and comparisons between racial-ethnic groups or between registries. Another commonly used concept is the overall survival, which, unlike the cancer-specific survival, uses death due to any causes as the event of interest.

There are two types of measures for net survival: cause-specific survival and relative survival (Cronin and Feuer, 2000; Schaffar et al., 2015, 2017). Cause-specific survival is calculated by specifying the cause of death, where patients who die of causes other than cancer of interest are considered to be censored. Although detailed medical records may be available to ascertain the cause of death information in clinical trials, the cause of death in population-based survival data is primarily based the death certificate, thus, is often unreliable or not available. Therefore, cause-specific survival is much less appealing in population-based cancer survival analysis. The other measure of net survival, i.e., relative survival, is often used as a better alternative. Relative survival is calculated as the ratio of the observed overall survival of the cancer patients to the expected survival from the comparable cancer-free population. The expected survival is estimated from the general population life tables defined by sex, single calendar year and single year of age, for each country. Even though relative survival might not be directly relevant from a patient's perspective, it is particularly useful for studying temporal trends in cancer patient survival and comparing populations where expected survival may vary, which is important from a public health perspective.

Let $S_O(t)$ be the observed overall survival function for the cancer patients and $S_E(t)$ be the expected survival function in a cancer-free group in the general population that is comparable to the cancer patients with respect to age, sex, calendar year and possible other covariates. The relative survival function is calculated as

$$S(t) = S_O(t)/S_E(t). \tag{8.1}$$

The relative survival function $S(t)$ can be interpreted as the proportion of patients who would have survived up to time t if the cancer of interest is the only possible cause of death. It is easy to see that the overall survival can be written as $S_O(t) = S_E(t)S(t)$, which implies that the overall survival is the result of two independent competing risks of deaths due to cancer of

TABLE 8.1
A random sample of 10 patients of the individually-listed colorectal cancer survival data.

Sex	Year of diagnosis	AJCC Stage	Survival Time (month)	Event	Expected Hazard
Male	2005	III	129	0	0.0412
Female	2010	I	61	0	0.0611
Female	2004	IV	18	1	0.0030
Male	2009	III	81	0	0.0564
Female	2009	II	77	0	0.0112
Male	2009	III	14	1	0.0896
Male	2005	IV	62	1	0.0309
Male	2005	I	126	1	0.0060
Female	2010	IV	3	1	0.2969
Male	2008	II	13	1	0.0068

interest and other causes. The relative survival function can be modeled as the parametric or semiparametric survival models or the cure models described in early chapters.

Let

$$\lambda_O(t) = -\frac{d\log S_O(t)}{dt}, \lambda_E(t) = -\frac{d\log S_E(t)}{dt} \text{ and } \lambda(t) = -\frac{d\log S(t)}{dt}$$

be the corresponding hazard functions for the deaths due to any causes, cancer of interest and other causes. Equation (8.1) implies an additive hazards model. That is, the overall hazard $\lambda_O(t)$ of the cancer patients is the sum of the expected hazard $\lambda_E(t)$ and the excess hazard $\lambda(t)$ associated with a diagnosis of the cancer:

$$\lambda_O(t) = \lambda_E(t) + \lambda(t). \tag{8.2}$$

The additive hazards model is the commonly used model for the population-based survival analysis (Hakulinen and Tenkanen, 1987; Dickman et al., 2004).

The population-based cancer survival data are usually organized into two types of format, i.e., individually-listed survival data or grouped survival data. When survival times and covariates are available for each individual, the data format is called individually-listed or case-listing survival data. Suppose that there are n subjects diagnosed with cancer of interest. The individually-listed survival data with expected hazard rates are denoted by $(t_i, \delta_i, \boldsymbol{x}_i, \lambda_{Ei})$ for the ith subject, where t_i is the overall survival time for any causes, δ_i is the indicator of death, $\boldsymbol{x}_i$ is the vector of covariates and λ_{Ei} is the expected hazard rate of dying at time t_i from any causes if the subject is cancer free. Table 8.1 shows the individually-listed survival data for a random sample of 10 colorectal cancer patients diagnosed in the year 2004 from the SEER program.

For the patient with covariates $\boldsymbol{x}$, let $S_O(t|\boldsymbol{x}), S_E(t|\boldsymbol{x})$ and $S(t|\boldsymbol{x})$ be the overall survival function, expected survival function and relative survival function, respectively. Let $f_O(t|\boldsymbol{x}), f_E(t|\boldsymbol{x})$ and $f(t|\boldsymbol{x})$ be the corresponding density functions. The likelihood function for the individually-listed relative survival data can be written as

$$L(\boldsymbol{\theta}) = \prod_{i=1}^{n} \left\{ f_O(t_i|\boldsymbol{x}_i)^{\delta_i} S_O(t_i|\boldsymbol{x}_i)^{1-\delta_i} \right\}, \tag{8.3}$$

where $\boldsymbol{\theta}$ is a vector of the parameters in the model for the relative survival. Since

$$f_O(t|\boldsymbol{x}) = -\frac{dS_O(t|\boldsymbol{x})}{dt} = -\frac{d\{S(t|\boldsymbol{x})S_E(t|\boldsymbol{x})\}}{dt} = S_E(t|\boldsymbol{x})f(t|\boldsymbol{x}) + f_E(t|\boldsymbol{x})S(t|\boldsymbol{x})$$

and $\lambda_E(t|\boldsymbol{x}) = f_E(t|\boldsymbol{x})/S_E(t|\boldsymbol{x})$, the likelihood function in (8.3) can be expressed as

$$L(\boldsymbol{\theta}) \propto \prod_{i=1}^{n} \left\{ \left[\lambda_E(t_i|\boldsymbol{x}_i) S(t_i|x_i) + f(t_i|\boldsymbol{x}_i) \right]^{\delta_i} S(t_i|\boldsymbol{x}_i)^{1-\delta_i} \right\},$$

where the expected hazard for the ith individual $\lambda_E(t_i|\boldsymbol{x}_i) = \lambda_{Ei}$ is a known constant from the life tables. In Table 8.1, the expected hazards for the colorectal cancer patients are shown in the last column.

Because the population-based cancer survival data may consist of records for thousands or even millions of patients, the survival times are usually grouped or rounded into discrete intervals $I_j = [t_{j-1}, t_j), j = 1, ..., J$ where $t_0 = 0$ and t_J is the time of the end of follow-up. For the convenience of reporting and analysis, the intervals are usually equally spaced, e.g., monthly or annual intervals. The cancer population are first stratified by patient characteristics (covariates) like race, sex, historical stage etc. For each stratum, the survival data are then organized into a life table (Spika et al., 2017). For the interval I_j, the number of subjects alive in the beginning of interval is denoted by n_j, the number of deaths due to any causes during the interval is denoted as d_j and the number of subjects lost to followup is denoted as l_j. Based on actuarial assumption, the adjusted number of people at risk in the beginning of interval I_j is $r_j = n_j - 0.5l_j$. A sample of grouped survival data for patients diagnosed with AJCC stage IV colorectal cancer are shown in Table 8.2. For grouped survival data, the nonparametric estimates of relative survival function have been describe by Cronin and Feuer (2000).

We assume that the number of deaths due to any causes, d_{xj} at interval I_j in the stratum with covariates $\boldsymbol{x}$, follows a binomial distribution, i.e.,

$$d_{\boldsymbol{x}j} \sim \text{Binomial}(r_{\boldsymbol{x}j}, p_j(\boldsymbol{x})),$$

where

$$p_j(\boldsymbol{x}) = P(t < t_j | t \geq t_{j-1}, \boldsymbol{x}) = 1 - \frac{S_O(t_j|\boldsymbol{x})}{S_O(t_{j-1}|\boldsymbol{x})} = 1 - \frac{S_E(t_j|\boldsymbol{x})S(t_j|\boldsymbol{x})}{S_E(t_{j-1}|\boldsymbol{x})S(t_{j-1}|\boldsymbol{x})}$$

TABLE 8.2
Group survival data for AJCC stage IV colorectal cancer patients diagnosed in the year 2004.

		Alive		Lost to	Observed Survival %		Expected Survival %		Relative Survival %	
Sex	Interval	at start	Died	Followup	Interval	Cumulative	Interval	Cumulative	Interval	Cumulative
M	1	2968	1465	8	50.6	50.6	96.7	96.7	52.3	52.3
	2	1495	581	6	61.1	30.9	97.6	94.4	62.5	32.7
	3	908	339	1	62.6	19.3	97.8	92.3	64.1	21.0
	4	568	181	0	68.1	13.2	97.9	90.4	69.6	14.6
	5	387	106	2	72.5	9.6	97.7	88.2	74.3	10.8
	6	279	49	0	82.4	7.9	97.4	86.0	84.6	9.2
	7	230	31	3	86.4	6.8	97.3	83.6	88.9	8.1
	8	196	22	2	88.7	6.0	97.1	81.2	91.4	7.4
	9	172	29	0	83.1	5.0	96.9	78.6	85.8	6.4
	10	143	9	3	93.6	4.7	96.8	76.1	96.7	6.2
	11	131	7	5	94.6	4.4	96.8	73.7	97.7	6.0
F	1	2752	1460	10	46.9	46.9	96.6	96.6	48.5	48.5
	2	1282	495	2	61.4	28.7	98.0	94.7	62.6	30.4
	3	785	262	1	66.6	19.1	98.1	93.0	67.9	20.6
	4	522	145	3	72.1	13.8	98.1	91.2	73.6	15.2
	5	374	96	1	74.3	10.3	97.9	89.3	75.9	11.5
	6	277	46	3	83.3	8.5	97.7	87.3	85.2	9.8
	7	228	28	0	87.7	7.5	97.7	85.3	89.8	8.8
	8	200	21	0	89.5	6.7	97.6	83.2	91.7	8.1
	9	179	10	6	94.3	6.3	97.5	81.1	96.7	7.8
	10	163	9	2	94.4	6.0	97.4	79.0	97.0	7.6
	11	152	7	10	95.2	5.7	97.2	76.8	98.0	7.4

is the probability of death from any causes. Assuming constant hazard within each interval, the interval expected survival probabilities

$$E_j(\boldsymbol{x}) = S_E(t_j|\boldsymbol{x})/S_E(t_{j-1}|\boldsymbol{x}) = 1 - \exp\left\{-\lambda_{Ej}(t_j - t_{j-1})\right\}.$$

The values of $E_j(\boldsymbol{x})$ are known constants from the life tables. The observed data for grouped relative survival data consist of $\{\boldsymbol{x}, d_{\boldsymbol{x}j}, r_{\boldsymbol{x}j}, E_j(\boldsymbol{x}), j = 1, ..., J\}$. The likelihood function can be written as

$$L(\boldsymbol{\theta}) = \prod_{\boldsymbol{x}} \prod_{j=1}^{J} \left\{ p_j(\boldsymbol{x})^{d_{\boldsymbol{x}j}} (1 - p_j(\boldsymbol{x}))^{r_{\boldsymbol{x}j} - d_{\boldsymbol{x}j}} \right\}. \tag{8.4}$$

In fact, this is a special type survival data with both interval and right censoring. Let

$$m_{\boldsymbol{x}j} = \begin{cases} r_{\boldsymbol{x}j} - (r_{\boldsymbol{x},j+1} + d_{\boldsymbol{x},j+1}) = \frac{1}{2}(l_{\boldsymbol{x}j} + l_{\boldsymbol{x},j+1}) & \text{if } j < J \\ r_{\boldsymbol{x}J} & \text{if } j = J \end{cases} \tag{8.5}$$

be the number of subjects interval-censored in during interval I_j. Then the likelihood function in (8.4) can be written as

$$L(\boldsymbol{\theta}) \propto \prod_{\boldsymbol{x}} \prod_{j=1}^{J} \left\{ S(t_j|\boldsymbol{x})^{m_{\boldsymbol{x}j}} \left[S(t_{j-1}|\boldsymbol{x}) - S(t_j|\boldsymbol{x}) E_j(\boldsymbol{x}) \right]^{d_{\boldsymbol{x}j}} \right\}. \tag{8.6}$$

8.3 Parametric Cure Models for Net Survival

For many cancers, if the patients are diagnosed in early stages and treated successfully, they may become long-term survivors and eventually being cured from cancer. From the perspective of population-based survival, the mortality of the subgroup with long-term survival may experience the same mortality rate as in general cancer-free population, i.e, the excess hazard $\lambda(t)$ in equation (8.2) is equal to zero after some time point. This group of patients are considered being "statistically cured". This is a population-level definition of cure and does not necessarily imply that the cancer is eradicated in their bodies. One of the most often used cure models in population-based cancer studies is the mixture cure model (Yu et al., 2004a; Lambert et al., 2010) discussed in Section 2.2. When incorporating relative survival, the overall survival function from the mixture cure model can be written as

$$S(t|\boldsymbol{x}) = \pi_c(\boldsymbol{x}) + (1 - \pi_c(\boldsymbol{x}))S_u(t|\boldsymbol{x}), \tag{8.7}$$

where π_c is the proportion of the patients being cured, while the remainder, $1 - \pi_c(\boldsymbol{x})$, are uncured and $S_u(t|\boldsymbol{x})$ is the cancer-specific survival function for the uncured patients. Note that we use the notation $\pi_c(\boldsymbol{x}) = 1 - \pi(\boldsymbol{x})$ for cure fraction, where $\pi(\boldsymbol{x})$ is the proportion of non-cured patients in Equation (2.1). A parametric distribution, e.g., a Weibull distribution, may be used for $S_u(t|\boldsymbol{x})$ (Ying and Heitjan, 2008; Cancho et al., 2012).

Another parametric cure model used in population-based cancer studies is the non-mixture cure model (Tsodikov, 1998a, 2001) discussed in Section 2.4, which estimates an asymptote for the survival function as the cure proportion. The survival function for the non-mixture model can be written as

$$S(t|\boldsymbol{x}) = \pi_c(\boldsymbol{x})^{F^H(t|\boldsymbol{x})} \tag{8.8}$$

where $\pi_c(\boldsymbol{x})$ is the cure rate and $F^H(t|\boldsymbol{x})$ is a proper distribution function, as for the mixture model, a Weibull, extended Gamma or generalized F distribution can be used for $F^H(t|\boldsymbol{x})$.

8.3.1 Flexible Parametric Survival Model

By integrating equation (8.2), we obtain that

$$\Lambda_O(t) = \Lambda_E(t) + \Lambda(t) \tag{8.9}$$

where $\Lambda_O(t) = \int_0^t \lambda_O(u)du$ is the overall cumulative hazard, $\lambda_E(t) = \int_0^t \lambda_E(u)du$ the expected cumulative hazard and $\Lambda(t) = \int_0^t \lambda(u)du$ is the cumulative excess hazard. Andersson et al. (2011) and Andersson and Lambert (2012) proposed a class of flexible parametric survival models for the logarithm of the cumulative excess hazard based on restricted cubic spline functions:

$$\log\{\Lambda(t)\} = R(r, \delta_0) = \delta_{00} + \delta_{01}v_1(r) + \cdots + \delta_{0,J-1}v_{J-1}(r), \tag{8.10}$$

where $r = \log(t)$, J is the number of knots and $v_1(r), ..., v_J(r)$ are the basis functions with $v_j(r)$ defined as

$$v_j(r) = \begin{cases} r & j = 1 \\ (r-\tau_j)_+^3 - \rho_j(r-\tau_1)_+^3 - (1-\rho_j)(r-\tau_J)_+^3 & j = 2, ..., J-1 \end{cases},$$

where $u_+ = \max(0, u)$ and $\tau_1, ..., \tau_J$ are the locations of the knots, and $\rho_j = (\tau_J - \tau_j)/(\tau_J - \tau_0)$. Because the cumulative excess hazard $\Lambda(t)$ is a relatively stable function compared to the instantaneous hazard function $\lambda(t)$, the estimates for the log cumulative excess hazard scale instead of the log excess hazard scale tend to have less variability.

Up to the first knot, all spline variables except v_1 are zero, so the log cumulative excess hazard is forced to be linear before first knot τ_1. A vector of covariates $\boldsymbol{x} = (x_1, ..., x_p)$ may be included for the modeling of $\Lambda(t)$, where

$$\log \Lambda(t|\boldsymbol{x}) = R(t, \delta_0) + \boldsymbol{\beta}'\boldsymbol{x}. \tag{8.11}$$

This is a proportional hazards model for the excess hazards $\Lambda(t)$. Non-proportional excess hazards models with time-dependent covariate effects are also popular in population-based cancer studies and can be implemented by including interactions between covariates and splines for time. Since the time-dependent effects usually do not require as many knots as the baseline cumulative excess hazard, new spline parameters may be used for each time-dependent effect, and separate knot positions can be chosen for each new covariate with a time-dependent effect. Let $\boldsymbol{z} = (z_1, ..., z_q)$ be the vector of time-dependent covariates. The inclusion of time dependent covariates $\boldsymbol{z}$ yields the model

$$\log \Lambda(t|\boldsymbol{x}, \boldsymbol{z}) = R(t, \delta_0) + \boldsymbol{\beta}^{'}\boldsymbol{x} + \sum_{i=1}^{q} R(r, \delta_i) z_i, \tag{8.12}$$

where q is the number of time-dependent covariate effects, and the spline function for the ith time-dependent effect $R(r, \delta_i)$ can be defined similar as equation (8.10). Above flexible parametric models do not explicitly include the cure component, but they provide a basis for the flexible parametric cure model.

8.3.2 Flexible Parametric Cure Model

The statistical cure is reached when the excess hazard rate is zero and hence, the cumulative excess hazard will be constant after this time. By forcing the log cumulative excess hazard in the flexible parametric survival model to not only be linear but also to have zero slope after the last knot, the model explicitly allows the estimation of cure rate. The model can be formulated by calculating the spline variables "backwards", treating the knots in reversed order, and set the restriction that the linear spline variable be zero. The basis spline functions for the flexible parametric cure model are defined as

$$v_j(r) = (\tau_{J-j} - r)_+^3 - \rho_j(\tau_J - r)_+^3 - (1 - \rho_j)(\tau_1 - r)_+^3, j = 1, ..., J - 1, \tag{8.13}$$

where $\rho_j = (\tau_{J-j} - \tau_1)/(\tau_J - \tau_1)$. The relative survival function from the flexible parametric survival model, with splines calculated backwards and with restriction on the parameter for the linear spline variable ($\delta_{01} = 0$) is defined as

$$S(t) = \exp\left\{-\exp\left(\delta_{00} + \delta_{02}v_2(r) + \cdots + \delta_{0,J-1}v_{J-1}(r)\right)\right\}. \tag{8.14}$$

Let $F^H(t) = \exp\left(\delta_{02}v_2(r) + \cdots + \delta_{0,J-1}v_{J-1}(r)\right)$. The flexible parametric cure model can be seen as a special case of a non-mixture cure model with the cure probability π_c and

$$S(t) = \pi_c^{F^H(t)},$$

where $\pi_c = \exp(-\exp(\delta_{00}))$. The flexible parametric cure model can be written as a proportional excess hazards model when there is no time-dependent effect. Fixed covariates $\boldsymbol{x}$ are included in the cure probability as

$$\pi_c(\boldsymbol{x}) = \exp(-\exp(\delta_{00} + \boldsymbol{x}^{'}\boldsymbol{\beta})).$$

This is a special case of the non-mixture cure model with complimentary log-log link function for the cure probability. In general, time-dependent covariates $\boldsymbol{z}$ can also be included in Equation (8.14). The relative survival function can be written as

$$S(t|\boldsymbol{x}, \boldsymbol{z}) = \exp\{-\Lambda(t|\boldsymbol{x}, \boldsymbol{z})\}, \tag{8.15}$$

where $\Lambda(t|\boldsymbol{x}, \boldsymbol{z})$ is defined as equation (8.12). The constraint of a zero effect for the linear spline term has to be incorporated for each spline function $R(r, \delta_i)$. All spline variables take the value 0 from the point of the last knot τ_J, which means that the constant parameter δ_{00} is the log cumulative excess hazard at and beyond the last knot for the reference group with $\boldsymbol{x} = \boldsymbol{z} = 0$, and can therefore be used to estimate the cure rate. Andersson et al. (2011) recommended using orthogonal splines, e.g., Gram-Schmidt orthogonalization, around the last knot. The orthogonalization allows direct predictions of cure from the constant parameters. All parameters are estimated using maximum likelihood estimation on individual level data (Lambert and Royston, 2009). The latency survival function for uncured patients can be estimated in the same way as for the non-mixture cure model discussed in Section 2.4.1, and the median survival time for the uncured can be estimated using a Newton-Raphson algorithm in a similar way as Lambert (2007).

8.3.3 Software Implementations

The mixture cure model of grouped survival data has been implemented in a stand-alone software CANSURV (Yu et al., 2005). The R packages of fitting cure model for individually-listed relative survival data include `rstpm2` and `flexsurvcure`. The `flexsurvcure` package was discussed in Section 2.6 and it fits the parametric cure models. `rstpm2` fits the flexible parametric cure models. Both the parametric cure models and flexible cure models are popular for modeling population-based survival data. However, there are some differences in the actual model specifications. The usual parametric cure model considers only fully parametric models, e.g., Weibull, lognormal etc, while the flexible parametric cure model uses restricted spline functions to estimate the cumulative hazard function for the latency distribution for the uncured patients. The flexible cure models only use the complimentary log-log link function for cure rate, while the parametric cure models may use both logistic or complimentary log-log link functions. For the mixture cure model, fixed covariates can be included in both the incidence and latency components of the mixture cure model because the two components have distinct clinical meanings. For the non-mixture cure model, fixed covariates are typically used in the cure rate only.

The R package `rstpm2` implements the generalized survival models (Liu et al., 2017, 2018b), where $g(S(t|x)) = \eta(t, x)$ for a link function g, survival $S(t)$ at time t with covariates $\boldsymbol{x}$ and a linear predictor $\eta(t, x)$. It can be used to fit the flexible parametric cure model as described in Section 8.3.2. The main function for fitting the generalized survival models are `stpm2` for parametric models possibly with clustered data, and `pstpm2` for penalized models with the option of clustered data as well (Clements and Liu, 2019). The syntax for `stpm2` is:

```
stpm2(formula, data, smooth.formula = NULL, df = 3, tvc = NULL,
     link.type=c("PH","PO","probit","AH","AO"), theta.AO=0,
     bhazard = NULL, robust = FALSE, cluster = NULL,
     frailty = !is.null(cluster) & !robust,
     RandDist=c("Gamma","LogN"),
     ...)
```

The `formula` includes a `Surv` object on the left-hand side and covariates other than the time variable on the right-hand side. The penalized function is not included in `pstpm2`. The time effects can be specified in several ways, among which the most general way is to use `smooth.formula`. This specification may include interactions between time and covariates. For example, `smooth.formula=~nsx(log(time),df=3)+x:nsx(log(time),df=2)` specifies a baseline natural spline smoother of the `log(time)` with three degrees of freedom, with an interaction between a covariate `x` and a natural spline smoother of `log(time)` with `df=2`. In addition, one may use `smooth.formula=~x:log(time)` for a log-linear interaction between a covariate `x` and `log(time)`.

The type of the link function is specified with the `link.type` argument. The link functions include the complimentary log-log link for the PH model, the logit link for the PO model, the probit link, the log link for the additive hazards (denoted as AH in the program, which is different from AH used elsewhere in this book) model and the the general Aranda-Ordaz (AO) link function (Aranda-Ordaz, 1981). The AO link function is specified as

$$g(\mu) = \log\left(\frac{\mu^{-\theta_{AO}} - 1}{\theta_{AO}}\right).$$

This link functions include the logit and complimentary log-log links as special cases and are widely used for proportions. For the AO link, the fixed value of ψ is specified using the `theta.AO` argument. For relative survival, a vector for the baseline hazards can be specified using the `bhazard` argument. A vector for the clusters can be specified with the `cluster` argument. The calculation of robust standard errors can be specified with the `robust=TRUE` argument. If the `robust` option is FALSE, then a frailty or random effects model is used, with either a default Gamma `RandDist="Gamma"` or a normal `RandDist="LogN"` frailty.

The default specification for the additive hazards model is

```
rstpm2(Surv(time,event)~x, data=data, link.type="AH")
```

If natural splines are used for the baseline time effect and a constant hazard for a unit change is assumed in the covariate x, an equivalent specification is

```
stpm2(Surv(time,event)~1, data=data, link.type="AH",
     smooth.formula=~nsx(time,df=3)+x:time)
```

where there is default smoother for time and an interaction between linear `x` and linear `time`. The regression coefficient for `x:time` can be interpreted as the additive rate for a unit change in `x`. The syntax for fitting the penalized models with `pstpm2` is very similar. For details, see Clements (2019).

Another R package for fitting parametric cure models is `flexsurvcure`, which is as a wrapper around `flexsurvreg` (Jackson, 2016). For a parametric mixture cure model, it is assumed that the cured subjects experience no excess mortality compared to the background mortality of cancer-free population and the excess mortality for the remaining individuals is modeled by parametric models. By contrast, a parametric non-mixture model rescales an existing parametric distribution such that the probability of net survival approaches the cure fraction as time approaches infinity. The syntax of using the `flexsurvcure` function is

```
flexsurvcure(formula, data, weights, bhazard, subset, dist,
             na.action, link = "logistic", mixture = T, ...)
```

The `formula` specifies the association between covariates and a survival object `Surv`. The `Surv` objects may include `right, counting, interval1` or `interval2` censored survival data. When there are no covariates, one may simply use `Surv(time, dead) ~ 1`. By default, covariates are placed on the `theta` parameter of the distribution, representing the cure fraction, through a linear model with a selected link function. Covariates can be placed on parameters of the base distribution by using the name of the parameter as a `function` in the formula. For example, in a Weibull model, the following expresses the `scale` parameter in terms of `age` and `stage`, and the `shape` parameter in terms of `sex` and `stage`:

```
Surv(time, dead) ~ age + stage + shape(sex) + shape(stage)
```

However, if the names of some ancillary parameters clash with any potential functions in the formulae, e.g., `I()`, or `factor()`, then those functions will not work in the formula. Alternatively, the safer way to include covariates in ancillary parameters is to use the `anc` argument to `flexsurvreg`. Note that unlike the function `survreg`, the function `strata()` is ignored in the function `flexsurvcure`, so that any covariates surrounded by `strata()` are applied to the location parameter.

The `data` argument specifies the data set including covariates and time and censoring variables. If not given, the variables should be in the working environment. `weights` and `bhazard` are optional variables for case weights and expected hazards for relative survival models, respectively. The `subset` argument is a logical vector specifying the subset of `data`. The `dist` specifies the latency distributions, which include `gengamma`, `genf`, `weibull`, `lnorm` etc. For details, see the manual for R package `flexsurv`. `na.action` is a missing data filter function and `link` is a string representing the link function to use for the cure fraction with the default `logistic`. The `mixture` argument takes the value of `TRUE/FALSE` to specify whether a mixture model should be fitted with default `TRUE`. The other augment to be passed to `flexsurvreg` can be specified using `...`.

8.4 Testing the Existence of Statistical Cure

When relative survival is used as the measure of net survival, the cure rate is defined as proportion of cancer patients who have similar survival experience with the general cancer-free population. For cancers that are curable, the relative survival curve often appears to reach a plateau with sufficient follow-up time. This plateau implies that relative survival is close to or even greater than 1. In other words, the excess hazard rate due to cancer is close to 0. At the point from which the cancer patients no longer experience excess mortality, we refer to the group as being "statistically cured". It is important to note that this definition of cure is from a population perspective, and it does not provide information on an individual's cure status. An individual may be considered "medically cured" if cancer is eradicated from his or her body. However, it is difficult to confirm medical cure and such information is unavailable in population-based cancer studies. Thus, in the analysis considered here, we are only interested in statistical cure from a population perspective.

Based on the mixture cure model, Maller and Zhou (1996) derived a likelihood ratio test to examine the existence of cure. The asymptotic null distribution of the likelihood-ratio test statistic takes a 50-50 mixture of a chi-squared distribution and the probability mass at zero when the latency distribution for uncured patients has a gamma distribution. Peng et al. (2001) examined the performance of the test under different parametric assumptions for the latency distribution. The likelihood ratio test of cure is most appropriate when a substantial number of subjects are censored toward the end of the study so that the survival curve reaches a plateau. Detailed discussions of the tests can be found in Section 6.2.

In the context of cancer survival, the likelihood ratio test requires accurate information on cause of death, so that deaths due to causes other than the cancer of interest are not attributed to cancer and thus treated as censored. In addition, the likelihood-ratio test is based on a parametric assumption of the latency distribution. When the underlying latency distribution is misspecified, the test may have an erroneous type I error rate (Peng and Zhang, 2008a). In this section, we briefly describe a nonparametric one-sample log-rank test for population-based relative survival data (Yu, 2012). The goal of the test is to examine whether the survival of cancer patients is non-inferior (equivalent) to that of the general population within a prespecified non-inferiority margin.

8.4.1 Testing Hypothesis of Non-Inferiority of Survival

We consider one sample survival data without stratification or covariate $\boldsymbol{x}$. As described in Section 8.2, the population-based survival data are usually organized as life tables. For the jth intervals $I_j = [t_{j-1}, t_j)$, the relative survival data consist of $\{(n_j, d_j, l_j, E_j), j = 1, ..., J\}$, where n_j is the number of people alive at the beginning of interval I_j, d_j is the number of patients dying from all causes, l_j is the number of patients lost to follow-up during interval I_j and $E_j = S_E(t_j)/S_E(t_{j-1})$ is the expected survival probability during interval I_j. Let $r_j = n_j - 0.5l_j$ be the number of subject at risk during interval I_j based on the actuarial assumption and p_j be the probability of dying during interval I_j given that a patient is alive at the beginning of interval I_j and can be calculated as

$$p_j = P(T < t_j | T \geq t_{j-1}) = 1 - \frac{S_O(t_j)}{S_O(t_{j-1})}, \quad j = 1, ..., J. \tag{8.16}$$

Let $p_j^E = 1 - E_j$ be the expected probability of death from all causes for the cancer-free population. Then the excess probability of death due to cancer is $p_j - p_j^E$. Survival of cancer patients is supposed to be inferior to that of the cancer-free population, so it is expected that $p_j \geq p_j^E$. Hence, the existence of cure implies the non-inferiority of the survival of cancer patients within a prespecified margin Δ.

Let $p_j^\Delta = p_j^E + \Delta$ be the expected hazard within the non-inferiority margin Δ. We may consider a one-sided non-inferiority hypothesis

$$H_0 : p_j \geq p_j^\Delta \text{ for all } j \quad \text{vs } H_1 : p_j < p_j^\Delta, \text{ for } j \geq \tau, \tag{8.17}$$

where τ is the time when the excess mortality is below the non-inferiority margin Δ. Usually Δ is a small positive value that defines a clinically meaningful difference in survival. When $\Delta = 0$, rejecting the null hypothesis means that the survival of cancer patients is the same as that of the cancer-free population, which implies the existence of statistical cure. In order to guarantee that survival is non-inferior to the survival of the cancer-free population after τ, a sufficient condition is that the hazard rates of cancer death after diagnosis of cancer are non-increasing after τ. This assumption is reasonable based on the follow-up time of 30 years from the SEER survival data (Howlader et al., 2011) as the majority of cancer cases are diagnosed after the age of 45 and the life expectancy is about 80 years.

8.4.2 A Minimum Version of One-Sample Log-Rank Test

Because the hypothesis testing depends on the unknown τ, the resulting null and alternative hypotheses are not fixed. Therefore, the intended hypothesis testing is different from the traditional one. Here we describe a minimum version of a one-sample log-rank test for testing the non-inferiority of survival.

One sample log-rank test (Gail and Ware, 1979; Woolson, 1981) has been used to compare the survival of a cohort with a known survival curve. The test statistic is given by

$$T_1 = \frac{\sum_{j=1}^{J}(d_j - D_j)}{\sqrt{\sum_{j=1}^{J} v_j}}, \tag{8.18}$$

where $D_j = r_j p_j^{\Delta}$ is the expected number of deaths under the null hypothesis of non-inferiority during interval I_j and $v_j = r_j p_j^{\Delta}(1 - p_j^{\Delta})$. For a large sample size, the log-rank statistic T_1 follows a standard normal distribution. Sposto et al. (1997) proposed a partially grouped log-rank test for continuous survival data to examine the equivalence of two survival distributions after a known cutoff time τ. The proposed test is a one-sided test where the alternative hypothesis is that the survival of cancer patients is worse than that of the cancer-free population, while the null hypothesis is that the cancer patient's survival is non-inferior to that for the general population within a prespecified margin after an unknown cutoff time.

The usual log-rank test assigns equal weight to each interval. Suppose that differences in survival between cancer patients and the general population begin to diminish after some initial time period and then remain a small positive value. Because our focus is on the equivalence of survival in the late periods, it would be ideal to give relatively more weight to the differences in the late periods. As we expect that cancer patients tend to have excess mortality rate in early time after diagnosis, no weight should be given to the events during the initial period.

Let $U_j = d_j - D_j, j = 1, ..., J$, $L_k = \sum_{j=k}^{J} U_j$ and $V_k = \sum_{j=k}^{J} v_j$. The log-rank statistics after excluding the survival data in the first $k - 1$ intervals are defined as

$$T_k = \frac{L_k}{\sqrt{V_k}} = \frac{\sum_{j=k}^{J}(d_j - D_j)}{\sqrt{\sum_{j=k}^{J} v_j}}, k = 1, ..., J. \tag{8.19}$$

We have the following two propositions regarding to the joint distribution of $(T_1, ..., T_J)$ under the null and alternative hypothesis.

Theorem 8.4.1 *Under the null hypothesis of inferior survival, the asymptotic joint distribution of the log-rank test statistics is multivariate normal (MVN), i.e.,* $(T_1, ..., T_J)' \sim MVN(\mathbf{0}, \mathbf{\Sigma})$, *where the* (k, l) *element of the covariance matrix* $\sigma_{kl} = \sqrt{V_l / V_k}$ *for* $k < l$.

Proof 8.4.1 *Under the null hypothesis of inferiority of survival for all intervals, the log-rank statistic* L_k *has an asymptotic normal distribution with mean 0 and variance* $V_k = \sum_{j=k}^{J} v_j, j = 1, ..., J$. *As linear combinations of* L_1, ..., L_J, *the joint distribution for the test statistics* $T_1, ..., T_J$ *is MVN and the* *marginal distributions are standard normal. Because* $U_1, ..., U_J$ *are mutually independent, the covariance of* L_k *and* L_l *for* $k > l$ *is*

$$\begin{aligned} Cov(L_k, L_l) &= Cov\left(\sum_{j=l}^{J} U_j, \sum_{j=k}^{J} U_j\right) = Cov\left(\sum_{j=l}^{J} U_j, \sum_{j=k}^{l-1} U_j + \sum_{j=l}^{J} U_j\right) \\ &= Var(L_l) = V_l. \end{aligned}$$

Therefore, the asymptotic covariance between T_k *and* T_l *is*

$$\sigma_{kl} = Cov(T_k, T_l) = Cov\left(\frac{L_k}{\sqrt{V_k}}, \frac{L_l}{\sqrt{V_l}}\right) = \frac{V_l}{\sqrt{V_k V_l}} = \sqrt{V_l / V_k}.$$

Theorem 8.4.2 *Let* $\mu_k^* = \sum_{j=k}^{J} r_j (p_j - p_j^{\Delta})$, $v_j^* = r_j p_j (1 - p_j)$ *and* $V_k^* = \sum_{j=k}^{J} v_j^*$. *Under the alternative hypothesis* $H_1 : p_j < p_j^{\Delta}$ *for* $j \geq \tau$, *the asymptotic joint distribution of the test statistics* $(T_1, ..., T_J)' \sim MVN(\boldsymbol{\mu}^*, \boldsymbol{\Sigma}^*)$, *where* $\boldsymbol{\mu}^* = (\mu_1^* / \sqrt{V_1^*}, ..., \mu_J^* / \sqrt{V_J^*})$ *and* $\boldsymbol{\Sigma}^*$ *is the covariance matrix with* (k, l) *entry* $\sigma_{kl}^* = V_l^* / \sqrt{V_k V_l}$.

Proof 8.4.2 *Under the alternative hypothesis, the expectation and variance for the number of deaths at interval* j *are* $D_j^* = r_j p_j$ *and* $v_j^* = r_j p_j (1 - p_j)$. *The log-rank statistic* L_k *has an asymptotic normal distribution with mean* $\mu_k^* = \sum_{j=k}^{J} (D_j^* - D_j)$ *and variance* $V_k^* = \sum_{j=k}^{J} v_j^*$. *Therefore, the test statistic* T_k

$$T_k = \frac{L_k}{\sqrt{V_k}} = \frac{L_k - \mu_j^*}{\sqrt{V_k^*}} \sqrt{\frac{V_k^*}{V_k}} + \frac{\mu_j^*}{\sqrt{V_k}} \sim N\left(\frac{\mu_j^*}{\sqrt{V_k}}, \frac{V_k^*}{V_k}\right).$$

Similar to the covariance under the null hypothesis in Theorem 8.4.1, the covariance between L_k *and* L_l *for* $k < l$ *can be calculated as*

$$Cov(L_k, L_l) = Var(L_l) = V_l^*.$$

Therefore, the covariance between T_k *and* T_l *for* $k < l$ *is*

$$Cov(T_k, T_l) = Cov\left(\frac{L_k}{\sqrt{V_k}}, \frac{L_l}{\sqrt{V_l}}\right) = \frac{V_l^*}{\sqrt{V_k V_l}}.$$

Based on the definition of T_k in (8.19), a negative value of T_k means that the observed survival for the cancer patients is better than that for the general population. If survival of cancer patients is indeed noninferior to that for the general population, it is expected that the minimum of $T_1, ..., T_j$ should be smaller than a threshold value after a certain period of time. Therefore, the test statistic for the non-inferiority of survival can be defined as the minimum of the log-rank test statistics

$$T = \min(T_1, ..., T_J). \tag{8.20}$$

Based on the MVN distribution for $(T_1, ..., T_J)$ specified in Theorem 8.4.1, the p-value of the non-inferiority test of survival is calculated as

$$p = \mathrm{P}[\min(T_1, ..., T_J) < t] = 1 - \mathrm{P}(T_1 \geq t, ..., T_J \geq t),$$

where t is the observed value of the test statistic T. The p-value can be computed based on the MVN distribution for $(T_1, ..., T_J)$ using the `pmvnorm` function in the R package `mvtnorm`.

The power can be defined as

$$\beta = \mathrm{P}(H_0 \text{ is rejected}|H_1 \text{ is true}).$$

The power can be calculated as the proportion of rejecting the null hypothesis using the Monte Carlo method when the survival data is generated from the alternative hypothesis. In addition to the existence of cure (non-inferiority of survival), the time of reaching non-inferiority τ is also of interest. When the null hypothesis is rejected, an ad-hoc estimate of τ is defined as

$$\hat{\tau} = \mathrm{argmin}_k\{T_k, k = 1, ..., J\}.$$

Note that the estimator $\hat{\tau}$ is dependent on the size of p_j^{Δ} and ultimately on the size of the clinically meaningful difference Δ. When the value of Δ is closer to 0, the criterion of survival non-inferiority is more stringent and the time to reach non-inferiority would be longer or even unattainable. The asymptotic property of the estimator $\hat{\tau}$ is difficult to derive, one can use simulation to study its empirical property.

The above test is about the existence of cure or non-inferiority of late survival, rather than differences in late survival. The data may provide strong evidence of cure when the null hypothesis is rejected based the test of non-inferiority (8.17). A common issue about the interpretation of hypothesis testing arises when failing to reject the null hypothesis because there is not enough power to demonstrate non-inferiority due to limited number of subjects or follow-up time. Failing to reject the null hypothesis does not necessarily mean the absence of cure. It is almost impossible that the cancer patients and general population have exactly the same hazard rates when the sample size of cancer patients is large.

Note that the non-inferiority test of survival is different from the test of cure of Maller and Zhou (1995), referred to as the MZ test, in several respects. First, the non-inferiority test is intended to test whether non-inferiority of survival is achieved during the observation period. The MZ test examines whether cure exists, which may occur in the infinite future, based on observed data. It is possible that cure exists but does not occur during the observation period. In fact, based on the formulation of the mixture cure model, the excess hazard is always positive until t goes to infinity. Second, the non-inferiority test is nonparametric and does not require specifications of survival models for cancer patients, whereas the MZ test of cure is based on parametric mixture cure models. The asymptotic distribution of the MZ test statistic is developed when the latency distribution is a Gamma distribution. For other latency distributions, the MZ test statistic may not follow the same distribution. Third, the non-inferiority test is more flexible, and it includes the test of cure as a special case when the non-inferiority margin $\Delta = 0$. For many cancers that impose a long-term excess risk, it is more reasonable to test that the excess hazard is below a certain positive margin.

The test statistics $T_k, k = 1, ..., J$, and their minimum T are based on log-rank tests, which assign the same weight to each interval. It is well known that the log-rank test is optimal when the hazard ratio of the intervention group versus the control group is constant as a function of follow-up time. However, this is unlikely to be the case in many cancer survival studies. For example, for testing non-inferiority of survival, it is expected that the weighted log-rank test that places greater weights on long-term survivors would be more powerful than the usual log-rank test with equal weights. Weighted log-rank tests have been proposed to compare survival distributions of two groups (Fleming and Harrington, 1991). By adding weights w_j to the log-rank statistics T_k in (8.19), the weighted log-rank test can be calculated as

$$T_k(w) = \frac{L_k(w)}{\sqrt{V_k(w)}} = \frac{\sum_{j=k}^{J} w_j(d_j - E_j)}{\sqrt{\sum_{j=k}^{J} w_j^2 v_j}}, k = 1, ..., J, \tag{8.21}$$

where w_j are positive weights corresponding to the jth interval. Fleming and Harrington (1991) introduced the family of tests $G^{\rho,\nu}$ with the weight functions $w_j = S_O(t_j)^{\rho}\{1 - S_O(t_j)\}^{\nu}$ for $\rho \geq 0$ and $\nu \geq 0$. With different weights, the weighted log-rank tests are optimal under certain alternative hypotheses. Four members of this family are commonly used: $G^{0,0}, G^{1,0}, G^{0,1}$ and $G^{1,1}$. They cover a wide range of possible differences in the survival distributions, and the weight function $G^{0,0}$ leads to the unweighted log-rank test. Specifically, the four types of weight are designed to detect constant difference, early difference, late difference, and middle difference, respectively. Based on Theorem 8.4.1 for log-rank tests, we have the following corollary for weighted log-rank tests.

Corollary 8.4.1 *Let* $V_k(w) = \sum_{j=k}^{J} w_j v_j^2$*. Under the null hypothesis of excess mortality, the asymptotic distribution of the weighted log-rank test statistics is multivariate normal (MVN), i.e.,* $(T_1(w), ..., T_J(w))' \sim MVN(\mathbf{0}, \mathbf{\Sigma}(w))$*, where the* (k, l) *entry of the covariance matrix* $\sigma_{kl}(w) = \sqrt{V_l(w)/V_k(w)}$ *for* $k < l$*.*

When the weighted log-rank tests are used, the corresponding test of non-inferiority of survival becomes

$$T(w) = \min(T_1(w), ..., T_J(w)),$$

where $T_k(w), k = 1, ..., J$, are the weighted log-rank tests (8.21). The tests with weight $G^{0,0}$ and $G^{0,1}$ have been shown to have a higher power of demonstrating cure and maintain the Type 1 error rate closer to the target α level. The test with weight $G^{0,0}$ is recommended because of its simplicity. Additional simulation also shows that the MZ likelihood ratio test has a low power of testing non-inferiority of survival for the population-based cancer survival data and the nonparametric log-rank test is the preferred method for demonstrating non-inferiority (cure) of cancer survival.

8.5 Applications

The SEER program began collecting data on cancer cases on January 1, 1973, in the states of Connecticut, Iowa, New Mexico, Utah, and Hawaii and the metropolitan areas of Detroit and San Francisco-Oakland. Since then, the SEER Program has been expanded to cover numerous additional areas. The population-based cancer survival data from the SEER Program can be extracted from the SEER*Stat software. For each survival session that generate the survival data, the output from the SEER*Stat includes a data file and a dictionary file. The SEER 18 registries include cancer cases diagnosed from 2000 through the current data year from 18 registries in the United States. For illustration, we extract the colorectal cancer survival data for SEER18 program with the SEER*Stat software. The data include 185,047 colorectal cancer patients who are diagnosed between 2004 and 2010. The covariates include sex (0=Male, 1=Female), American Joint Committee on Cancer (AJCC) stage (0=Stage I, 1=Stage II, 2=Stage III, 3=Stage IV), year of diagnosis (0=2004, ...,6=2010). The reference group is the males diagnosed with Stage I colorectal cancer in the year 2004. The survival times are recorded as annual intervals. The end of the follow-up is 2015 and the maximum follow-up is 11 years. The percentages of colorectal cancer patients by sex and AJCC stage are shown in Table 8.3. The percentage of men with colorectal cancer is slightly higher with 51.4%.

TABLE 8.3
Percentages of colorectal cancer patients by sex and AJCC stage.

	AJCC Stage				
Sex	I	II	III	IV	All stages
Male	13.1	13.3	13.7	11.3	51.4
Female	11.8	13.2	13.2	10.4	48.6
Both	24.9	26.5	26.9	21.7	100.0

8.5.1 Weibull Mixture Cure Model for Grouped Survival Data

The mixture cure model to the grouped survival data has been in a standard-alone software package CANSURV software (Yu et al., 2005). CANSURV fits several popular parametric models and parametric mixture cure models to relative survival data. A logistic model is used to model the cure rate

$$\text{logit}[\pi_c(\boldsymbol{x})] = \boldsymbol{x}^{'}\boldsymbol{\gamma}, \tag{8.22}$$

where $\boldsymbol{\gamma}$ is the vector of coefficients. The latency distribution $S_u(t|\boldsymbol{x})$ are parametric, e.g, lognormal and loglogistic and Weibull, distributions. CANSURV uses a location-scale parametrization for the parametric distributions, i.e.,

$$S_u(t|\boldsymbol{x}) = \begin{cases} 1-\Phi\left(\frac{\log t-\mu(\boldsymbol{x})}{\sigma}\right) & \text{Lognormal} \\ \left\{1+\exp[\frac{\log t-\mu(\boldsymbol{x})}{\sigma}]\right\}^{-1} & \text{Loglogistic} \\ \exp\left\{-\exp\left[\frac{\log t-\mu(\boldsymbol{x})}{\sigma}\right]\right\} & \text{Weibull,} \end{cases} \tag{8.23}$$

where $\mu(\boldsymbol{x}) = \boldsymbol{x}^{'}\boldsymbol{\beta}$ is the location parameter and σ is the scale parameter. The location parameter $\mu(\boldsymbol{x})$ is related to the median survival time of the uncured patients. That is, the median survival time is $\exp(\mu(\boldsymbol{x}))$ for the lognormal and loglogistic distributions and $\exp(\mu(\boldsymbol{x}))(\log 2)^{\sigma}$ for the Weibull distribution.

The parameter estimates of Weibull mixture cure model for the colorectal cancer relative survival data are shown in Table 8.4. Sex and AJCC stage are used as a categorical variable and the year of diagnosis as a continuous variable. The top section shows the parameter estimates of the logistic model for cure rate π_c. We see that females have significantly higher cure rate than male. The cure rate decreases significantly as the AJCC stage increases and the cure rate remains stable with respect to the year of diagnosis. The estimated and observed relative survival rates for patients that are diagnosed in the year 2000 are shown in Figure 8.1. The estimated relative survival rates are very close to the observed survival rates, indicating a good model fit. The estimated cure fractions and median survival time for the uncured patients are shown in Table 8.5. There are statistically significant differences in cure rate and median survival time between male and female. However, the actual differences are not clinically important. For example, the differences of cure rates between males and females are at most 5.1% and the differences of median survival times for the uncured patients are all within 0.6 year.

8.5.2 Analysis of Individually-Listed Colorectal Cancer Relative Survival Data

The relative survival data can also be presented as individually listed where each row corresponds the record for a cancer patient. We consider the random sample of 10 subjects of the individually-listed colorectal cancer survival data

TABLE 8.4
Parameter estimates of mixture cure models for colorectal cancer relative survival data.

Parameter	Estimate	Std. Error	Wald χ^2	P-value
	Cure π_c			
Intercept	1.745	0.063	759.706	<0.001
Sex				
Male				
Female	0.205	0.025	65.670	<0.001
AJCC Stage				
Stage I				
Stage II	-1.225	0.081	227.919	<0.001
Stage III	-2.027	0.068	882.711	<0.001
Stage IV	-4.593	0.066	4839.418	<0.001
Year of diagnosis	-0.006	0.007	0.659	0.417
	Location parameter μ			
Intercept	1.389	0.094	216.186	<0.001
Sex				
Male				
Female	-0.137	0.015	85.159	<0.001
AJCC Stage				
Stage I				
Stage II	0.589	0.110	28.516	<0.001
Stage III	0.378	0.097	15.296	<0.001
Stage IV	-0.974	0.094	106.156	<0.001
Year of diagnosis (2004-2010)	0.023	0.004	34.933	<0.001
	Scale parameter σ			
$\log(\sigma)$	0.154	0.007	483.084	<0.001

in Table 8.1. The survival time is recorded monthly and the event indicator is a binary variable for death, the expected hazard is the hazard function of death for the matched cancer-free population.

Both mixture and non-mixture cure models for individually-listed relative survival data have been implemented in the R package `flexsurvcure`. The R code for fitting the Weibull mixture cure model for the colorectal cancer data is

```
flexsurvcure(Surv(Survival.Time, Event) ~ Sex + Stage + Year,
             data = CSD,
             bhazard = Expected_Hazard,
             dist = "weibull",
             mixture = TRUE,
             anc = list(scale = ~Sex + Stage + Year)
             )
```

The data set name is `CSD` and the covariates include `Sex`, `Stage` and `Year`. The overall survival time is `Survival.Time` and indicator of death is `Event`. The

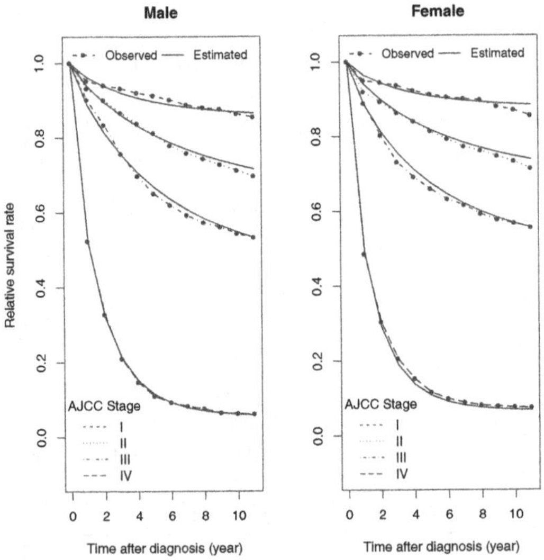

FIGURE 8.1
Comparison of the observed relative survival rates and the estimates from the mixture cure model.

TABLE 8.5
Estimates of cure rate and median survival time for the uncured patients.

		AJCC Stage			
Sex	Parameter	I	II	III	IV
Male	Cure rate (%)	85.1	62.7	43.0	5.5
	Median survival time for the uncured	2.6	4.7	3.8	1.0
Female	Cure rate (%)	87.5	67.4	48.1	6.6
	Median survival time for the uncured	2.3	4.1	3.3	0.9

expected hazard rate is `Expected_Hazard`. The Weibull mixture cure model is specified by `dist="Weibull"` and `mixture=TRUE`. The Weibull survival function in R functions `flexsurv` and `flexsurvreg` is

$$S_u(t|\boldsymbol{x}) = \exp\left[-\left(\frac{t}{b(\boldsymbol{x})}\right)^a\right]$$

where a is the shape parameter and $b(\boldsymbol{x}) = \exp(\boldsymbol{x}'\boldsymbol{\beta})$ is the scale parameter. All three covariates are used to predict the cure fraction by argument `Surv(Survival.Time, Event) ~ Sex + Stage + Year`. The three covariates are used for the scale parameter $b(\boldsymbol{x})$ by argument `anc=list(scale = ~Sex + Stage + Year)`. The output for the Weibull mixture cure model is shown in Figure 8.2. The parameter estimate for `Sex` in the logistic model for cure rate is 0.245 with 95% confidence interval (0.198,

```
Estimates:
                  data mean  est       L95%      U95%      se        exp(est)  L95%      U95%
theta                   NA    0.82316   0.79892   0.84504        NA        NA        NA        NA
shape                   NA    0.90068   0.89316   0.90827   0.00386        NA        NA        NA
scale                   NA    8.30994   6.73543  10.25253   0.89067        NA        NA        NA
Sex                0.48558    0.24544   0.19847   0.29241   0.02396   1.27818   1.21953   1.33965
StageII            0.26538   -1.07390  -1.25632  -0.89148   0.09307   0.34167   0.28470   0.41005
StageIII           0.26900   -1.74901  -1.91261  -1.58541   0.08347   0.17395   0.14770   0.20486
StageIV            0.21673   -4.32210  -4.48460  -4.15959   0.08291   0.01327   0.01128   0.01561
Year               2.98284   -0.00585  -0.01834   0.00664   0.00637   0.99416   0.98182   1.00666
scale(Sex)         0.48558   -0.13273  -0.15949  -0.10597   0.01365   0.87570   0.85257   0.89945
scale(StageII)     0.26538    0.00278  -0.22870   0.23425   0.11810   1.00278   0.79557   1.26396
scale(StageIII)    0.26900   -0.31932  -0.53277  -0.10587   0.10890   0.72664   0.58698   0.89954
scale(StageIV)     0.21673   -1.67860  -1.88898  -1.46823   0.10733   0.18663   0.15123   0.23033
scale(Year)        2.98284    0.02072   0.01379   0.02765   0.00354   1.02093   1.01388   1.02803

N = 185047,  Events: 101724,  Censored: 83323
Total time at risk: 947834.9
Log-likelihood = -243291.5, df = 13
AIC = 486609
```

FIGURE 8.2
Output from the Weibull mixture cure model for the colorectal cancer data by flexsurvcure.

0.292). This means that female (`Sex=1`) has much higher cure rate than male (`Sex=0`). The cure rate also decreases significant as cancer stage increases from Stage I to Stage IV. The results are consistent with those from the CANSURV analysis for the grouped relative survival data.

The R code for fitting the Weibull non-mixture cure model using `flexsurvcure` is

```
flexsurvcure(Surv(Survival.Time,Event)~Sex+Stage+Year,
             bhazard=Expected_Hazard,
             mixture=FALSE,
             data=CSD,
             dist="weibull")
```

Note that the covariates `Sex`, `Stage` and `Year` are only used in the logistic regression for cure rate. The output is shown in Figure 8.3. The parameter estimates for `Sex` is 0.044 with 95% confidence interval (0.011, 0.077). This means that females have statistically significantly higher cure rate than males. We also see that patients with higher AJCC stages have lower cure rates. The results are consistent with those from the mixture cure model in Figure 8.2.

The R code for fitting the flexible non-mixture cure model using `rstpm2` is

```
stpm2(Surv(Survival.Time,Event)~Sex+Stage+Year,
      data=CSD,
      bhazard=CSD$Expected_Hazard,
      df=5,
      cure=TRUE)
```

where `df=6` is the degrees of freedom for the baseline smoothers for the cumulative hazard function. The covariates `Sex`, `Stage` and `Year` are used in the regression for cure rate. The output is shown in Figure 8.4. The parameter estimates for the three covariates are all highly significant. Note that a default log-log link function is used in the regression for cure. The signs of the parameter estimates for the flexible cure model are reversed from the signs for the non-mixture Weibull cure model in Figure 8.3.

8.5.3 Testing the Existence of Cure for Colorectal Cancer Patients

We apply the one-sample log-rank test to the relative survival data for colorectal cancer patients who are diagnosed in the year 2004. The excess probability of death due to cancer for the four cancer stages are shown in Figure 8.5. The horizontal reference line corresponds to excess mortality probability of 0.02 per year. We see that the excess mortality for the Stage I colorectal cancer patients drops below 0.02 shortly after diagnosis, while the excess mortality for the Stage IV patients drop sharply after diagnosis, however, is still above 0.02 after 10 years. The tests of non-inferiority, shown in Table 8.6, convey

```
Estimates:
           data mean  est       L95%      U95%      se        exp(est)  L95%      U95%
theta            NA   0.85505   0.84693   0.86281        NA       NA        NA        NA
shape            NA   0.94427   0.93564   0.95297   0.00442       NA        NA        NA
scale            NA   6.22450   5.95559   6.50556   0.14026       NA        NA        NA
Sex         0.48558   0.04448   0.01149   0.07746   0.01683   1.04548   1.01156   1.08054
StageII     0.26538  -0.96483  -1.02530  -0.90436   0.03085   0.38105   0.35869   0.40480
StageIII    0.26900  -1.77775  -1.83486  -1.72063   0.02914   0.16902   0.15964   0.17895
StageIV     0.21673  -5.61983  -5.72059  -5.51908   0.05141   0.00363   0.00328   0.00401
Year        2.98284   0.02247   0.01410   0.03083   0.00427   1.02272   1.01420   1.03132

N = 185047,  Events: 101724,  Censored: 83323
Total time at risk: 947834.9
Log-likelihood = -243505, df = 8
AIC = 487026
```

FIGURE 8.3
Output from the non-mixture cure model for the colorectal cancer data by flexsurvcure.

```
Coefficients:
                                              Estimate Std. Error   z value      Pr(z)
(Intercept)                                 -6.1665425  0.0302223 -204.0397 < 2.2e-16 ***
Sex                                         -0.0036000  0.0087170   -0.4130    0.6796
StageII                                      0.8423773  0.0273385   30.8129 < 2.2e-16 ***
StageIII                                     1.4791410  0.0254415   58.1388 < 2.2e-16 ***
StageIV                                      3.2419960  0.0245560  132.0248 < 2.2e-16 ***
Year                                        -0.0152129  0.0021961   -6.9272 4.292e-12 ***
nsx(log(Survival.Time), df = 5, cure = TRUE)1 3.3135535  0.0169434  195.5655 < 2.2e-16 ***
nsx(log(Survival.Time), df = 5, cure = TRUE)2 3.6952632  0.0170303  216.9817 < 2.2e-16 ***
nsx(log(Survival.Time), df = 5, cure = TRUE)3 2.0291759  0.0091888  220.8320 < 2.2e-16 ***
nsx(log(Survival.Time), df = 5, cure = TRUE)4 6.6091385  0.0347154  190.3803 < 2.2e-16 ***
nsx(log(Survival.Time), df = 5, cure = TRUE)5 3.4602196  0.0145999  237.0027 < 2.2e-16 ***
---
Signif. codes:  0 *** 0.001 ** 0.01 * 0.05 . 0.1   1

 -2 log L: 483631.8
```

FIGURE 8.4
Output from the non-mixture cure model for the colorectal cancer data by stpm2.

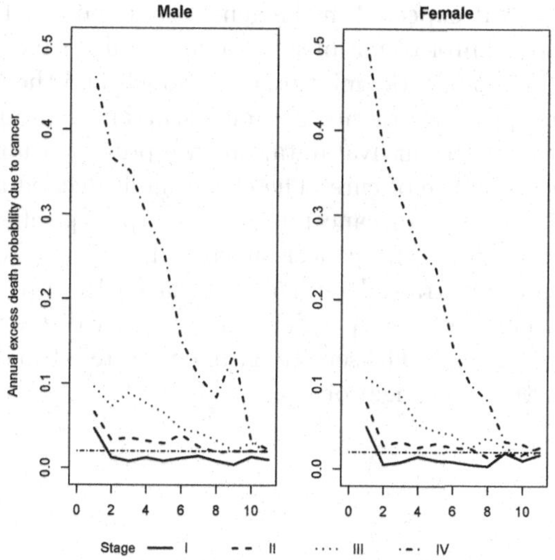

FIGURE 8.5
Excess probability of death due to colorectal cancer.

TABLE 8.6
Test of non-inferiority of survival for colorectal cancer patients

	Male		Female	
Stage	p-value	$\hat{\tau}$	p-value	$\hat{\tau}$
I	<0.001	2	<0.001	2
II	0.823	NR	0.622	NR
III	0.776	NR	0.703	NR
IV	0.917	NR	0.887	NR

similar results. The survival for Stage I patients is non-inferior to the cancer-free population in two years after diagnosis. However, the non-inferiority of survival is not reached (NR) for Stage II-IV patients even after 10 years of diagnosis.

8.6 Summary

The interest in estimating the probability of cure has been increasing in cancer survival analysis as the curability of many cancer diseases is becoming a reality. For the population-based cancer survival analysis, the cure is achieved when the mortality (hazard) rate in the diseased group of individuals returns to the same level as that expected in the general population. The cure rate is a useful measure to monitor trends of survival for curable cancers. There are two main types of cure models: the mixture cure models and the non-mixture cure models. In this chapter, we describe parametric and flexible cure models for the population-based cancer survival data, and we present a nonparametric log-rank test for the existence of cure. The cure time is defined as the time when the excess mortality due to cancer is within a pre-specified non-inferiority margin. We use the colorectal cancer survival data from the SEER program as an application to illustrate the use of R packages. However, the estimates of cure rate may depends on the specification of latency distribution and follow-up time (Yu et al., 2004a). The sensitivity of cure rate estimates from different models needs further investigations.

9

Design and Analysis of Cancer Clinical Trials

9.1 Introduction

Cancer is a heterogeneous disease and differs greatly among different patients and even within the same type of tumor. Survival rates may vary greatly between different cancer types and remain poor for some cancers, while some treatments can have serious side effects (ICR, 2014). Exciting advances are paving the way to better treatments and possibly more cures. Although it is difficult to achieve cure for most advanced solid tumors, many types of cancer, e.g., leukemia, lymphoma, testicular cancers, may have long-lasting durable remission. Because of the progress of early diagnosis and cancer treatment, many cancer patients become long-term survivors, even though one cannot be sure that cancer eventually goes away after treatment. In this chapter, we refer the "cure" as long-term remission, meaning there is still a slight chance that disease may come back. But, in general, a person who stays cancer free five years after a diagnosis has better odds of recovery.

Targeted cancer therapies are often highly effective initially, but tumors may develop resistance later. A recent breakthrough in cancer treatment is the development of cancer immunotherapy. Cancer immunotherapy stimulates the patient's immune system to fight tumors, attempting to restore the immune system to the robustness of its youth. An exciting phenomenon of cancer immunotherapy is the durability of antitumour responses, with some patients achieving cancer remission for many years (Harris et al., 2016; Del Paggio, 2018). Because long-term durable tumor control seems achievable with the cancer immunotherapy, the concept of "clinical cure" is emerging. Wolchok et al. (2017) presented the progression-free survival (PFS) and overall survival (OS) for advanced melanoma patients treated with ipilimumab, nivolumab and the combination therapy from a Phase III clinical trial (Checkmate-067 study). For illustration, we consider the survival for patients treated with nivolumab and ipilimumab monotherapies. The PFS and OS data were reconstructed from the Kaplan-Meier plots from the published clinical trial analysis using the algorithm described by Guyot et al. (2012). The PFS and OS Kaplan-Meier curves for the reconstructed individual survival data are shown in Figures 9.1 and 9.2, respectively. The median progression-free survival was 6.9 months with 95% confidence interval 5.1 to 9.7 months in the nivolumab group, as compared with 2.9 months (95% confidence interval 2.8

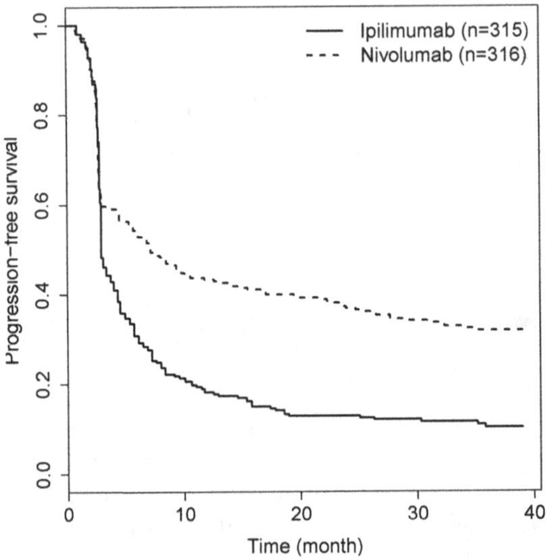

FIGURE 9.1
Kaplan-Meier curves of the reconstructed PFS data for ipilimumab and nivolumab in Checkmate-067 study.

to 3.2 months) in the ipilimumab group (Figure 9.1). The hazard ratio for PFS was 0.55 with 95% confidence interval 0.45 to 0.66 with nivolumab versus ipilimumab. The overall 3-year survival rate was 52% in the nivolumab group, as compared with 34% in the ipilimumab group. The median overall survival time reaches 37.6 months (95% confidence interval 29.1 months to not reached) in the nivolumab group and 19.9 months (95% confidence interval 16.9 to 24.6 months) in the ipilimumab group (Figure 9.2). The hazard ratio for death was 0.65 (95% confidence interval 0.53 to 0.80) with nivolumab versus ipilimumab.

This clearly shows that the existence of long-term survivors after the treatment of immunotherapy. The statistical methods and techniques described in previous chapters can be applied to survival data with long-term survivors from cancer clinical trials. Some design issues for clinical trial with cure have been discussed in Wu (2018). In this chapter, we present some recent development in the application of cure modeling in the statistical design and planning and hypothesis testing in cancer clinical trials. We focus on the discussions in the context of immuno-oncology clinical trials.

Endpoints are measurable clinical and biological findings that are used for the development and assessment of treatment options (Fiteni et al., 2014). In the treatment of cancer, endpoints can be classified into two categories: patient-centered clinical endpoints including OS and health-related quality of life (QoL), and tumor-centered clinical endpoints such as PFS. Surrogate

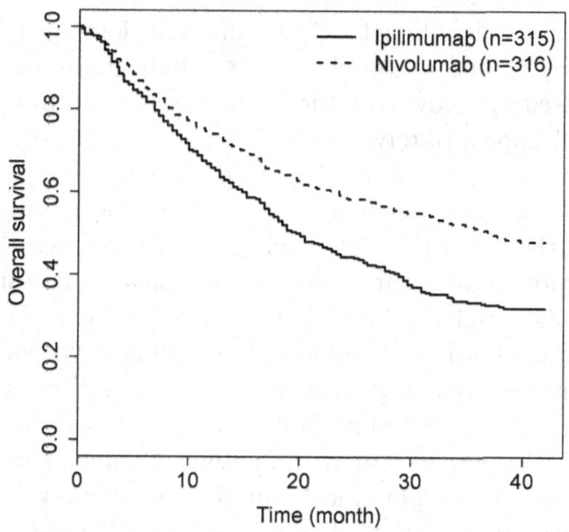

FIGURE 9.2
Kaplan-Meier curves of the reconstructed OS data for ipilimumab and nivolumab in Checkmate-067 study.

endpoints are tumor-centered clinical endpoints that can be used as substitutes for patient-centered clinical endpoints, particularly OS. The choice of endpoints in oncology trials is a major problem. The published Consolidated Standards of Reporting Trials (CONSORT) best-practice guidelines encourage reporting clearly defined primary and secondary outcome measures. OS is the gold standard of endpoints, but as increasing numbers of effective salvage treatments become available for many types of cancer, much larger numbers of patients are included; this requires a longer follow-up period and increases the cost of clinical trials.

9.2 Testing Treatment Effects in the Presence of Cure

The conventional trial designs and endpoints did not capture the novel patterns of responses in immuno-oncology trials (Hoering et al., 2017). Long-term survival and delayed clinical benefit are two common phenomena. Stable disease or responses can occur after conventional progressive disease owing to clinically insignificant new lesions in the presence of other responsive lesions and to a reduction in total tumor burden. As such, discontinuation of immuno-oncology therapies at the first sign of progressive disease might not always be appropriate. In addition, durable stable disease might represent meaningful antitumor activity in patients who do not meet the criteria for an objective response. Because the clinical benefit of immuno-oncology agents might extend beyond that of traditional cytotoxic agents, alternative statistical methods should be considered to allow treatment efficacy of immuno-oncology therapies to be assessed appropriately.

Several immuno-oncology therapies have shown a delayed clinical effect likely due to their mechanism of action (Anagnostou et al., 2017). Importantly, a delay in the separation of survival curves violates the fundamental assumption of proportional hazards for typical clinical trial design and analysis methods, which might reduce the statistical power of a study to differentiate between two treatment arms. In some patients, long-term survival might be achievable with immuno-oncology therapies, which is reflected by a plateau in survival curves with sufficiently long follow-up.

Su and Zhu (2018) demonstrated the potential value of weighted log-rank tests and argued that the weighted log-rank test should play a more important role in confirmatory clinical trials. The unweighted log-rank test is frequently used to detect a potential treatment effect in randomized clinical trials with time-to-event endpoints. It is asymptotically the most powerful test under the proportional hazards setting, but it has been shown to lose power substantially when the proportional hazards assumption is violated (Schoenfeld, 1981). Weighted log-rank tests with various fixed and adaptive weight functions have been proposed in the literature to increase the power of a trial when non-proportional hazards are expected e.g., (Fleming and Harrington, 2011; Xu et al., 2017; Yang and Prentice, 2009). In particular, the $G^{\rho,\nu}$ family of weights proposed by Fleming and Harrington (2011) allows the flexibility to assign greater weights to either early or late failure times as controlled by the two parameters ρ and ν. The $G^{\rho,\nu}$ family of weights are given by

$$w_j = \hat{S}(t_j)^{\rho}(1 - \hat{S}(t_j))^{\nu}, \tag{9.1}$$

with $\rho \geq 0$ and $\nu \geq 0$ and $\hat{S}(t_j)$ the Kaplan-Meier estimate of survival for the pooled data. The weights with $\rho = 1$ and $\nu = 0$ are used to detect early treatment effects and the weights with $\rho = 0$ and $\nu = 1$ are mainly for detecting late treatment effects. The most powerful weighted log-rank test assigns the weights proportionally to the magnitude of the log-hazard ratio (Schoenfeld, 1981).

Delayed separation of survival curves has been frequently observed in clinical trials with time-to-event endpoints, but the adoption of weighted log-rank tests has been limited. In cases where there are both a strong biological rationale and some clinical evidence to support a delayed treatment effect, we would encourage the consideration of pre-specifying a weighted log-rank test for the primary analysis with the log-rank test being a sensitivity analysis. Clinical evidence may be generated from either trials of other treatments with a similar mechanism of action or completed trials with the same treatment. In Figures 9.1 and 9.2, the survival curves showed little separation during the first 3 months of treatment. Therefore, a weighted log-rank test may be appropriate for analysis of PFS and OS data for the Checkmate-067 trial.

We encourage clinical trial practitioners to consider a weighted log-rank test when both the mechanism of action and existing clinical evidence point to a potential delayed treatment effect. With an appropriately chosen weight function the loss of power should be fairly minimal under the proportional hazards setting, and the gain in power can be substantial in the presence of non-proportional hazards. Even if the preference is to follow the precedence of using the log-rank test in confirmatory trials, a weighted log-rank test may be pre-specified as an important sensitivity analysis to help better characterize the potential benefit of a new treatment.

9.2.1 Comparison of Log-Rank Type Tests

In a typical oncology clinical trial, let t^* be the event time and c be the censoring time. The event status indicator $\delta = 1$ for events and $\delta = 0$ for right-censored times and the observed survival time $t = \min(t^*, c)$. Let x denote the group indicator, where $x = 0$ for the control group and $x = 1$ for the treatment group. The following hypothesis testing is frequently considered in oncology clinical trials:

$$\begin{aligned} H_{0\lambda} &: \lambda(t|x=0) = \lambda(t|x=1), \text{ for all } t, \\ H_{1\lambda} &: \lambda(t|x=0) \neq \lambda(t|x=1), \text{ for some } t, \end{aligned}$$

where $\lambda(t|x)$ is the hazard function for group x. Callegaro and Spiessens (2017) compared the power and effect size of different log-rank type tests under non-proportional hazards assumptions. Here, we consider a few popular log-rank type statistics.

Suppose there are n subjects in the trial. Let t_i be the observed survival time and δ_i be the event indicator and let x_i be the group indicator for the ith subject, $i = 1, \ldots, n$. Let $N_i(t) = \delta_i I(t_i \leq t)$ and $Y_i(t) = I(t_i \geq t)$ be the failure and at-risk processes for the ith subject. The weighted log-rank test statistic can then be written as

$$L = \sum_{i=1}^{n} \int_0^{\tau} W(t)\{x_i - \bar{x}(t)\} \mathrm{d}N_i(t), \tag{9.2}$$

where τ is the end of follow-up and $\bar{x}(t) = \sum_{i=1}^{n} x_i Y_i(t) / \sum_{i=1}^{n} Y_i(t)$. The weighted log-rank statistic can also expressed as

$$T_w = \frac{\sum_{j=1}^{J} w_j (d_{1j} - E_j)}{\sqrt{\sum_{j=1}^{J} w_j^2 V_j}}, \tag{9.3}$$

where d_{1j} is the number of events observed in treatment group at the event time t_j, E_j and V_j are the mean and the variance of d_{1j} under the null hypothesis and w_j is the weight function. If the weights are constant, then T_w is the classic unweighted log-rank test. Under the null hypothesis, the weighted log-rank test statistic is asymptotically normally distributed.

Qiu and Sheng (2008) proposed a powerful and robust two-stage (TS) procedure to compare two hazard rate functions. In Stage 1, the unweighted log-rank test is used to test the overall treatment effect at α_1 level. If the log-rank test is significant, then the null hypothesis of no difference is rejected; otherwise a new log-rank test is used to test the crossing hazards at the α_2 level. They developed weights such that the weighted log-rank test is asymptotically independent of the unweighted test. The adaptive weights are derived based on the estimated crossing point and to maximize the weighted log-rank statistic. In Stage 2, bootstrap is used to estimate the p-value at significance level $\alpha_2 = (\alpha - \alpha_1)/(1 - \alpha_1)$. The TS method is implemented in the R package `TSHRC` (Sheng et al., 2017).

Yang and Prentice (2009) proposed another adaptive weighted log-rank test. The adaptive weights are derived from a flexible hazard model (Yang and Prentice, 2005):

$$\lambda(t|x = 1) = \frac{\theta_E \theta_L}{\theta_E + (\theta_L - \theta_E) S(t|x = 0)} \lambda(t|x = 0),$$

where $S(t|x = 0)$ is the survival function for the control group and θ_E, θ_L represent the short-term and long-term hazard ratios, respectively. This model includes the proportional hazards model ($\theta_E = \theta_L$) and the proportional odds model ($\theta_L = 1$) as special cases. The proposed method may also accommodate the non-proportional-hazards cases, e.g., the crossing hazards and crossing survivor functions. Yang and Prentice (2009) also proved that the adaptive log-rank test is asymptotically equivalent to the unweighted log-rank test under the proportional hazards alternatives. The Yang and Prentice (YP) method is implemented in the R package `YPmodel`.

The weighted and adaptive log-rank tests have been shown to have higher power than the unweighted log-rank tests when the proportional hazards assumption is not satisfied (Callegaro and Spiessens, 2017). However, the use of unequal weights implies survival for a certain period, e.g., late survival difference, is more important than the other, e.g., early survival difference. In addition, the weighted log-rank tests only show the overall effects of treatment in the whole study period. For some oncology clinical trials, the early overlap of the Kaplan-Meier curves between two groups suggests that the treatment does not exhibit its full effect early on but also creates no harm to the patients. A natural hypothesis of a desirable treatment would consist of two components, namely (i) the treatment is non-inferior to the control during the whole study period and (ii) the treatment is superior to the control group after a pre-defined change point. We thus protect patients from being harmed by the treatment and also provide researchers a proper conclusion in the sense that the alternative hypothesis truly reflects a change point in the hazard ratio. To address this issue, Sit et al. (2016) formulated an intersection union test (Berger et al., 1996). Specifically, the overall null hypothesis

$H_0 = H_{10} \cup H_{20}$, where

$$\begin{aligned} H_{10} &: \lambda_1(t)/\lambda_0(t) \geq \Delta_{10} \text{ for } t \in [0, \tau], \\ H_{20} &: \lambda_1(t)/\lambda_0(t) \geq \Delta_{20} \text{ for } t \in [t_0, \tau]. \end{aligned}$$

where $\Delta_{10} > 1$ is the non-inferiority margin and $0 < \Delta_{20} \leq 1$ is the threshold of treatment efficacy. Usually, we set $\Delta_{20} = 1$. The overall alternative hypothesis $H_1 = H_{11} \cap H_{21}$, where

$$\begin{aligned} H_{10} &: \lambda_1(t)/\lambda_0(t) < \Delta_{10} \text{ for } t \in [0, \tau], \\ H_{20} &: \lambda_1(t)/\lambda_0(t) < \Delta_{20} \text{ for } t \in [t_0, \tau]. \end{aligned}$$

Therefore, a non-inferiority log-rank test can be used for H_{10} over the entire study duration $[0, \tau]$ and a superiority log-rank test for H_{20} after the pre-specified change point $[t_0, \tau]$. Under this construction, only when both hypotheses are rejected, we can conclude that the overall null hypothesis is rejected. Controlling each test as a α-level test for the intersection union test can maintain the overall type I error at α-level (Berger et al., 1996).

Selection of the non-inferiority and superiority margins $(\Delta_{10}, \Delta_{20})$ is necessary before implementing the proposed intersection union test. We need to determine how close the new treatment must be compared to the control group on the efficacy so to declare significant improvement. The ICH documents offer two guidelines for determining the corresponding margins (FDA, 2010): (1) the non-inferiority margins should be determined based on both statistical analysis of historical data and clinical judgement (2) the margin cannot exceed the minimum effect size that the active drug would be reasonably expected to produce compared with placebo, based on, if exist, past placebo-controlled trials under similar conditions.

A simulation study can be used to examine the unweighted and weighted log-rank tests (LR and WLR), the adaptive test (YP) (Yang and Prentice, 2009), the two-stage test (TS) (Qiu and Sheng, 2008) and the intersection-union test (IUT) (Sit et al., 2016). We consider the scenario with both delayed treatment effect and cure. The survival function of the control group is given by

$$S_0(t) = \pi_c + (1 - \pi_c)S_u(t),$$

where the survival function for the uncured patients $S_u(t) = \exp(-\theta t)$ and π_c is the cure rate. The survival function for the treatment group is given as

$$S_1(t) = \begin{cases} S_0(t) & t \leq t_0 \\ S_0(t_0)^{1-r} S_0(t)^r & t > t_0 \end{cases},$$

where t_0 is the delayed treatment effect onset time. When $\pi_c = 0$ and $t_0 = 0$, r is the hazard ratio between the treatment and control groups. In the simulation, we assume that for the control group, the cure rate $\pi_c = 0.05$ or 0.1, and latency distribution is exponential with hazard rate $\lambda_0(t) \equiv \lambda_0 = 1$ or 2. We also assume that the delayed onset time t_0=0.5 or 0.75 years and the

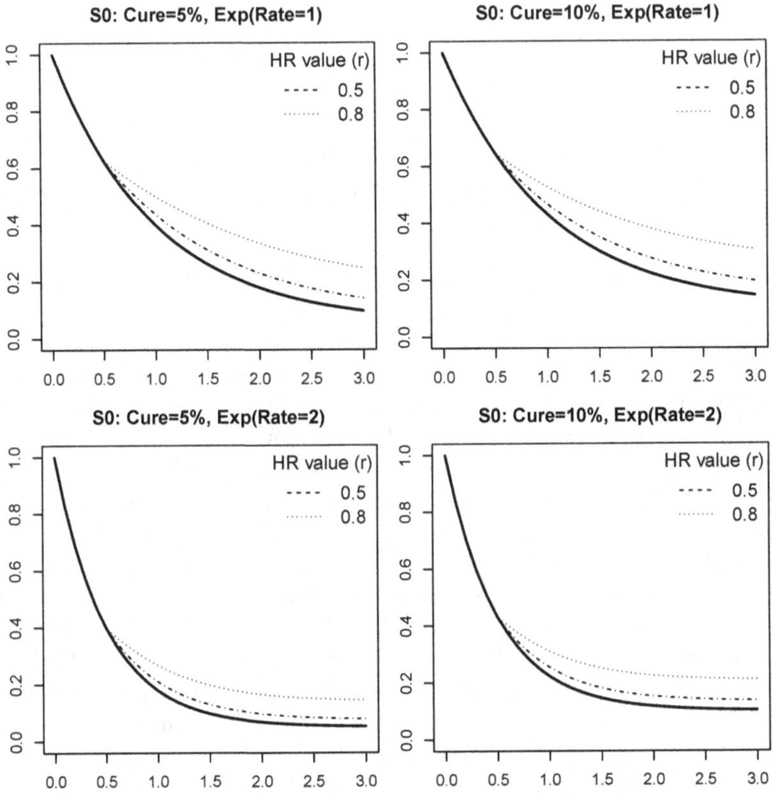

FIGURE 9.3
Survival curves in the simulation for the comparison of tests.

hazard ratio of treatment $r = 0.5$ or 0.8 after the onset of treatment effect. The survival curves used in the simulation are shown in Figure 9.3. In addition, we set the number of subjects $n = 100$ or 200 in each of the two groups, the censoring times generated from the uniform distribution to create about 10% censoring, and the maximum follow-up time $\tau = 3$ year. The power of different tests is shown in Table 9.1. We see that the TS and YP tests tend to be more powerful than the unweighted log-rank test. The IUT has less power than the YP test, but the non-inferiority test may protect that patients from overall inferiority.

9.2.2 Sample Size for the Weighted Log-Rank Test under the Proportional Hazards Cure Model

When designing oncology clinical trials with cure or long-term survivors, the traditional sample size calculation methods may not be adequate because the

TABLE 9.1
Comparison of the power of the log-rank type tests and the IUT

					WLR		Adaptive		IUT Δ_{20}	
λ_0	cure	r	n	LR	Early	Late	TS	YP	1.05	1.15
1	0.05	0.5	100	0.895	0.687	0.944	0.881	0.924	0.891	0.913
1	0.05	0.5	200	0.995	0.927	0.998	0.996	0.998	0.996	0.997
1	0.05	0.8	100	0.191	0.123	0.213	0.174	0.213	0.144	0.177
1	0.05	0.8	200	0.345	0.202	0.389	0.302	0.371	0.305	0.348
1	0.1	0.5	100	0.864	0.668	0.920	0.848	0.902	0.858	0.884
1	0.1	0.5	200	0.990	0.920	0.997	0.990	0.996	0.993	0.994
1	0.1	0.8	100	0.192	0.136	0.210	0.179	0.218	0.142	0.176
1	0.1	0.8	200	0.316	0.208	0.354	0.282	0.340	0.271	0.311
2	0.05	0.5	100	0.725	0.343	0.896	0.767	0.829	0.698	0.763
2	0.05	0.5	200	0.951	0.580	0.996	0.971	0.985	0.961	0.972
2	0.05	0.8	100	0.142	0.084	0.191	0.150	0.170	0.082	0.118
2	0.05	0.8	200	0.241	0.117	0.326	0.242	0.271	0.182	0.238
2	0.1	0.5	100	0.675	0.347	0.860	0.722	0.778	0.650	0.714
2	0.1	0.5	200	0.942	0.619	0.994	0.964	0.979	0.954	0.967
2	0.1	0.8	100	0.138	0.086	0.182	0.150	0.159	0.077	0.110
2	0.1	0.8	200	0.231	0.126	0.322	0.229	0.263	0.170	0.216

cured patients are not taken into account. In this section, we show some recent developments in sample size calculation for the weighted log-rank test under the mixture cure models. The survival function for the mixture cure model is defined as

$$S(t|x) = \pi_c(x) + (1 - \pi_c(x))S_u(t|x) \tag{9.4}$$

for two groups: a control group with $x = 0$ and a treatment group with $x = 1$. Let $\pi_x = \pi_c(x)$ be the cure rate and let $\lambda_x(t) = \lambda_u(t|x)$ denote corresponding hazard function for the uncured patients in group x. The latency and the incidence parts of the mixture cure model are further specified as

$$\lambda_1(t) = \exp(\eta)\lambda_0(t) \text{ and } \mathrm{logit}(\pi_1) = \mathrm{logit}(\pi_0) + \gamma, \tag{9.5}$$

where η is the log-hazard ratio of treatment versus control for the uncured patients, and γ is the log-odds ratio of the cure rates. Even though the latency hazard function follows the PH assumption, the overall hazard function, which is given by

$$\lambda(t|x) = \frac{\frac{1-\pi_0}{1-\pi_0+\pi_0\exp(\gamma x)}[S_u(t|x=0)]^{\exp(\eta x)}}{\frac{\pi_0\exp(\gamma x)}{1-\pi_0+\pi_0\exp(\gamma x)} + \frac{1-\pi_0}{1-\pi_0+\pi_0\exp(\gamma x)}[S_u(t|x=0)]^{\exp(\eta x)}}\lambda_0(t)\exp(\eta x),$$

does not satisfy the proportional hazards assumption when $\pi_c(x) \not\equiv 0$.

Under this model, the null hypothesis of interest is

$$H_0 : \pi_0 = \pi_1 \text{ and } \lambda_0(t) = \lambda_1(t), \tag{9.6}$$

or equivalently

$$H_0 : \eta = \gamma = 0. \tag{9.7}$$

Three alternative hypotheses are considered

$$\begin{aligned} H_{1A} : &\quad \eta \neq 0, \gamma \neq 0, \\ H_{1B} : &\quad \eta \neq 0, \gamma = 0, \\ H_{1C} : &\quad \eta = 0, \gamma \neq 0. \end{aligned} \tag{9.8}$$

Because the parameters η and γ represent short-term and long-term effects on survival, the three alternative hypotheses represent differences of survival in the whole study period, differences of short-term survival only, and differences of long-term survival only, respectively.

Suppose that the weighted log-rank tests are used to test the hypothesis (9.7). Wang et al. (2012b) considered a series of local alternatives

$$H_{1A,n} : \eta = \eta^*/\sqrt{n}, \gamma = \gamma^*/\sqrt{n}$$

for fixed positive constants η^* and γ^*. If the censoring process is independent of the failure time and treatment allocation, the sample size is given by

$$n = \frac{(Z_{1-\alpha} + Z_{1-\beta})^2 \int_0^\tau w^2(t) S_C(t) f_0(t) \mathrm{d}t}{p(1-p)(1-\pi_0)\left\{\int_0^\tau w(t) m(t) S_C(t) f_0(t) \mathrm{d}t\right\}^2}, \tag{9.9}$$

where $S_C(t)$ is the common survival function for the censoring times in both groups, p is the proportion of patients in the treatment group, $f_0(t) = \mathrm{d}S_0(t)/\mathrm{d}t$ is the density function of failure time for the uncured patients in the control group, and $m(t) = \pi_0\{\gamma + \Lambda_0(t)\}/S_0(t) - \eta$ with $\Lambda_0(t) = -\log S_u(t|x = 0)$ and $S_0(t) = \pi_0 + (1 - \pi_0) S_u(t|x = 0)$. The sample size calculation for the local alternatives have implemented in R package `NPHMC` (Cai et al., 2014).

Xiong and Wu (2017) pointed out that there are two potential issues relating to the approach of sample size calculation on the basis of a series of local alternatives. The theoretical issue is that the accuracy of the formula derived under the local alternatives is not guaranteed when the alternative departures from the null. The practical issue is that the alternative hypothesis in application is always fixed, and does not change as the sample size changes. Thus, it is expected that the formula performs well only when the alternative is close to the null. Their simulation study showed that the sample size formula based on the local alternatives becomes questionable when the alternative departs reasonably away from the null. Under the fixed alternatives H_{1A} - H_{1C} in (9.8), they proposed the following sample size calculation method

$$n = \frac{(Z_{1-\alpha} + Z_{1-\beta})^2 \int_0^\tau w^2(t) q_1(t) S_C(t) f_0(t) \mathrm{d}t}{p(1-p)(1-\pi_0)(1-\pi_0+\pi_0 e^{\gamma})\left\{\int_0^\tau w(t) q_2(t) S_C(t) f_0(t) \mathrm{d}t\right\}^2}, \tag{9.10}$$

where

$$q_1(t) = \frac{q(t)\{p(1-\pi_0+\pi_0 e^{\gamma})+(1-p)\theta[S_0(t)]^{\theta-1}\}}{[p+(1-p)q(t)]^2},$$

$$q_2(t) = \frac{q(t)\{\theta[S_0(t)]^{\theta-1}[q(t)(1-\pi_0+\pi_0 e^{\gamma})]^{-1}-1\}}{p+(1-p)q(t)},$$

$$q(t) = \frac{\pi_0 e^{\gamma}+(1-\pi_0)[S_0(t)]^{\theta}}{[\pi_0 e^{\gamma}+(1-\pi_0)][\pi_0+(1-\pi_0)S_0(t)]},$$

and $\theta = \exp(\eta)$ is the hazard ratio of the treatment.

One may assume subjects are accrued over an accrual period of duration t_a and an additional follow-up time t_f that gives a total study duration of $\tau = t_a + t_f$. For simplicity, we assume that the only censoring is administrative censoring at time τ and that there is no loss to follow-up. Various distributions have been used for the patient accrual (enrollment). For example, the uniform enrollment during $[0, t_a]$, the survival function for the censoring times is given by

$$S_C(t) = \begin{cases} 1 & \text{if } t \le t_f \\ (t_a + t_f - t)/t_a & \text{if } t_f \le t \le t_a + t_f \\ 0 & \text{if otherwise} \end{cases}.$$

The survival functions $S_C(t)$ corresponding other patient enrollment distributions are specified in Table 1 of Cai et al. (2014). The integration for the sample size calculation can be calculated by numeric integrations, for example, by using the R function `integrate`. The Weibull distribution is assumed for the latency distribution with $S_0(t) = \exp(-\lambda_0 t^a)$. Under these assumptions, this sample size calculation method is implemented in an R function (Xiong and Wu, 2017) below.

```
sample.size.WLR<-function(shape, lambda0, pi0, pi1, p, ta, tf, HR,
                          alpha, power, rho=0, nu=0){
       z0=qnorm(1-alpha/2)
       z1=qnorm(power)
       tau=ta+tf
       delta=1/HR

       gamma=log(pi1/(1-pi1))-log(pi0/(1-pi0))
       q=function(t) {
         num=pi0*exp(gamma)+(1-pi0)*S0(t)^delta
         den=(pi0*exp(gamma)+(1-pi0))*(pi0+(1-pi0)*S0(t))
         num/den
       }
       S0=function(t){exp(-lambda0*t^shape)}
       h0=function(t){shape*lambda0*t^(shape-1)}
       S.C=function(t){1-punif(t, tf, tau)}

       w=function(t) {
         S0.Star=function(t) { pi0+(1-pi0)*S0(t) }
```

```
        S1.Star=function(t) { pi1+(1-pi1)*(S0(t))^delta }
        S.pool=p*S0.Star(t)+(1-p)*S1.Star(t)
        if (is.na(rho) | is.na(nu)) {
              w.t=1
        } else {
              w.t=(S.pool^rho)*((1-S.pool)^nu)
        }
        w.t
      }

      q1=function(t){
              den=(p+(1-p)*q(t))^2
              num=q(t)*(p*(1-pi0+pi0*exp(gamma))+(1-p)*delta*S0(t)
              ^(delta-1))
              num/den
      }
      q2=function(t){
              den=p+(1-p)*q(t)
              num=q(t)*(delta*S0(t)^(delta-1)/(q(t)*(1-pi0+pi0*exp
              (gamma)))-1)
              num/den
      }
      f1=function(t){w(t)^2*q1(t)*S.C(t)*S0(t)*h0(t)}
      f2=function(t){w(t)*q2(t)*S.C(t)*S0(t)*h0(t)}
      A=integrate(f1, 0, tau)$value
      B=integrate(f2, 0, tau)$value
      nX=(z0+z1)^2*A/(p*(1-p)*(1-pi0)*(1-pi0+pi0*exp(gamma))*B^2)
      m=function(t){pi0*(gamma-log(delta)*log(S0(t)))/(pi0+(1-pi0)
      *S0(t))-log(delta)}
      g1=function(t) w(t)^2*S.C(t)*S0(t)*h0(t)
      g2=function(t) w(t)*m(t)*S.C(t)*S0(t)*h0(t)
      C=integrate(g1, 0, tau)$value
      D=integrate(g2, 0, tau)$value
      nW=(z0+z1)^2*C/(p*(1-p)*(1-pi0)*D^2)
      sample.size=ceiling(c(nX, nW))
      sample.size
}
```

The syntax of the R function is

```
sample.size.WLR(shape, lambda0, pi0, pi1, HR, p, ta, tf, alpha,
power, rho=0, nu=0),
```

where `shape` is the parameter a, `lambda0` is λ_0, `pi0` is π_0, `pi1` is π_1, `HR` is θ, `p` is p, which is $p = 0.5$ under the typical 1:1 randomization, `ta` is t_a, `tf` is t_f, `alpha` is the type I error rate α, `power` is the power desired, `rho` and `nu` are ρ and ν in the Fleming-Harrignton weight function (9.1). The output from this function includes sample sizes from the two methods by Wang et al. (2012b) and Xiong and Wu (2017).

9.2.3 Power and Sample Size in the Presence of Delayed Onset of Treatment Effect and Cure

The power and sample size calculation for immuno-oncology clinical trials need to deal with the delayed onset of treatment effects. If a cure fraction is present in the trials, most of the existing methods do not consider the existence of cure or long-term survivors and the tests may have a low power to detect the true treatment effect. In this section, we describe a new weighted log-rank test to detect the treatment effect under a piecewise PH mixture cure model with a random delay time (Liu et al., 2018a).

Suppose that the treatment variable is denoted as x, where $x = 0$ for the control group and $x = 1$ for the treatment group. Let $\lambda_x(t)$, $\Lambda_x(t)$, $S_x(t)$ be the hazard function, cumulative hazard function, and survival function for group x. Considered the following four survival models:

- PH model: The PH model assumes that $S_1(t) = S_0(t)^r$, where r is the constant hazard ratio.

- Piecewise PH (PPH) model with change-point τ. The change-point represents the onset time of the delayed treatment effect

$$S_1(t) = \begin{cases} S_0(t), & t \leq \tau \\ S_0(\tau)^{1-r} S_0(t)^r & t > \tau \end{cases} \tag{9.11}$$

- PHC model assumes that subjects in the x group are potentially cured from the cancer with a probability of π_x and the survival function for the uncured subjects is $S_{xu}(t)$. The overall survival functions for the control and treatment groups are

$$\begin{aligned} S_0(t) &= \pi_0 + (1 - \pi_0) S_{0u}(t), \\ S_1(t) &= S_0(t)^r = \pi_1 + (1 - \pi_1) S_{1u}(t), \end{aligned} \tag{9.12}$$

  where $\pi_1 = \pi_0^r$ and $S_{1u}(t) = [S_0(t)^r - \pi_0^r]/(1 - \pi_0^r)$. The PHC can be used when a cure rate is present but without delayed treatment onset time. More details of this cure model can be found in Section 2.4.

- Piecewise PHC model (PPHC) with a fixed delay time. This model assumes that the survival function $S_0(t)$ for the control group is specified in Equation (9.12) and the survival function for the treatment group is specified in Equation (9.11). The PPHC is a generalization of the PH, the PHC, and the PPH models. If $\pi_0 = 0$, it is reduced to the PPH model. If $\tau = 0$, it is reduced to the PHC model. If $\pi_0 = 0$ and $\tau = 0$, it is reduced to the PH model.

The PPHC is a flexible model that allows both delayed onset of treatment effect and cure. Furthermore, the delayed onset time τ for the treatment group may be a random variable. Given the delayed onset time τ, the conditional survival function $S_1(t|\tau)$ is

$$S_1(t|\tau) = S_0(t)I(t \leq \tau) + S_0(\tau)^{1-r}S_0(t)^r I(t > \tau). \tag{9.13}$$

Let $G_\tau(\tau)$ be the survival function for the random delay time. The marginal survival function for the treatment group is

$$S_1(t) = S_0(t)G_\tau(t) - S_0(t)^r \int_0^t S_0(\tau)^{1-r} dG_\tau(\tau),$$

where $S_0(t)$ is the overall survival function in the control group as specified in (9.12). Let $(\tau_{\min}, \tau_{\max})$ denote the range of the possible values of τ. Based on the PPHC with random delay time, the survival functions for the control and treatment groups are identical, i.e., $S_1(t) = S_0(t)$ when $t \leq \tau_{\min}$ and take the proportional hazards form, i.e., $S_1(t) = S_0(t)^r E_\tau(S_0(\tau)^{1-r})$ when $t > \tau_{\max}$. Between $\tau_{\min}$ and $\tau_{\max}$, the hazard ratio changes from 1 to r gradually, instead of a sudden jump as in the PPHC with a fixed delay time.

For the treatment group, let n_1 denote the number of patients, $N_{1i} = N_{1i}(t)$ and $Y_{1i} = Y_{1i}(t)$ be the respective counting process and at-risk process of the ith patient, $N_1 = \sum_1^{n_1} N_{1i}$ and $Y_1 = \sum_1^{n_1} Y_{1i}$, and $p_1 = p_1(t)$ be the at risk probability function. In the control group, $n_0, N_{0i}, Y_{0i}, N_0, Y_0$ and p_0 are similarly defined. In the pooled sample, let $n = n_0 + n_1$ be the total number of patients, Λ be the pooled cumulative hazard function, $N = N_1 + N_0$ and $Y = Y_1 + Y_0$, and p be the pooled at risk probability function. The weighted log-rank test statistic is defined as

$$T_w = L_w/\sqrt{V_w}, \tag{9.14}$$

where

$$L_w = n^{-\frac{1}{2}} \int \frac{w(t)}{Y}\left(Y_0 dN_1 - Y_1 dN_0\right), \; V_w = \frac{1}{n}\int w(t)^2 \frac{Y_0 Y_1}{Y^2} dN.$$

Under the null hypothesis H_0: $S_1(t) = S_0(t)$, the weighted log-rank statistic is asymptotic normal $T_w \sim N(0,1)$. Under the local alternatives H_1: $\log(\Lambda_1/\Lambda_0) = o(1)$, which means that the ratio of the two cumulative hazard functions is bounded, it can be shown that the proposed weights are nearly optimal under mild assumptions and that the test statistic is approximately distributed as

$$T_w \sim N(\sqrt{n}\mu/\sqrt{V_w}, 1),$$

where

$$\mu = \int w(t)c(1-c)\frac{p_0 p_1}{p} d(\Lambda_1 - \Lambda_0), V_w = \int w(t)^2 c(1-c)\frac{p_0 p_1}{p} d\Lambda,$$

$\Lambda(t)$ is the cumulative hazard of the pooled data and $c = n_1/n$ is the proportion of patients in the treatment group. For the simplicity of notation, the argument t is omitted from the functions $p_0(t), p_1(t), p(t), \Lambda_1(t), \lambda_2(t)$ and $\Lambda(t)$. Let $S_C(t)$ be the survival function for the censoring times. It is clear that $S(t) = (1-c)S_0(t) + cS_1(t)$, $p = (1-c)p_0 + cp_1$, $p_1 = S_1 S_C$, and $p_0 = S_0 S_C$. The power function for a total sample size n is given by

$$\text{Power}(n) = P(T_w < Z_{1-\alpha})$$

and the sample size is given by

$$N_w(\beta) = \frac{V_w(Z_{1-\alpha} + Z_{1-\beta})^2}{\mu^2}, \tag{9.15}$$

where α is the Type 1 error rate and β is the type II error rate.

Because the weighted log-rank test statistic T_w is invariant with respect to a constant change in weight, one may assume $\max w(t) = 1$. The optimal weight w_O is defined as the weight that minimizes the sample size for any given type I error rate of α and type II error rate of β. Although the optimal weight may not exist or may be difficult to computer in general, Liu et al. (2018a) showed that the sample size formula (9.15) is satisfactory when the condition $\log(\Lambda_1/\Lambda_0) = o(1)$ holds. The Cauchy-Schwarz Inequality implies that

$$\begin{aligned}
\left|\frac{\mu}{\sqrt{V_w}}\right| &= \left|\frac{\int w(t)c(1-c)\frac{p_0p_1}{p}d(\Lambda_1 - \Lambda_0)}{\sqrt{\int w(t)^2 c(1-c)\frac{p_0p_1}{p}d\Lambda}}\right| \\
&= \left|\frac{\int w(t)\sqrt{\lambda}\frac{\lambda_1-\lambda_0}{\sqrt{\lambda}}c(1-c)\frac{p_0p_1}{p}dt}{\sqrt{\int w(t)^2\lambda c(1-c)\frac{p_0p_1}{p}dt}}\right| \\
&\leq \sqrt{\int \frac{(\lambda_1-\lambda_0)^2}{\lambda}c(1-c)\frac{p_0p_1}{p}dt},
\end{aligned} \tag{9.16}$$

where λ is the hazard function of the pooled survival data. The equality holds if and only if $w = K(\lambda_1 - \lambda_0)/\lambda$ for a constant K. Therefore, the optimal weight $w_O = K(\lambda_1 - \lambda_0)/\lambda$.

In practice, because the hazard functions λ_0, λ_1 and λ for the control, treatment and pooled groups cannot be reliably estimated, the optimal weight is difficult to obtain. In the presence of both delayed onset of treatment effect and cure, the cumulative distribution function, $F_\tau(t) = 1 - G_\tau(t)$, of the random delay onset time τ is suggested to use as the weight. The main reason is that F_τ is a close approximation of the optimal weight w_O. There are two additional advantages of using F_τ as the weight. First, F_τ can be estimated from historical data using the proposed PPHC. Second, the weight based on F_τ is intuitive as a larger weight is used for stronger treatment effect at time t. The sample size based on the F_τ weight is given as

$$N_{F_\tau}(\beta) = \frac{(Z_\alpha + Z_\beta)^2 \int F_\tau^2 p_0 p_1/p d\Lambda}{c(1-c)\left(\int F_\tau p_0 p_1/p d(\Lambda_1 - \Lambda_0)\right)^2}. \tag{9.17}$$

The performance of F_τ as a good approximation of the optimal weight is confirmed in simulation (Liu et al., 2018a).

The following is the R function implements the sample size calculation:

```
DelayCureSampleSize<-function(accural=30, followup=16,
cure=0.2, shape=1, scale=12/log(2),
HR.post.delay=0.7, delay.start=0, delay.end=9,
TypeI=0.05, TypeII=0.1,
beta.a=1, beta.b=1, quad.points=50,
SC=function(t){min (46-t, 30)/30},
Wt=function(t){pbeta((t)/9, shapel=1, shape2=1)})
{
        #### derived parameters, etc
        boundary<-unique(c(delay.start, delay.end, followup,
        followup+accural, 0))
        boundary<-boundary[order(boundary)]
        boundary.low<-boundary[-length(boundary)]
        boundary.upp<-boundary[-1]
        boundary.mat<-cbind(boundary.low, boundary.upp)
        delay.span<-delay.end-delay.start

        #### gauss-Legendre quadrature
        #### g is the integrand to integrate over [0, t]
        GQ<-gauss.quad(n=quad.points, kind="legendre")
        GQ.int<-function(g, limits=c(0,1)) {
                upp<-limits[2]
                low<-limits[1]
                sum(sapply(GQ$nodes, function(s) {
                        g((upp-low)*s/2+(upp+low)/2)*(upp-low)/2})*
                        GQ$weights)
        }

        #### utility functions: so, fo, si, f1, Sc, Stau
        S0<-function(t) {
                cure+(1-cure)*pweibull(t, shape=shape, scale=scale,
                lower.tail=FALSE)
        }
        f0<-function(t) {
                (1-cure)*dweibull(t, shape=shape, scale=scale)
        }

        ##fo and so has to be globally smooth
        Stau<-function(t) {
                pbeta((t-delay.start)/delay.span, shapel=beta.a,
                shape2=beta.b, lower.tail=FALSE)
        }
        ftau<-function(t) {
                dbeta((t-delay.start)/delay.span, shapel=beta.a,
                shape2=beta.b)/delay.span
```

```
        }
        int.grand4S1<-function (tau) {
                S0(tau)^(1-HR.post.delay)*ftau(tau)
        }
        S1<-function(t) {
                S0(t)*Stau(t)+S0(t)^HR.post.delay*GQ.int(int.
                grand4S1, c(0, min(t,delay.end)))
        }
        f1<-function(t) {
                f0(t)*Stau(t) + f0(t)*HR.post.delay*
                S0(t)^(HR.post.delay-1)*GQ.int(int.grand4S1, c(0,
                min(t,delay.end)))
        }
        S.all<-function(t) { (S0(t)+S1(t))/2 }
        f.all<-function(t) { (f0(t)+f1(t))/2 }
        num.int.grand<-function(t) {
                (1-Stau(t))^2*S0(t)*S1(t)*(S.all(t)^(-2))*SC(t)*f.
                all(t)
        }
        den.int.grand<-function(t) {
                (1-Stau(t))*S0(t)*S1(t)/S.all(t)*SC(t)*(f1(t)/S1(t)-
                f0(t)/S0(t))
        }
        int.num<-sum(apply(boundary.mat, 1, function (vec.tmp)
        GQ.int(num.int.grand, limits=vec.tmp)))
        int.den<-sum(apply(boundary.mat, 1, function (vec.tmp)
        GQ.int(den.int.grand, limits=vec.tmp)))

        #### sample size
        4*int.num*(qnorm(TypeI/2)+qnorm (TypeII))^2/int.den^2
}
```

The input parameters may be the design input parameters or be estimated from historical data. For example, `accural` and `followup` are the patient enrollment duration and study duration, `cure` is the target cure rate, `shape` and `scale` are the shape and scale parameters of the Weibull latency distribution, `HR.post.delay` is pre-specified hazard ratio after delayed treatment onset time, `delay.start` and `delay.end` specify the range of delay onset time in month, `TypeI` and `TypeII` are the Type 1 and 2 error rates, `beta.a`, `beta.b` and `Wt` are the parameters and functions that specify the distribution of random delayed onset time and `SC` is the function for the censoring times.

9.3 Some Design Issues in Clinical Trials with Cure

9.3.1 Cure Modeling in Real-Time Prediction

Many cancer clinical trials determine the interim and final analyses times based on the occurrence of a pre-specified number of events. For example, a cancer trial could be designed to have 80% statistical power with 300 deaths, with planned interim analyses after the 100th and 200th deaths, and a final analysis when the 300th death occurs (Bagiella and Heitjan, 2001). Because the times of occurrence of these landmark events are random, it is desirable to have a tool for predicting these milestones for proper logistical planning. A number of statistical models have been proposed for the prediction of event numbers in clinical trials with survival endpoints (Ying et al., 2004; Ying and Heitjan, 2008; Donovan et al., 2006, 2007). These models assume that all subjects will eventually experience the event if follow-up time is sufficiently long (Heitjan et al., 2015; Zhang and Long, 2012). For the clinical trials where cure or long-term survival is possible, ignoring the possibility of cure may lead to biases in event prediction, because a fraction of surviving patients would be predicted to experience events even though they are no longer susceptible.

To address the issue of bias in event prediction based on the conventional survival models, Chen (2016) proposed to use cure models. At each prediction time, the parametric mixture cure model with the best model fit is selected and used to predict the future events for all the subjects who would be enrolled in the future and do not yet have an event at the analysis time. Based on a real immuno-oncology clinical trial, Chen (2016) demonstrated that the predictions based on the mixture cure models are much closer to the target. Because of the identifiability issue (Li et al., 2001) of parametric mixture cure model, the estimation based on limited follow-up time may be unreliable and the extrapolation of survival beyond the study follow-up time are highly variable. In this section, we describe a real-time Bayesian prediction method introduced by Ying et al. (2017). It uses mixture cure modeling and currently accumulating trial data to construct the accrual/survival model and then to predict and simulate the future course of a trial.

Consider a simple scenario of two-arm randomized clinical trial where all patients are enrolled at time 0 and join the trial according to a Poisson process with a constant rate of μ per unit of time and are randomized 1:1 between the two study arms. Each participant can either i) develop the event of interest, ii) remain in the trial without occurrence of the event, or iii) become lost to follow-up. At current calendar time $t_0 > 0$, one intends to make predictions about the future course of the trial. A typical goal is to predict the calendar time T^* at which the D^*th event will occur. Let x be the indicator of treatment arms, where $x = 0$ for the control group and $x = 1$ for the treatment group.

In the presence of cure, one may use a parametric mixture cure model where

$$S(t|x) = \pi_c(x) + (1 - \pi_c(x))S_u(t|x), \tag{9.18}$$

where $\pi_c(x)$ is the cure probability that can be modeled with a logistic regression, and $S_u(t|x) = \exp\left(-(t/\beta_x)^{\alpha_x}\right)$, $\alpha_x > 0$, $\beta_x > 0$, is the Weibull survival function for the uncured patients from arm x. We also assume that the time to loss to follow-up in arm x independently follows a Weibull model with arm-specific scale and shape parameters.

If $\pi_c(x) \equiv 0$, i.e., there is no cured fraction, a Bayesian prediction method can be implemented in the following way (Ying et al., 2004). The first step in the prediction modeling is to specify priors for the enrollment rate and the parameters of the Weibull event time and time to loss to follow-up distributions in each arm. For example, if the time unit is month, one may assume a gamma prior for the accrual rate, i.e., Gamma$(m, 1)$, where m is the expected number of patients recruited per month. The shape and scale parameters for the Weibull distribution may be derived from historical data. To create predictions at time t_0, one needs to compute the posterior density of the parameters using the data accrued up to that time. Based on the posterior density of parameters,

1. Sample a set of parameters from the posterior using importance sampling or some other methods.
2. Conditional on the sampled parameters, generate a data set from the predictive distribution of the enrollment, survival and loss-to-follow-up times:
   (a) Simulate the event and loss-to-follow-up times for participants who are enrolled and on study but have not yet experienced an event.
   (b) If the total enrollment goal has not yet been reached, simulate the enrollment, event, and loss times for a hypothetical set of participants who have not yet been enrolled.
   (c) Determine each subject's date of failure (real or simulated), and rank the event dates among subjects who either have had an event or are predicted to have an event.
   (d) Identify the date of the landmark time T^*.

Each replication of steps 1 and 2 generates a draw from the predictive distribution of the landmark time T^*. Repeating them many times, one can predict the landmark time as, for example, the median of the simulated distribution of T^*, with 95% prediction interval.

If $\pi_c(x) > 0$, the overall prediction procedure remains the same as described above, except that the cure status for the censored and not-yet-enrolled subjects is generated from a Bernoulli distribution with the estimated cure probability. Specifically, for a subject in arm x who was enrolled at calendar time τ_0, and did not experience an event by analysis time $t_0 \geq \tau_0$, let Y be the cure status, where $Y = 0$ being cured. The conditional cure probability for the subject in arm x is

$$P(Y = 0|T > t_0, x) = \frac{\pi_c(x)}{\pi_c(x) + (1 - \pi_c(x))S_u(t|x)}. \qquad (9.19)$$

For a subject who is simulated to be cured, the event time is imputed as infinity. If a subject is simulated as not cured, the event time is generated from $S_u(t|x)$ for a new subject, or from $S_u(t|x)$ conditional on the event time being at least t_0 for an existing censored subject.

For a cured subject, we set the event time to infinity. However, this is not reasonable if the endpoint is overall survival. Rather, we interpret the infinite event time as that the subject dies at a more advanced age, potentially from another disease than the one under study. The possibility of infinite event times has important ramifications for prediction algorithms, because in a given set of imputed event times it is possible that the predicted time of the event landmark T^* will itself be infinite. This would occur if we were attempting to predict the time of the D^*th event, but the set of imputed event times had fewer than D^* finite event times. Thus, in a given simulated predictive distribution it is possible for the upper limit of the prediction interval, the median prediction, and even the lower limit of the prediction interval to be infinite. In fact, it has been shown by simulation that using the mixture cure model yields better predictions for event counts when there is cure or when the survival curves become plateau. However, the average width of the prediction intervals of event counts based on the mixture cure model tends to be wider.

9.3.2 Futility Analysis of Survival Data with Cure

The accumulating results of clinical trials can be monitored for a variety of reasons. The primary reason is typically to help protect patient safety. If the interim results show that patients under the treatment are exposed with unnecessary risk, the protocol can be amended to mitigate that risk, or the clinical trial should be terminated. There is also often a strong ethical imperative or economic incentive to stop a trial as soon as efficacy has been established. One additional reason for stopping a clinical trial prematurely, which is somewhat more controversial than safety or efficacy is futility (He et al., 2012), i.e., the inability of the trial to achieve its objectives. The main goals of stopping for futility are to preserve resources that could be spent on more promising research, and to prevent patients from being exposed to ineffective experimental treatments unnecessarily (Snapinn et al., 2006; Lachin, 2005) .

It is important to distinguish between operational and statistical aspects of futility assessment. Operational aspects that might cause a clinical trial to be futile include slow recruitment of patients or slow accumulation of primary endpoints. However, we on statistical futility, in which the final results are unlikely to be statistically significant based on the interim results. From statistical perspective, stopping for futility is closely related to stopping for early efficacy. While stopping for efficacy implies early rejection of the null hypothesis and stopping for futility implies early rejection of alternative hypothesis. There are two fundamental approaches for assessing futility. The first approach is to calculate the probability of a statistically significant of the final result conditional on the interim results. If this probability is below a predefined threshold, the trial is terminated. We refer to this approach as the conditional approach, and further divide it into a frequentist method of stochastic curtailment based on the conditional power and a fully Bayesian method of predictive power and predictive probability. The second approach is the group sequential futility stopping boundaries defined by the β-spending function, either in isolation or in combination with group sequential efficacy boundaries. We describe in this section the conditional power calculation in the futility analysis for survival data with cure.

9.3.2.1 Conditional Power for Mixture Cure Models

Bernardo and Ibrahim (2000) proposed several futility stopping rules based on the mixture cure model. They adapted the asymptotic results by Ewell and Ibrahim (1997) to group sequential clinical trial designs for survival data with cure. Here we review the calculation of conditional power for the futility analysis.

Consider a trial in which subjects are randomized to one of two treatment arms and patients in both groups have a positive probability of being cured. We are interested in testing whether the cure rates and the survival distributions for those not cured in the two groups are equal, i.e., we are interested in the hypothesis

$$H_0 : S_1(t) = S_2(t) \text{ vs } H_1 : S_1(t) \neq S_2(t),$$

where $S_j(t) = \theta_j + (1-\theta_j)S_{uj}(t)$ is the survival distribution for treatment j, $j = 1, 2$. Consider a general class of local alternatives for the mixture cure rate model

$$\begin{aligned} S_{uj}(t) &= 1 - [1 - \exp\{(-1)^j\psi\}(1-\theta_0)]F_C^*(t) \\ &\quad - \exp\{(-1)^j\psi\}(1-\theta_0)[1 - 1 - F_{\bar{C}}^*(t)\exp\{(-1)^j\tau\}] \quad (9.20) \end{aligned}$$

where $F_C^*(t)$ and $F_{\bar{C}}^*(t)$ are the distribution functions for time to failure combined over both treatment groups among the cured and non-cured patients, respectively, the parameters ψ, τ and θ_0 are defined as follows:

$$\begin{aligned} \psi &= \frac{1}{2}\log\left(\frac{1-\theta_1}{1-\theta_1}\right), \\ \tau &= \frac{1}{2}\log\left(\frac{\Lambda_{u2}(t)}{\Lambda_{u1}(t)}\right), \\ \theta_0 &= 1 - [(1-\theta_1)(1-\theta_2]^{\frac{1}{2}}, \end{aligned}$$

and $\Lambda_{uj}(u)$ is the cumulative hazard function corresponding to $S_{uj}(t)$. Here we assume that the cumulative hazards $\Lambda_{u1}(t)$ and $\Lambda_{u2}(t)$ are proportional. So τ is a scalar. When $\psi = \tau = 0$, these alternative hypotheses reduce to the null hypothesis

$$1 - S_1(t) = 1 - S_2(t) = \theta_0 F_C^*(t) + (1-\theta_0) F_{\tilde{C}}^*(t), \tag{9.21}$$

which represents equality of the two survival distributions for both treatment arms. If we let $F_{\tilde{C}}^*(t) \to 0$, then we obtain a sub-distribution for the cure rate model under the null hypothesis.

Let n be the total number of events combined over both treatment groups. Assume there exists a sequence of real numbers $\alpha_n, \beta_n, n = 1, 2, ..,$ such that $\sqrt{n}\alpha_n \to \psi$ and $\sqrt{n}\beta_n \to \tau$ as $n \to \infty$. Under the sequence of local alternatives

$$\begin{aligned} S_{uj}(t) &= 1 - [1 - \exp\{(-1)^j \alpha_n\}(1-\theta_0)] F_C^*(t) \\ &\quad - \exp\{(-1)^j \alpha_n\}(1-\theta_0)\left[1 - \{1 - F_{\tilde{C}}^*(t)\}^{\exp\{(-1)^j \beta_n\}}\right], \end{aligned} \tag{9.22}$$

it can be shown that as $n \to \infty$, the normalized log-rank statistic converges to a normal distribution with mean $(\sqrt{n}\mu)/\sigma$ and unit variance, where

$$\mu = p(1-p)\int_0^\infty K(u|\psi, \tau, \theta_0) S_0(u) G_0(u) du, \tag{9.23}$$

$$K(u|\psi, \tau, \theta_0) = \frac{2(\theta_0 - 1) f_{\tilde{C}}^*(u)}{1 - (1-\theta_0) F_{\tilde{C}}^*(u)} \left\{ \tau + \frac{\psi + \tau\theta_0 \log(1 - F_{\tilde{C}}^*(u))}{1 - (1-\theta_0) F_{\tilde{C}}^*(u)} \right\}, \tag{9.24}$$

$$\sigma = p(1-p)\int_0^\infty f_0(u) G_0(u) du, \tag{9.25}$$

and p is the probability of assignment to treatment group, $S_0(u)$ denotes the survivor function under the null hypothesis, $f_0(u)$ is the density function of the failure times corresponding to $S_0(u)$, $f_{\tilde{C}}^*(u)$ is the density function of the failure times corresponding to $F_{\tilde{C}}^*(u)$, and $G_0(u)$ is the common survivor function of the censoring time for both treatment groups. These asymptotic results are valid under any parametric model for the non-cured group. Under the null hypothesis of equality of cure rates and survival distributions, $\mu = 0$. The preceding hypotheses can be reformulated as $H_0 : \mu = 0$ versus $H_1 : \mu \neq 0$. The value of μ represents differences in the cure rates and the latency survival distributions between the two treatment groups.

For K planned interim analyses, let $Z_k, k = 1, \ldots, K$ denote the normalized log-rank statistic at the kth interim analysis. The following theorem provides the distribution of the test statistics under the local alternatives specified in (9.22) (Bernardo and Ibrahim, 2000):

Theorem 9.3.1 *Let n_k denote the number of events at the kth interim analysis. Under the class of local alternatives specified in (9.22), $(Z_1, Z_2, \ldots, Z_K)$ follow a multivariate normal distribution with mean $(\sqrt{n_1}\mu/\sigma, \ldots, \sqrt{n_K}\mu/\sigma)$, unit variances and covariances equal to $\sqrt{n_k/n_{k'}}$ for $k < k'$.*

The proof of Theorem 9.3.1 uses the fact that $(\sqrt{n_1}Z_1, \sqrt{n_2}Z_2, \ldots, \sqrt{n_K}Z_K)$ can be written as partial sums with independent increments under the specified sequence of local alternatives for the cure rate model, which is the key idea in obtaining asymptotic normality. Proof of the asymptotic normality of these partial sums is a direct extension of that given in Ewell and Ibrahim (1997) and thus is omitted here for brevity. The result in Theorem 9.3.1 allows us to derive the stopping rules for three different sequential methods, namely conditional power, predictive power and repeated confidence intervals procedures. An implicit assumption in the application of Theorem 9.3.1 to these sequential methods is that the study follows a type II censoring mechanism since the value of n_K has to be known in advance. However, when other types of random censoring are in effect, the expected number of events at the end of the study, which is calculated at the design stage, can be used to estimate n_K. The prediction of number of events has been described in Section 9.3.1.

For the conditional power method, the trial is stopped at the kth interim in favor of the alternative hypothesis whenever the power upon completion of the trial given the value of Z_k is greater than some specified value, say p_E. Conversely, the trial is stopped early in favor of the null hypothesis whenever the conditional power at the kth interim analysis is less than some other specified value, p_F. Based on the asymptotic distribution of $(Z_1, Z_2, \ldots, Z_K)$ from Theorem 9.3.1, the conditional power at the kth analysis is

$$P_k(\mu) = 1 - \Phi\left(\frac{\sigma\sqrt{n_K}z_{1-\alpha} - \sigma\sqrt{n_k}Z_k - (n_K - n_k)\mu}{\sigma\sqrt{n_K - n_k}}\right),$$

where $z_{1-\alpha}$ is the standard normal $(1-\alpha)\times 100$th percentile. Let μ_0 and μ_1 be the values of μ in equation (9.23) under the null and alternative hypotheses, respectively. The conditional power method can be used formally as a stopping rule for the one-sided testing problem:

- stop the trial at the kth interim in favor of the alternative hypothesis if $P_k(\mu_0) > p_E$,
- stop the trial at the kth interim in favor of the null hypothesis if $P_k(\mu_1) < p_F$.

Setting the value of $\mu_0 = 0$, the stopping boundaries become:

- stop early in favor of H_1 if

$$Z_k > \sqrt{\frac{n_K}{n_k}}z_{1-\alpha} + \sqrt{\frac{n_K - n_k}{n_k}}z_{p_E}$$

- stop early in favor of H_0 if

$$Z_k < \sqrt{\frac{n_K}{n_k}}z_{1-\alpha} - \sqrt{\frac{n_K - n_k}{n_k}}z_{1-p_F} - \frac{n_K - n_k}{\sqrt{n_k}}\frac{\mu_1}{\sigma}.$$

Bayesian predictive inference is another method that can be used to decide if a trial may be stopped early. The idea is to calculate an average conditional power, which uses either the current posterior distribution or an elicited prior distribution as the weight function. This average conditional power is referred to as the predictive power.

9.3.2.2 Conditional Power for Non-Mixture Cure Models

Kuehnapfel et al. (2017) proposed the conditional power and unconditional power for futility analysis based on the following non-mixture cure model or the PHC model:

$$S(t|x) = \pi_c(x)^{F^H(t|x)},$$

where x is the group label with $x = 1$ for the control group and $x = 2$ for the treatment group, $\pi_c(x)$ is the cure rate for group x, and $F^H(t|x)$ is a proper parametric distribution function. The exponential, Weibull and gamma distributions have been considered for $F^H(t|x)$. We only focus on the exponential distribution with $F^H(t|x) = 1 - \exp(-\lambda_x t)$,, where λ_x is the rate parameter. Let $S_i(t) = S(t|x = i)$ and $F_i^H(t) = F^H(t|x = i)$. The corresponding hazard function $h_i(t)$ of $S_i(t)$ is

$$h_i(t) = -\lambda_i \exp(-\lambda_i t) \log(\pi_i),$$

and the hazard ratio between the two groups is

$$\theta(t) = \frac{\lambda_2}{\lambda_1} \exp\{-(\lambda_2 - \lambda_1)t\} \frac{\log(\pi_2)}{\log(\pi_1)}.$$

The time independence of the hazard ratio or the proportional hazards only holds if $\lambda_1 = \lambda_2$. The corresponding hazard ratio is $\theta = \log(\pi_2)/\log(\pi_1)$.

To compare the two treatment groups, we can test the following hypothesis

$$H_0 : \theta = 1 \text{ vs } H_1 : \theta \neq 1.$$

Let t_{ij} and δ_{ij} be the observed time and censoring indicator for subject j, $j = 1, \ldots, n_i$ in group i. A test statistic for the hypothesis is (Anderson, 2000)

$$W = \log(\hat{\theta}) = \log(-\log(\hat{\pi}_2)) - \log(-\log(\hat{\pi}_1)) = \log \frac{D_2}{O_2'} - \log \frac{D_1}{O_1'}, \quad (9.26)$$

where $D_i = \sum_{j=1}^{n_i} \delta_{ij}$ is the number of deaths in group i and

$$O_i' = \sum_{j=1}^{n_i} \{1 - \exp(-\hat{\lambda}_i t_{ij})\}. \quad (9.27)$$

The asymptotic power function of the test is given by

$$T_\theta = 1 + \Phi\left(\frac{z_{\frac{\alpha}{2}}\sigma_0 + \mu_0 - \mu_1}{\sigma_1}\right) - \Phi\left(\frac{z_{1-\frac{\alpha}{2}}\sigma_0 + \mu_0 - \mu_1}{\sigma_1}\right), \quad (9.28)$$

where Φ is the cumulative distribution for the standard normal distribution, z_α is the α quantile and

$$\begin{aligned}\mu_0 &= 0,\\ \sigma_0^2 &= 2[n\{1-\pi_1(1+\log^2\pi_1)\}]^{-1},\end{aligned}$$

are the mean and variance under the null distribution and

$$\begin{aligned}\mu_1 &= \log\theta,\\ \sigma_1^2 &= \{n[1-\pi_1(1+\log^2\pi_1)]\}^{-1}+\{n[1-\pi_1^\theta(1+(\theta\log\pi_1)^2)]\}^{-1}\end{aligned}$$

are the mean and variance under the alternative distribution.

The available data at interim analysis are denoted as $(D_1, O_1^{'}, D_2, O_2^{'})$. Let D_i^* denote the number of deaths and let $O_i^{'*}$ be a function of the future observation time of group i counted from time of interim analysis until final analysis of the study in analogy to the definition of $O_i^{'}$ in equation (9.27). The conditional test statistic can be defined similarly to equation (9.26),

$$W^* = \log\frac{D_2+D_2^*}{O_2^{'}+O_2^{'*}} - \log\frac{D_1+D_1^*}{O_1^{'}+O_1^{'*}}.$$

It can be shown (Kuehnapfel et al., 2017) that the asymptotic conditional power function can be calculated as (9.28) with the corresponding mean and variances:

$$\begin{aligned}\mu(\theta) &= \log\Delta_2 - \log\Delta_1,\\ \sigma^2(\theta) &= \frac{1}{n^*}\left[\{1-\exp(-\Delta_1)(1+\Delta_1^2)\}^{-1}+\{1-\exp(-\Delta_2)(1+\Delta_2^2)\}^{-1}\right],\end{aligned}$$

where n^* denotes the remaining sample size, i.e., the total sample size n minus the observed number of patients so far,

$$\begin{aligned}\Delta_1 &= \frac{d_1-\log(\pi_1)EO_1^{'*}}{o_1^{'}+EO_1^{'*}},\\ \Delta_2 &= \frac{d_2-\theta\log(\pi_1)EO_2^{'*}}{o_2^{'}+EO_2^{'*}},\end{aligned}$$

and $EO_i^{'*}$ is the expectation of future observation time, $O_i^{'*}$, of group i at the interim analysis.

The unconditional and conditional power formulae for the non-mixture models were implemented in the R package `cp`. The function `ConPwrExp` contains the formulae for the exponential model without any cure fraction while the functions for the non-mixture models are `ConPwrNonMixExp` for exponential survival, `ConPwrNonMixWei` for Weibull survival and `ConPwrNonMixGamma` for Gamma survival functions, respectively. A function for the comparison of these four models on the basis of AIC is also implemented using function

`CompSurvMod`. The conditional power based on the exponential model can be calculated using `ConPwrExpAndersen` function. The output from the model fit includes a summary of survival data of the interim analysis, AICs, parameter estimates, and estimates for the conditional power for the chosen model. Plots of the Kaplan-Meier curves and estimated parametric survival curves are provided.

As an example, the syntax of the function that calculates the conditional power for the non-mixture Weibull model is

```
ConPwrNonMixWei(data = test, cont.time = 12, new.pat = c(2.5, 2.5),
                theta.0 = 0.75, alpha = 0.05,
                disp.data = TRUE, plot.km = TRUE)
```

where `data` is the name of data frame that consists of at least three columns with the group in the first, survival status in the second and event time in the third column; `cont.time` is the trial duration after interim analysis; `new.pat` is a two-dimensional vector which consists of numbers of new patients being recruited at each time unit and corresponding study arm; `theta.0` is the clinically relevant difference assumed for initial power planning; `alpha` is the significance level for conditional power calculations, which usually takes the value of 0.05; `disp.data` is a logical value indicating whether all results of calculations should be displayed and the default value is FALSE; `plot.km` is a logical value indicating whether Kaplan-Meier curves and estimated survival curves assuming the exponential model should be plotted.

9.4 Applications

In this section, we apply the statistical methods described previously to the reconstructed overall survival data from the Checkmate-067 study, a Phase III trial for patients with advanced melanoma. The Checkmate-067 study was briefly introduced in Section 9.1. It is a double-blind randomized, controlled trial to investigate the effects of the combination therapy with nivolumab plus ipilimumab or the nivolumab monotherapy versus the ipilimumab monotherapy. The patients with previously untreated advanced melanoma are randomized into the three groups with 1:1:1 ratio. The two primary endpoints are progression-free survival and overall survival. For illustration, we only analyze the overall survival data for the two monotherapy arms. The trial was conducted at 137 sites in 21 countries, and the enrollment process began in July 2013 and ended in March 2014. The database was locked on May 24, 2017, resulting a minimum follow-up of 36 months for all patients alive. Among the 945 patients who underwent randomization, 316 patients were in the nivolumab group and 315 were in the ipilimumab group. The primary analysis of overall survival was conducted at 28 months of follow-up. An updated analysis of overall survival was presented by Wolchok et al. (2017).

The overall survival data for two monotherapy groups are reconstructed from the published figures using the algorithm developed by (Guyot et al., 2012). The steps for reconstructing data are as follows:

1. Save the figure with the Kaplan-Meier curves in jpeg format.
2. Extract the survival curves into numerical data for survival function.
3. Manually create the file with number of patient at-risk at specific time points.
4. The individual survival data are reconstructed from the survival function data and the patient at-risk data in Steps 3 and 4 using an R package `reconstructKM` (Sun, 2019).

For a comprehensive evaluation of the performances of the data reconstruction, see Wan et al. (2015). We first applied the Weibull mixture cure model to the reconstructed overall survival data. The overall survival function is specified

$$S(t|x) = 1 - \pi(x) + \pi(x)\exp\left\{-\left(\frac{t}{\exp(\beta_0 + \beta_1 x)}\right)^a\right\}, \tag{9.29}$$

where the shape parameter is a and the scale parameter is $\exp(\beta_0 + \beta_1 x)$ and the cure fraction

$$1 - \pi(x) = \frac{\exp(\gamma_0 + \gamma_1 x)}{1 + \exp(\gamma_0 + \gamma_1 x)}, \tag{9.30}$$

x is the categorical variable (factor) for the treatment group (Ipilimumab and Nivolumab). The parameter estimates are obtained using R package `flexsurvcure` with the following syntax

```
cure.model.estimates<-flexsurvcure(Surv(time, event)~group,
              data=checkmate067.data,
              link="logistic", dist="weibull",
              mixture=T, anc=list(scale=~treatment))
```

where `group` takes the value of `Nivolumab` or `Ipilimumab`. The reference group is `Ipilimumab`. The output of the mixture cure model estimates `cure.model.estimates` is shown in Figure 9.4.

The parameter estimates and the variance-covariance matrix of $(\gamma_0, \log(a), \beta_0, \gamma_1, \beta_1)$ can be obtained using `cure.model.estimates$coefficients` and `cure.model.estimates$cov`. They are summarized in Table 9.2. The p-values of the parameters are calculated based on the normal approximation. The estimated cure rates are 0.269 and 0.434 for the ipilimumab and nivolumab groups, respectively. The difference in cure rates is 0.165. We see that the estimate of γ_1 is 0.732 with standard error 0.224, which is highly significant with p-value $= 0.001$. This indicates the difference of cure rates between the two treatment groups are highly statistically significant. The difference of survival for the uncured patients between the two groups are measured by β_1.

```
> flexsurvcure(Surv(time, event)~group, data=checkmate067.data, link="logistic", dist="weibull", mixture=T,
+ anc=list(scale=~group))

Call:
flexsurvcure(formula = Surv(time, event) ~ group, data = checkmate067.data,
dist = "weibull", link = "logistic", mixture = T, anc = list(scale = ~group))

Estimates:
                     data mean      est     L95%     U95%       se exp(est)   L95%     U95%
theta                       NA   0.2690   0.2050   0.3445       NA       NA       NA       NA
shape                       NA   1.1993   1.0739   1.3393   0.0676       NA       NA       NA
scale                       NA  17.7970  14.7903  21.4149   1.6804       NA       NA       NA
groupNivolumab          0.5008   0.7323   0.2939   1.1708   0.2237   2.0799   1.3417   3.2244
scale(groupNivolumab)   0.5008   0.0784  -0.1962   0.3530   0.1401   1.0815   0.8218   1.4233

N = 631,  Events: 365,  Censored: 266
Total time at risk: 15090.92
Log-likelihood = -1699.885, df = 5
AIC = 3409.77
```

FIGURE 9.4
Output from the mixture cure model for reconstructed CheckMate-067 overall survival data.

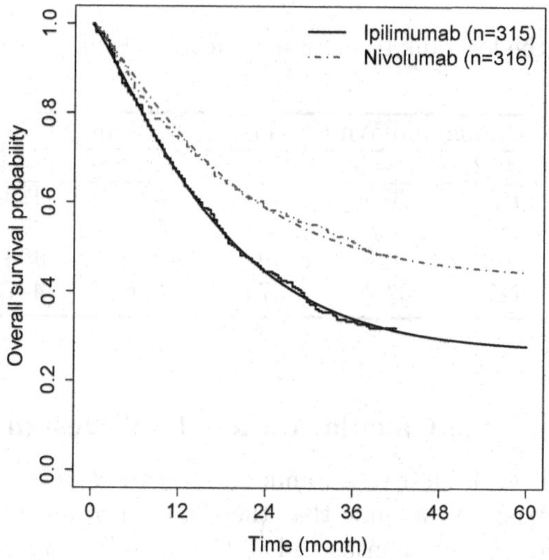

FIGURE 9.5
Estimated survival curves from the Weibull mixture cure model (smooth curves) and Kaplan-Meier survival curves (non-smooth curves) to the overall survival data in the Checkmate-067 study.

The estimate of β_1 is 0.078 with standard error 0.140, which is not statistically significant with p-value $= 0.576$. The corresponding hazard ratio of death for the uncured patients with nivolumab versus ipilimumab is given by $HR = \{\exp(\beta_1)\}^{-a} = \exp(-a\beta_1) = 0.91$, which is close to 1. Therefore, the difference of overall survival between the nivolumab and the iplimumab groups are mainly due to the differences in cure rates. The estimated survival curves from the Weibull mixture cure model are shown in Figure 9.5. We see that the estimated survival curves are close to the Kaplan-Meier survival estimates of the observed overall survival data. This shows that the mixture cure model provides a good fit to the overall survival data in the Checkmate-067 study.

TABLE 9.2
Parameter estimates of the Weibull mixture cure model for the Checkmate-067 overall survival data.

Name	Parameter	Estimate	SE	p-value
`theta`	γ_0	-0.999	0.182	<0.001
`shape`	$\log(a)$	0.182	0.056	0.001
`scale`	β_0	2.879	0.094	<0.001
`groupNivolumab`	γ_1	0.732	0.224	0.001
`scale(groupNivolumab)`	β_1	0.078	0.140	0.576

TABLE 9.3
Sample sizes for the log-rank tests for a clinical trial similar to the Checkmate-067 study.

		Xiong and Wu (2017)			Wang et al. (2012b)		
ρ	ν	$\tau_f = 28$	$\tau_f = 36$	$\tau_f = 44$	$\tau_f = 28$	$\tau_f = 36$	$\tau_f = 44$
0	0	417	375	355	480	429	405
0	1	481	428	404	541	477	448
1	0	465	426	408	539	493	472
1	1	447	397	374	506	447	420

9.4.1 Sample Size Calculation for Trial Design

Suppose that we will design a randomized two-arm trial similar to the Checkmate-067 trial. We assume that the randomization ratio is 1:1 and patient recruitment time is 8 months and additional follow-up time is 36 months, which is similar to the study duration in the Checkmate-067 study. We calculate the sample sizes of the Fleming and Harrington's weighted log-rank tests $G^{\rho,\nu}$ with $\alpha = 0.05$ and power 0.90. The weights are determined by ρ and ν, where the unweighted log-rank test corresponds to $\rho = \nu = 0$. The sample sizes for different values of ρ and ν and follow-up times τ_f are shown in Table 9.3. We can see that the unweighted log-rank test has the smaller sample sizes of 375 and 429 with a follow-up time of 28 months. The method of Xiong and Wu (2017) yields a smaller sample size. The actual sample sizes for the two mono-therapy arms are 633 for the Checkmate-067 study with a minimum follow-up of 36 months.

Based on the Kaplan-Meier plots of the overall survival data in Figure 9.2, we notice that the survival curves for the two monotherapy arms start to separate after about 4 months, indicating a delayed treatment onset time. We apply the method of Liu et al. (2018a) discussed in Section 9.2.3 to calculate the sample size for the weighted log-rank test with consideration of both delayed treatment onset time and cure rate. We assume that the survival function for the nivolumab arm follows equation (9.11) and the survival function for the control (ipilimumab) arm is $S_0(t) = \exp(-\lambda_0 t^a)$ and the delayed treatment effect onset time $\tau/\tau_{max} \sim \text{Beta}(1,1)$ with $\tau_{\max} = 6$ months. The parameter estimates of the mixture cure model with delayed onset of treatment effect is shown in Table 9.4. The cure rate for the control group is 0.278. The delayed treatment effect onset time is 2.826 months and the hazard ratio of the nivolumab is 0.652 after the effect onset. The estimated survival function from the mixture cure model with delayed onset time is shown in Figure 9.6. We see that the model fit is good to the overall survival data.

The sample size for the weighted log-rank test can be calculated using the R function described in Section 9.2.3. Based on the parameter estimates in Table 9.4, the syntax of the R code for the sample size is specified as

TABLE 9.4
Parameter estimates of the mixture cure model with delayed onset time.

Parameter	mean	sd	95% CI	
λ	0.030	0.006	0.020	0.043
a	1.220	0.074	1.077	1.364
π_0	0.278	0.029	0.218	0.337
r	0.652	0.077	0.500	0.812
τ	2.826	2.229	0.083	5.951

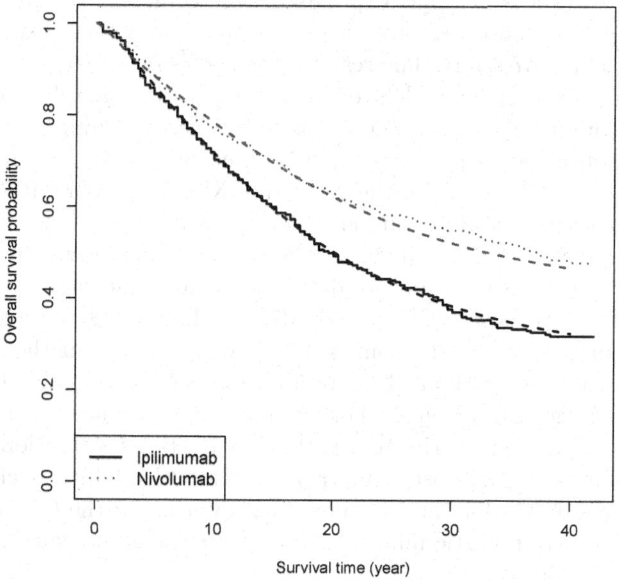

FIGURE 9.6
Estimated survival curves from the Weibull mixture cure model with delay onset time (smooth curves) and Kaplan-Meier survival curves (non-smooth curves) to the overall survival data in the Checkmate-067 study.

```
DelayCureSampleSize(accural=8, followup=36,
      cure=0.278, shape=1.220, scale=exp(2.890),
      HR.post.delay=0.652, delay.start=0, delay.end=6,
      TypeI=0.05, TypeII=0.1,
      beta.a=1, beta.b=1, quad.points=50,
      SC=function(t){1-pexp(t, rate=1/exp(4))},
      Wt=function(t){pbeta(t/6, shapel=1, shape2=1)})
```

In the R function, we set the Type 1 error 0.05 and power 0.9, and assume the accrual time is 8 months and the follow-up time is 36 months. The delayed

TABLE 9.5
Sample sizes with respect to different delayed treatment effect onset times $\tau_{\max}$.

	$\tau_{\max}$						
Censoring distribution	0	1	2	3	4	5	6
No censoring	380	388	398	410	423	438	453
Exponential(Rate=54.6)	495	508	525	545	567	590	616

onset time $\tau/\tau_{\max}$ is Beta(1,1) with $\tau_{\max} = 6$. The scale parameter for the Weibull distribution is $a^{-1/\gamma} = \exp(2.890)$. The censoring distribution SC is estimated from the censoring times in the reconstructed overall survival data in the Checkmate-067 study. The resulting sample size is 616.

To examine the impact of delayed onset time on the sample size, we vary the range of onset time $\tau_{\max}$. The sample size corresponding to no delayed onset time is obtained by setting $\tau_{\max}$ to a value close to 0. To compare with the sample size results based on the method of Xiong and Wu (2017), we consider the scenarios of no censoring and an exponential censoring distribution with rate parameter $\exp(4) = 54.6$. The results are summarized in Table 9.5. When there is no censoring and no delay onset time, the target sample size is 380, which is very close to sample size 375 for the unweighted log-rank test with follow-up time $\tau_f = 36$ months. If censoring occurs in the study, the sample size increases by about 30%. In addition, we see that the delay onset time leads to larger sample sizes. For example, the calculated sample size is 616 when the censoring distribution is the exponential distribution with rate 54.6 and maximum delay onset time $\tau_{\max} = 6$ months, which is close to the actual sample size 633 for the two monotherapy arms in the Checkmate-067 study and is a more realistic number that reflects the actual survival pattern and possible censoring issue.

9.4.2 Predicting Future Number of Events

As the enrollment phase is only 8 months, we consider a simple scenario by assuming all patients enter the trial at the same time (time 0). We assume that the interim analysis occurs at the middle point, i.e., 18 months after the treatment begins. We compare the performances of the Weibull mixture cure model and Weibull model for the prediction of future events at month 40 based on the interim data at month 18. As described in Section 9.3.1, we fit the Bayesian Weibull models with and without cure to the interim data at month 18.

For the reconstructed overall survival data, the number of events between months 18 and 40 is 117. The predicted number of events from the Weibull model is 125 with interquartile range (116, 135). The predicted number of events from the Weibull mixture cure model is 117 with interquartile range

(103, 128). As the Weibull mixture cure model provides a good fit to the overall survival data from the Checkmate-067 study, it is reasonable that the prediction based on the mixture cure model is much closer to the number of events from the reconstructed overall survival data.

In the actual Checkmate-067 study, 644 deaths are predicted at 28 months of follow-up for all three arms combined. The actual number of observed events is 467 deaths, which is larger than the prediction. This is probably due to the long-term survival rate (cure) of the overall survival.

9.5 Summary

In this chapter, we describe the use of cure models in the design and analysis of cancer clinical trials. Because of the breakthrough in cancer treatment and dissemination of cancer screening, many types of cancer are curable, especially in early stages. The usual unweighted log-rank tests may not be efficient in the presence of cured patients. The optimal weighted log-rank tests and the associated sample size calculation are presented for the clinical trial with delayed onset of treatment effect and cure. We also present some issues in the design and monitoring of clinical trial with cure. For the futility analysis, the conditional powers for the mixture and non-mixture cure models are presented. For the prediction of number of future events in the planning of clinical trial, the real-time prediction method based on the cure model shows better predictive performance. A reconstructed survival data set based on the Checkmate-067 study is used for illustration.

The cure model may also find many other applications in the evaluation of cancer treatment. For example, when the PH assumption is questionable, the survival functions for the two treatments may overlap or cross over. In this situation, some alternative measures of efficacy, e.g., restricted mean survival time (RMST) and lankmark survival, have been proposed. The cure model may be used to predict the RMST and lankmark survival based on the early clinical trial data. Another important component of the efficacy evaluation is the treatment effect in the real world. In the health economic assessment of a cancer treatment, relative survival may be estimated for the period that is observed in the trial, but also for the extrapolation period to obtain mean, incremental mean survival and corresponding uncertainty for an appraised method and its comparators. The cure model may be used for the survival extrapolation in the comparative analysis.

Bibliography

Odd O. Aalen. Modelling heterogeneity in survival analysis by the compound Poisson distribution. *The Annals of Applied Probability*, 2:951–972, 1992.

Mailis Amico and Ingrid Van Keilegom. Cure models in survival analysis. *Annual Review of Statistics and Its Application*, 5(1):311–342, 2018.

Valsamo Anagnostou, Mark Yarchoan, Aaron R/ Hansen, Hao Wang, Franco Verde, Elad Sharon, Deborah Collyar, Laura QM Chow, and Patrick M. Forde. Immuno-oncology trial endpoints: capturing clinically meaningful activity. *Clinical Cancer Research*, 23(17):4959–4969, 2017.

R.N. Anderson. A method for constructing complete annual U.S. life tables. *Vital and health statistics. Series 2, Data evaluation and methods research*, (129):1–28, 2000.

T. W. Anderson. On the distribution of the two-sample Cramér–von Mises criterion. *Annals of Mathematical Statistics*, 33:1148–1159, 1962.

Therese M. L. Andersson and Paul C. Lambert. Fitting and modeling cure in population-based cancer studies within the framework of flexible parametric survival models. *The Stata Journal*, 12:623–628, 2012.

Therese M. L. Andersson, Paul W. Dickman, Sandra Eloranta, and Paul C. Lambert. Estimating and modelling cure in population-based cancer studies within the framework of flexible parametric survival models. *BMC Medical Research Methodology*, 11(1):96, 2011.

Francisco J. Aranda-Ordaz. On two families of transformations to additivity for binary response data. *Biometrika*, 68(2):357–363, 1981.

Junichi Asano, Akihiro Hirakawa, and Chikuma Hamada. Assessing the prediction accuracy of cure in the Cox proportional hazards cure model: an application to breast cancer data. *Pharmaceutical Statistics*, 13(6):357–363, 2014.

B. Asselain, A. Fourquet, T. Hoang, A. D. Tsodikov, and A. Yu Yakovlev. A parametric regression model of tumor recurrence: an application to the analysis of clinical data on breast cancer. *Statistics & Probability Letters*, 29:271–278, 1996.

Emilia Bagiella and Daniel F. Heitjan. Predicting analysis times in randomized clinical trials. *Statistics in Medicine*, 20(14):2055–2063, 2001.

Sudipto Banerjee and Bradley P. Carlin. Parametric spatial cure rate models for interval-censored time-to-relapse data. *Biometrics*, 60(1):268–275, 2004.

Ole E. Barndorff-Nielsen and Bent Jørgensen. Some parametric models on the simplex. *Journal of Multivariate Analysis*, 39(1):106–116, 1991.

Lauren J. Beesley and Jeremy M. G. Taylor. Em algorithms for fitting multistate cure models. *Biostatistics*, 20(3):416–432, 2019.

Lauren J. Beesley, Jonathan W. Bartlett, Gregory T. Wolf, and Jeremy M. G. Taylor. Multiple imputation of missing covariates for the Cox proportional hazards cure model. *Statistics in Medicine*, 35(26):4701–4717, 2016.

Rudolf Beran. Nonparametric regression with randomly censored survival data. Technical report, University of California, Berkeley, CA, 1981.

Roger L. Berger, Jason C. Hsu, Walter W. Hauck, Sharon Anderson, Michael P. Meredith, Mark A. Heise, Jen pei Liu, Shein-Chung Chow, Donald J. Schuirmann, and J. T. Gene Hwang. Bioequivalence trials, intersection-union tests and equivalence confidence. *Statistical Science*, 11 (4):283–319, 1996.

J. Berkson and R.P. Gage. Survival curve for cancer patients following treatment. *Journal of the American Statistical Association*, 47(259):501–515, 1952.

Patricia Bernardo and Joseph G. Ibrahim. Group sequential designs for cure rate models with early stopping in favour of the null hypothesis. *Statistics in Medicine*, 19(22):3023–3035, 2000.

Aurelie Bertrand, Catherine Legrand, Raymond J. Carroll, Christophe De Meester, and Ingrid Van Keilegom. Inference in a survival cure model with mismeasured covariates using a simulation-extrapolation approach. *Biometrika*, 104(1):31–50, 2017.

J. Besag, J. York, and A. Mollié. Bayesian image restoration, with two applications in spatial statistics. *Annals of the Institute of Statistical Mathematics*, 43(1):1–20, 1991.

Nicky Best, M. K. Cowles, and Karen Vines. *CODA: Convergence diagnosis and output analysis software for Gibbs sampling output.* MRC Biostatistic Unit, Cambridge, UK, 1995.

Rebecca A. Betensky and David A. Schoenfeld. Nonparametric estimation in a cure model with a random cure times. *Biometrics*, 57:282–286, 2001.

J. W. Boag. Maximum likelihood estimates of the proportion of patients cured by cancer therapy. *Journal of the Royal Statistical Society*, 11:15–53, 1949.

Christine Bouchardy, Elisabetta Rapiti, and Simone Benhamou. Cancer registries can provide evidence-based data to improve quality of care and prevent cancer deaths. *eCancer Medical Science*, 8, 2014.

G. E. P. Box and D. R. Cox. An analysis of transformations. *Journal of the Royal Statistical Society, Series B*, 26:211–252, 1964.

Vincent Bremhorst and Philippe Lambert. Flexible estimation in cure survival models using Bayesian P-splines. *Computational Statistics & Data Analysis*, 93:270–284, 2016.

David H. Brewster, Jan-Willem Coebergh, and Hans H. Storm. Population-based cancer registries: the invisible key to cancer control. *The Lancet Oncology*, 6(4):193–195, 2005.

Glenn W. Brier. Verification of forecasts expressed in terms of probability. *Monthly Weather Review*, 78:1–3, 1950.

P. Broët, P. Tubert-Bitter, Y. De Rycke, and T. Moreau. A score test for establishing non-inferiority with respect to short-term survival in two-sample comparisons with identical proportions of long-term survivors. *Statistics in Medicine*, 22:931–940, 2003.

P. Broët, Alexander Tsodikov, Yann de Rycke, and T. Moreau. Two-sample statistics for testing the equality of survival functions against improper semi-parametric accelerated failure time alternatives: an application to the analysis of a breast cancer clinical trial. *Lifetime Data Analysis*, 10:103–120, 2004.

Philippe Broët, Yann De Rycke, Pascale Tubert-Bitter, Joseph Lellouch, Bernard Asselain, and Thierry Moreau. A semiparametric approach for the two-sample comparison of survival times with long-term survivors. *Biometrics*, 57:844–852, 2001.

E. R. Brown and Joseph G. Ibrahim. Bayesian approaches to joint cure-rate and longitudinal models with applications to cancer vaccine trials. *Biometrics*, 59:686–693, 2003.

Chao Cai, Songfeng Wang, Wenbin Lu, and Jiajia Zhang. NPHMC: An R-package for estimating sample size of proportional hazards mixture cure model. *Computer Methods and Programs in Biomedicine*, 113(1):290–300, 2014.

Andrea Callegaro and Bart Spiessens. Testing treatment effect in randomized clinical trials with possible nonproportional hazards. *Statistics in Biopharmaceutical Research*, 9(2):204–211, 2017.

Vicente G. Cancho, Josemar Rodrigues, and Mario de Castro. A flexible model for survival data with a cure rate: a Bayesian approach. *Journal of Applied Statistics*, 38(1):57–70, 2011.

Vicente G. Cancho, Mário de Castro, and Josemar Rodrigues. A Bayesian analysis of the Conway–Maxwell–Poisson cure rate model. *Statistical Papers*, 53(1):165–176, 2012.

A. B. Cantor and J. J. Shuster. Parametric versus non-parametric methods for estimating cure rates based on censored survival data. *Statistics in Medicine*, 11:931–937, 1992.

Alan B. Cantor. Projecting the standard error of the Kaplan-Meier estimator. *Statistics in Medicine*, 20:2091–2097, 2001.

B.P. Carlin and T.A. Louis. *Bayes and Empirical Bayes Methods for Data Analysis, Second Edition*. Chapman & Hall/CRC Texts in Statistical Science. Taylor & Francis, 2010.

J.M.F. Carrasco, E.M.M. Ortega, and G.M. Cordeiro. A generalized modified Weibull distribution for lifetime modeling. *Computational Statistics & Data Analysis*, 53(2):450–462, 2008.

Chih-Chung Chang and Chih-Jen Lin. LIBSVM: A library for support vector machines. *ACM Transactions on Intelligent Systems and Technology (TIST)*, 2(3):1–27, 2011.

Nilanjan Chatterjee and Joanna Shih. A bivariate cure-mixture approach for modeling familial association in disease. *Biometrics*, 57:779–786, 2001.

Chyong-Mei Chen and Tai-Fang C. Lu. Marginal analysis of multivariate failure time data with a surviving fraction based on semiparametric transformation cure models. *Computational Statistics & Data Analysis*, 56:645–655, 2012.

Ming-Hui Chen, Joseph G. Ibrahim, and Debajyoti Sinha. A new Bayesian model for survival data with a surviving fraction. *Journal of the American Statistical Association*, 94(447):909–919, 1999.

Ming-Hui Chen, David P. Harrington, and Joseph G. Ibrahim. Bayesian cure rate models for malignant melanoma: a case-study of Eastern Cooperative Oncology Group trial E1690. *Journal of the Royal Statistical Society: Series C (Applied Statistics)*, 51(2):135–150, 2002.

Ming-Hui Chen, Joseph G. Ibrahim, and Debajyoti Sinha. A new joint model for longitudinal and survival data with a cure fraction. *Journal of Multivariate Analysis*, 91:18–34, 2004.

T.T. Chen. Predicting analysis times in randomized clinical trials with cancer immunotherapy. *BMC Medical Research Methodology*, 16:12, 2016.

Ying Qing Chen. Accelerated hazards regression model and its adequacy for censored survival data. *Biometrics*, 57:853–860, 2001.

Ying Qing Chen and Mei-Cheng Wang. Analysis of accelerated hazards models. *Journal of the American Statistical Association*, 95:608–618, 2000.

Sangbum Choi and Xuelin Huang. Maximum likelihood estimation of semiparametric mixture component models for competing risks data. *Biometrics*, 70(3):588–598, 2014.

Sangbum Choi, Xuelin Huang, and Yi-Hau Chen. A class of semiparametric transformation models for survival data with a cured proportion. *Lifetime data analysis*, 20(3):369–386, 2014.

Sangbum Choi, Xuelin Huang, and N. Cormier Janice. Efficient semiparametric mixture inferences on cure rate models for competing risks. *The Canadian Journal of Statistics*, 43:420–435, 2015.

Sangbum Choi, Liang Zhu, and Xuelin Huang. Semiparametric accelerated failure time cure rate mixture models with competing risks. *Statistics in Medicine*, 37(1):48–59, 2018.

Mark Clements. *Introduction to the rstpm2 package.* Karolinska Institutet, 2019. URL `https://cran.r-project.org/web/packages/rstpm2/vignettes/Introduction.pdf`.

Mark Clements and Xing-Rong Liu. *rstpm2: Generalized Survival Models*, 2019. URL `https://CRAN.R-project.org/package=rstpm2`. R package version 1.4.5.

P. Congdon. Bayesian modelling strategies for spatially varying regression coefficients: a multivariate perspective for multiple outcomes. *Computational Statistics and Data Analysis*, 51(5):2586–2601, 2007.

A. S. C. Conlon, J. M. G. Taylor, and Daniel J. Sargent. Multi-state models for colon cancer recurrence and death with a cured fraction. *Statistics in Medicine*, 33(10):1750–1766, 2014.

Freda Cooner, Sudipto Banerjee, and A. Marshall McBean. Modelling geographically referenced survival data with a cure fraction. *Statistical Methods in Medical Research*, 15(4):307–324, 2006.

Freda Cooner, Sudipto Banerjee, Bradley P. Carlin, and Debajyoti Sinha. Flexible cure rate modeling under latent activation schemes. *Journal of the American Statistical Association*, 102:560–572, 2007.

E. A. Copelan, J. C. Biggs, J. M. Thompson, P. Crilley, J. Szer, J. P. Klein, N. Kapoor, B. R. Avalos, I. Cunningham, K. Atkinson, K. Downs, G. S. Harmon, M. B. Daly, I. Brodsky, S. I. Bulova, and P. J. Tutschka. Treatment for acute myelocytic leukemia with allogeneic bone marrow transplantation following preparation with Bu/Cy. *Blood*, 78:838–843, 1991.

Fabien Corbiere and Pierre Joly. A SAS macro for parametric and semi-parametric mixture cure models. *Computer Methods and Programs in Biomedicine*, 85:173–180, 2007.

Fabien Corbiere, Daniel Commenges, Jeremy M. G. Taylor, and Pierre Joly. A penalized likelihood approach for mixture cure models. *Statistics in Medicine*, 28:510–524, 2009.

D. R. Cox and D. Oakes. *Analysis of Survival Data.* Chapman and Hall, New York, 1984.

Kathleen A. Cronin and Eric J. Feuer. Cumulative cause-specific mortality for cancer patients in the presence of other causes: a crude analogue of relative survival. *Statistics in medicine*, 19(13):1729–1740, 2000.

Martin Crowder. *Multivariate Survival Analysis and Competing Risks.* Chapman and Hall/CRC, 2012.

Dorota M. Dabrowska. Non-parametric regression with censored survival time data. *Scandinavian Journal of Statistics*, 14:181–197, 1987.

Dorota M. Dabrowska. Uniform consistency of the kernel conditional Kaplan-Meier estimate. *Annals of Statistics*, 17:1157–1167, 1989.

A. C. Davison and D. V. Hinkley. *Bootstrap Methods and Their Application.* Cambridge University Press, New York, 1997.

Mário de Castro, Vicente G. Cancho, and Josemar Rodrigues. A Bayesian long-term survival model parametrized in the cured fraction. *Biometrical Journal*, 51(3):443–455, 2009.

Daiane de Souza, Vicente G. Cancho, Josemar Rodrigues, and Narayanaswamy Balakrishnan. Bayesian cure rate models induced by frailty in survival analysis. *Statistical Methods in Medical Research*, 26 (5):2011–2028, 2017.

Joseph C. Del Paggio. Immunotherapy: cancer immunotherapy and the value of cure. *Nature Reviews Clinical Oncology*, 15(5):268, 2018.

A. P. Dempster, N. M. Laird, and D. B. Rubin. Maximum likelihood from incomplete data via the EM algorithm. *Journal of the Royal Statistical Society, Series B*, 39:1–38, 1977.

P. W. Dickman, A. Sloggett, M. Hills, and T. Hakulinen. Regression models for relative survival. *Statistics in Medicine*, 23(1):51–64, 2004.

P. Diggle, I. Sousa, and A. Chetwynd. Joint modelling of repeated measurements and time-to-event outcomes: the fourth Armitage lecture. *Statistics in Medicine*, 27:2981–2998, 2008.

Lore Dirick, Gerda Claeskens, and Bart Baesens. An akaike information criterion for multiple event mixture cure models. *European Journal of Operational Research*, 241(2):449–457, 2015.

Lore Dirick, Tony Bellotti, Gerda Claeskens, and Bart Baesens. Macroeconomic factors in credit risk calculations: including time-varying covariates in mixture cure models. *Journal of Business & Economic Statistics*, pages 1–14, 2017.

Qingli Dong, Yingwei Peng, and Peizhi Li. *Time to delisted for listed firms in Chinese stock markets: An analysis using a mixture cure model with time-varying covariates*, 2020. Under revision for Journal of the Operational Research Society.

J. M. Donovan, M. R. Elliott, and D. F. Heitjan. Predicting event times in clinical trials when treatment arm is masked. *Journal of Biopharmaceutical Statistics*, 16(3):343–356, 2006.

J. M. Donovan, M. R. Elliott, and D. F. Heitjan. Predicting event times in clinical trials when randomization is masked and blocked. *Clinical Trials*, 4(5):481–490, 2007.

Libby Ellis, Laura M. Woods, Jacques Estève, Sandra Eloranta, Michel P. Coleman, and Bernard Rachet. Cancer incidence, survival and mortality: explaining the concepts. *International Journal of Cancer*, 135(8):1774–1782, 2014.

B. S. Everitt. A Monte Carlo investigation of the likelihood ratio test for number of classes in latent class analysis. *Multivariate Behavioral Research*, 23:531– 538, 1988.

Marian Ewell and Joseph G. Ibrahim. The large sample distribution of the weighted log rank statistic under general local alternatives. *Lifetime Data Analysis*, 3(1):5–12, 1997.

Diane L. Fairclough. *Design and analysis of quality of life studies in clinical trials*. Chapman and Hall/CRC, 2010.

Jianqing Fan and Runze Li. Variable selection via nonconcave penalized likelihood and its oracle properties. *Journal of the American Statistical Association*, 96:1348–1360, 2001.

Jianqing Fan and Runze Li. Variable selection for Cox's proportional hazards model and frailty model. *Annals of Statistics*, 30(1):74–99, 2002.

Hong-Bin Fang, Gang Li, and Jianguo Sun. Maximum likelihood estimation in a semiparametric logistic/proportional-hazards mixture model. *Scandinavian Journal of Statistics*, 32:59–75, 2005.

V. T. Farewell. The use of mixture models for the analysis of survival data with long-term survivors. *Biometrics*, 38:1041–46, 1982.

V. T. Farewell. Mixture models in survival analysis: are they worth the risk? *The Canadian Journal of Statistics*, 14(3):257–262, 1986.

FDA. Guidance for industry non-inferiority clinical trials. *Center for Biologics Evaluation and Research (CBER)*, 2010.

Michael G. Findley and Tze Kwang Teo. Rethinking third-party interventions into civil wars: an actor-centric approach. *The Journal of Politics*, 68:828–837, 2006.

Jason P. Fine and Robert J. Gray. A proportional hazards model for the subdistribution of a competing risk. *Journal of the American Statistical Association*, 94:496–509, 1999.

F. Fiteni, V. Westeel, X. Pivot, C. Borg, D. Vernerey, and F. Bonnetain. Endpoints in cancer clinical trials. *Journal of Visceral Surgery*, 151(1): 17–22, 2014.

Thomas R. Fleming and David P. Harrington. *Counting processes and survival analysis*, volume 169. John Wiley & Sons, 2011.

T.R. Fleming and D. P. Harrington. *Counting Processes and Survival Analysis*, 1991.

Ana-Maria Forsea. Cancer registries in europe-going forward is the only option. *eCancer Medical Science*, 10, 2016.

Silvia Francisci, Riccardo Capocaccia, Enrico Grande, Mariano Santaquilani, Arianna Simonetti, Claudia Allemani, Gemma Gatta, Milena Sant, Giulia Zigon, Freddie Bray, et al. The cure of cancer: a European perspective. *European Journal of Cancer*, 45(6):1067–1079, 2009.

M. H. Gail and J. H. Ware. Comparing observed life table data with a known survival curve in the presence of random censorship. *Biometrics*, 35(2): 385–391, 1979.

John W. Gamel and Ian W. McLean. A stable, multivariate extension of the log-normal survival model. *Computers and Biomedical Research*, 27: 148–155, 1994.

D. Gamerman, A. R. B. Moreira, and H. Rue. Space-varying regression models: Specifications and simulation. *Computational Statistics and Data Analysis*, 42(3):513–533, 2003.

Theo Gasser and Hans-Georg Müller. Kernel estimation of regression functions. In *Smoothing Techniques for Curve Estimation*, pages 23–68. Springer, 1979.

A. Gelman and D.B. Rubin. Inference from iterative simulation using multiple sequences. *Statistical Science*, 7(4):457–472, 1992.

Thomas A. Gerds and Martin Schumacher. Consistent estimation of the expected brier score in general survival models with right-censored event times. *Biometrical Journal*, 48:1029–1040, 2006.

W. R. Gilks, S. Richardson, and D. Spiegelhalter. *Markov Chain Monte Carlo in Practice.* Chapman & Hall/CRC Interdisciplinary Statistics. Taylor & Francis, 1995.

A.I. Goldman. Survivorship analysis when cure is a possibility: a Monte Carlo study. *Statistics in Medicine*, 3(2):153–163, 1984.

A. Lawrence Gould, Mark Ernest Boye, Michael J. Crowther, Joseph G. Ibrahim, George Quartey, Sandrine Micallef, and Frederic Y. Bois. Joint modeling of survival and longitudinal non-survival data: current methods and issues. Report of the DIA Bayesian Joint Modeling Working Group. *Statistics in Medicine*, 34(14):2181–2195, 2015.

R. J. Gray and A. A. Tsiatis. A linear rank test for use when the main interest is in differences in cure rates. *Biometrics*, 45:899–904, 1989.

Chong Gu. *Smoothing Spline ANOVA Models*, volume 297. Springer Science & Business Media, 2013.

Yu Gu, Debajyoti Sinha, and Sudipto Banerjee. Analysis of cure rate survival data under proportional odds model. *Lifetime Data Analysis*, 17:123–134, 2011.

Patricia Guyot, A. E. Ades, Mario JNM Ouwens, and Nicky J. Welton. Enhanced secondary analysis of survival data: reconstructing the data from published kaplan-meier survival curves. *BMC Medical Research Methodology*, 12(1), 2012.

T. Hakulinen and L. Tenkanen. Regression analysis of relative survival rates. *Applied Statistics*, 36:309–317, 1987.

Stephen Hall, Karleen Schulze, Patti Groome, William Mackillop, and Eric Holowaty. Using cancer registry data for survival studies: the example of the Ontario Cancer Registry. *Journal of Clinical Epidemiology*, 59(1):67–76, 2006.

L. G. Hanin, M. Zaider, and A. Y. Yakovlev. Distribution of the number of clonogens surviving fractionated radiotherapy: a long-standing problem revisited. *International Journal of Radiation Biology*, 77:205–213, 2001.

Leonid Hanin and Li-Shan Huang. Identifiability of cure models revisited. *Journal of Multivariate Analysis*, 130:261–274, 2014.

W. Hardle and E. Mammen. Comparing nonparametric versus parametric regression fits. *The Annals of Statistics*, 21(4):1926–1947, 1993.

Wolfgang Härdle, Marlene Müller, Stefan Sperlich, and Axel Werwatz. *Nonparametric and semiparametric models*. Springer Science & Business Media, 2004.

Samuel J. Harris, Jessica Brown, Juanita Lopez, and Timothy A. Yap. Immuno-oncology combinations: raising the tail of the survival curve. *Cancer Biology & Medicine*, 13(2):171, 2016.

Pei He, Tze Leung Lai, and Olivia Y. Liao. Futility stopping in clinical trials. *Statistics and Its Interface*, 5(4):415–423, 2012.

D. F. Heitjan, Z. Ge, and G.-S. Ying. Real-time prediction of clinical trial enrollment and event counts: a review. *Contemporary Clinical Trials*, 45: 26–33, 2015.

Antje Hoering, Brian Durie, Hongwei Wang, and John Crowley. End points and statistical considerations in immuno-oncology trials: impact on multiple myeloma. *Future Oncology*, 13(13):1181–1193, 2017.

Philip Hougaard. *Analysis of Multivariate Survival Data*. Springer, New York, 2000.

N. Howlader, A.M. Noone, and M. Krapcho. *SEER Cancer Statistics Review, 1975-2008*, 2011.

Wei-Wen Hsu, David Todem, and KyungMann Kim. A sup-score test for the cure fraction in mixture models for long-term survivors. *Biometrics*, 72(4): 1348–1357, 2016.

Kathy L. Hudson and Francis S. Collins. The 21st century cures act — a view from the NIH. *New England Journal of Medicine*, 376(2):111–113, 2017.

David R. Hunter and Kenneth Lange. Computing estimates in the proportional odds model. *Annals of the Institute of Statistical Mathematics*, 54 (1):155–168, 2002.

J. L. Hutton and P. F. Monaghan. Choice of parametric accelerated life and proportional hazards models for survival data: asymptotic results. *Lifetime Data Analysis*, 8:375–393, 2002.

J. G. Ibrahim, H. Chu, and L. M. Chen. Basic concepts and methods for joint models of longitudinal and survival data. *Journal of Clinical Oncology*, 28: 2796–2801, 2010.

Joseph G. Ibrahim, Ming-Hui Chen, and Debajyoti Sinha. *Cure Rate Models*, pages 155–207. Springer, 2001.

ICR. Progress towards cancer cures. Technical report, The Institute of Cancer Research, London, 2014.

Ross Ihaka and Robert Gentleman. R: a language for data analysis and graphics. *Journal of Computational and Graphical Statistics*, 5(3):299–314, 1996.

Christopher H. Jackson. flexsurv: a platform for parametric survival modeling in R. *Journal of Statistical Software*, 70, 2016.

B. Yu James and Benjamin D. Smith. NCI SEER public-use data: applications and limitations in oncology research. *Oncology Research*, 2009.

Wenyu Jiang, Haoyu Sun, and Yingwei Peng. Prediction accuracy for the cure probabilities in mixture cure model. *Statistical Methods in Medical Research*, 26(5):2029–2041, 2017.

Zhezhen Jin, D. Y. Lin, L. J. Wei, and Zhiliang Ying. Rank-based inference for the accelerated failure time model. *Biometrika*, 90:341–353, 2003.

J. D. Kalbfleisch and R. L. Prentice. *The Statistical Analysis of Failure Time Data*. John Wiley & Sons, New York, 2nd edition, 2002.

Farin Kamangar, Graça M. Dores, and William F. Anderson. Patterns of cancer incidence, mortality, and prevalence across five continents: defining priorities to reduce cancer disparities in different geographic regions of the world. *Journal of Clinical Oncology*, 24(14):2137–2150, 2006.

E. L. Kaplan and P. Meier. Nonparametric estimation from imcomplete observations. *Journal of the American Statistical Association*, 53:457–481, 1958.

J. H. Kersey, D. Weisdorf, M. E. Nesbit, T. W. LeBien, W. G. Woods, P. B. McGlave, T. Kim, D. A. Vallera, A. I. Goldman, B. Bostrom, D. Hurd, and N. K. C. Ramsay. Comparison of autologous and allogeneic bone marrow transplantation for treatment of high-risk refractory acute lymphoblastic leukemia. *The New England Journal of Medicine*, 317:461–467, 1987.

J. M. Kirkwood, M. H. Strawderman, M. S. Ernstoff, T. J. Smith, E. C. Borden, and R. H. Blum. Interferon alfa-2b adjuvant therapy of high-risk resected cutaneous melanoma: the eastern cooperative oncology group trial EST 1684. *Journal of Clinical Oncology*, 14(1):7–17, 1996.

Lev B. Klebanov and Andrei Y. Yakovlev. A new approach to testing for sufficient follow-up in cure-rate analysis. *Journal of Statistical Planning and Inference*, 137:3557–3569, 2007.

John P. Klein and Per Kragh Andersen. Regression modeling of competing risks data based on pseudovalues of the cumulative incidence function. *Biometrics*, 61(1):223–229, 2005.

John P. Klein and Melvin L. Moeschberger. *Survival Analysis, Techniques for Censored and Truncated Data*. Spinger-Verlag, New York, 2nd edition, 2003.

Andreas Kuehnapfel, Fabian Schwarzenberger, and Markus Scholz. On the conditional power in survival time analysis considering cure fractions. *The International Journal of Biostatistics*, 13(1), 2017.

A.Y.C. Kuk and C.H. Chen. A mixture model combining logistic regression with proportional hazards regression. *Biometrika*, 79(3):531–541, 1992.

John M. Lachin. A review of methods for futility stopping based on conditional power. *Statistics in Medicine*, 24(18):2747–2764, 2005.

Xin Lai and Kelvin K. W. Yau. Long-term survivor model with bivariate random effects: applications to bone marrow transplant and carcinoma study data. *Statistics in Medicine*, 27:5692–5708, 2008.

Xin Lai and Kelvin K. W. Yau. Multilevel mixture cure models with random effects. *Biometrical Journal*, 51(3):456–466, 2009.

Lajmi Lakhal-Chaieb and Thierry Duchesne. Association measures for bivariate failure times in the presence of a cure fraction. *Lifetime Data Analysis*, 23(4):517–532, 2017.

K. F. Lam, Daniel Y. T. Fong, and O. Y. Tang. Estimating the proportion of cured patients in a censored sample. *Statistics in Medicine*, 24:1865–1879, 2005.

P. C. Lambert, P. W. Dickman, C. L. Weston, and J. R. Thompson. Estimating the cure fraction in population-based cancer studies by using finite mixture models. *Journal of the Royal Statistical Society: Series C (Applied Statistics)*, 59(1):35–55, 2010.

Paul C. Lambert. Modeling of the cure fraction in survival studies. *Stata Journal*, 7(3):351, 2007.

Paul C. Lambert and Patrick Royston. Further development of flexible parametric models for survival analysis. *The Stata Journal*, 9(2):265–290, 2009.

E. M. Laska and M. J. Meisner. Nonparametric estimation and testing in a cure model. *Biometrics*, 48:1223–1234, 1992.

N. J. Law, J. M. G. Taylor, and H. Sandler. The joint modelling of a longitudinal disease progression marker and the failure time process in the presence of cure. *Biostatistics*, 3:547–563, 2002.

E. Lesaffre, D. Rizopoulos, and R. Tsonaka. The logistic transform for bounded outcome scores. *Biostatistics*, 8:72–85, 2007.

M. N. Levine, V. H. Bramwell, K. I. Pritchard, B. D. Norris, L. E. Shepherd, H. Abu-Zahra, B. Findlay, D. Warr, D. Bowman, J. Myles,

A. Arnold, T. Vandenberg, R. MacKenzie, J. Robert, J. Ottaway, M. Burnell, C. K. Williams, and D. S. Tu. Randomized trial of intensive cyclophosphamide, epirubicin, and fluorouracil chemotherapy compared with cyclophosphamide, methotrexate, and fluorouracil in premenopausal women with node-positive breast caner. *Journal of Clinical Oncology*, 16:2651–2658, 1998.

Mark N. Levine, Kathleen I. Pritchard, Vivien H.C. Bramwell, Lois E. Shepherd, Dongsheng Tu, and Nancy Paul. Randomized trial comparing cyclophosphamide, epirubicin, and fluorouracil with cyclophosphamide, methotrexate, and fluorouracil in premenopausal women with node-positive breast cancer: Update of national cancer institute of canada clinical trials group trial MA.5. *Journal of Clinical Oncology*, 23:5166–5170, 2005.

Chin-Shang Li and Jeremy M. G. Taylor. Smoothing covariate effects in cure models. *Communications in Statistics*, 31(3):477–493, 2002a.

Chin-Shang Li and Jeremy M. G. Taylor. A semi-parametric accelerated failure time cure model. *Statistics in Medicine*, 21:3235–3247, 2002b.

Chin-Shang Li, Jeremy M. G. Taylor, and Judy P. Sy. Identifiability of cure models. *Statistics & Probability Letters*, 54:389–395, 2001.

Gang Li and Somnath Datta. A bootstrap approach to nonparametric regression for right censored data. *Annals of the Institute of Statistical Mathematics*, 53(4):708–729, 2001.

Peizhi Li, Yingwei Peng, Ping Jiang, and Qingli Dong. A support vector machine based semiparametric mixture cure model. *Computational Statistics*, 35:931–945, 2020.

Yi Li and Jin Feng. A nonparametric comparison of conditional distributions with nonnegligible cure fractions. *Lifetime Data Analysis*, 11:367–387, 2005.

Kung-Yee Liang and Scott L. Zeger. Longitudinal data analysis using generalized linear models. *Biometrika*, 73:13–22, 1986.

D. Y. Lin. Cox regression analysis of multivariate failure time data: the marginal approach. *Statistics in Medicine*, 13(21):2233–2247, 1994.

D. Y. Lin and Zhiliang Ying. Semiparametric analysis of the additive risk model. *Biometrika*, 81:61– 71, 1994.

D. Y. Lin, L. J. Wei, and Z. Ying. Checking the Cox model with cumulative sums of martingale-based residuals. *Biometrika*, 80:557–572, 1993.

Stuart R. Lipsitz, Keith B. G. Dear, and Lueping Zhao. Jackknife estimators of variance for parameter estimates from estimating equations with applications to clustered survival data. *Biometrics*, 50:842–846, 1994.

Shufang Liu, Chenghao Chu, and Alan Rong. Weighted log-rank test for time-to-event data in immunotherapy trials with random delayed treatment effect and cure rate. *Pharmaceutical Statistics*, 2018a.

Xiang Liu, Yingwei Peng, Dongsheng Tu, and Hua Liang. Variable selection in semiparametric cure models based on penalized likelihood, with application to breast cancer clinical trials. *Statistics in Medicine*, 31:2882–2891, 2012.

Xing-Rong Liu, Yudi Pawitan, and Mark S. Clements. Generalized survival models for correlated time-to-event data. *Statistics in Medicine*, 36(29): 4743–4762, 2017.

Xing-Rong Liu, Yudi Pawitan, and Mark Clements. Parametric and penalized generalized survival models. *Statistical Methods in Medical Research*, 27(5): 1531–1546, 2018b.

Ana López-Cheda, Ricardo Cao, M. Amalia Jácome, and Ingrid Van Keilegom. Nonparametric incidence estimation and bootstrap bandwidth selection in mixture cure models. *Computational Statistics & Data Analysis*, 105:144–165, 2017a.

Ana López-Cheda, M. Amalia Jácome, and Ricardo Cao. Nonparametric latency estimation for mixture cure models. *TEST*, 26(2):353–376, 2017b.

Thomas A. Louis. Finding the observed information matrix when using the EM algorithm. *Journal of the Royal Statistical Society, Series B*, 44(2): 226–233, 1982.

Wenbin Lu. Maximum likelihood estimation in the proportional hazards cure model. *Annals of the Institute of Statistical Mathematics*, 60(3):545–574, 2008.

Wenbin Lu. Efficient estimation for an accelerated failure time model with a cure fraction. *Statistica Sinica*, 20:661–674, 2010.

Wenbin Lu and Zhiliang Ying. On semiparametric transformation cure model. *Biometrika*, 91:331–343, 2004.

Thomas Lumley. *Survival curve estimation under complex sampling*. The University of Washington, 2010. http://r-survey.r-forge.r-project.org/survey/survcurve.pdf.

D. Lunn, D. Spiegelhalter, A. Thomas, and N. Best. The BUGS project: evolution, critique and future directions. *Statistics in Medicine*, 28(25): 3049–3067, 2009.

David J. Lunn, Andrew Thomas, Nicky Best, and David Spiegelhalter. WinBUGS-a Bayesian modelling framework: concepts, structure, and extensibility. *Statistics and Computing*, 10(4):325–337, 2000.

R. A. Maller and S. Zhou. Estimating the proportion of immunes in a censored sample. *Biometrika*, 79(4):731–739, 1992.

R. A. Maller and S. Zhou. Testing for sufficient follow-up and outliers in survival data. *Journal of the American Statistical Association*, 89:1499–1511, 1994.

R. A. Maller and S. Zhou. Testing for the presence of immune or cured individuals in censored survival data. *Biometrics*, 51:1197–1205, 1995.

Ross A. Maller and Xian Zhou. *Survival Analysis with Long-Term Survivors*. John Wiley & Son Ltd, 1996.

Meng Mao and Jane-Ling Wang. Semiparametric efficient estimation for a class of generalized proportional odds cure models. *Journal of the American Statistical Association*, 105:302–311, 2010.

K.V. Mardia. Multi-dimensional multivariate gaussian markov random fields with application to image processing. *Journal of Multivariate Analysis*, 24 (2):265–284, 1988.

Edson Z. Martinez, Jorge A. Achcar, Alexandre A. A. Jácome, and José S. Santos. Mixture and non-mixture cure fraction models based on the generalized modified weibull distribution with an application to gastric cancer data. *Computer Methods and Programs in Biomedicine*, 112(3):343–355, 2013.

Abdullah Masud, Wanzhu Tu, and Zhangsheng Yu. Variable selection for mixture and promotion time cure rate models. *Statistical Methods in Medical Research*, 27(7):2185–2199, 2018.

Isaac Meilijson. A fast improvement to the EM algorithm on its own terms. *Journal of the Royal Statistical Society, Series B*, 51:127–138, 1989.

Xiao-Li Meng and Donald B. Rubin. Using EM to obtain asymptotic variance-covariance matrices: the SEM algorithm. *Journal of the American Statistical Association*, 86:899–909, 1991.

M. L. Moeschberger and John P. Klein. A comparison of several methods of estimating the survival function when there is extreme right censoring. *Biometrics*, 41:253–259, 1985.

Jane Monaco, Jianwen Cai, and James Grizzle. Bootstrap analysis of multivariate failure time data. *Statistics in Medicine*, 24:3387–3400, 2005.

U. U. Müller and I. van Keilegom. Goodness-of-fit tests for the cure rate in a mixture cure model. *Biometrika*, 106(1):211–227, 2019.

E. A. Nadaraya. On estimating regression. *Theory of Probability and its Applications*, 9:141, 1964.

S. K. Ng and G. J. McLachlan. An EM-based semi-parametric mixture model approach to the regression analysis of competing-risks data. *Statistics in Medicine*, 22:1097–1111, 2003.

Mioara Alina Nicolaie, Jeremy M. G. Taylor, and Catherine Legrand. Vertical modeling: analysis of competing risks data with a cure fraction. *Lifetime Data Analysis*, 25(1):1–25, 2019.

Luis E. Nieto-Barajas and Guosheng Yin. Bayesian cure rate model accommodating multiplicative and additive covariates. *Statistics and Its Interface*, 2 (4):513–521, 2009.

Yi Niu and Yingwei Peng. Marginal regression analysis of clustered failure time data with long-term survivors. *Journal of Multivariate Analysis*, 123: 129–142, 2014.

Yi Niu, Lixin Song, Yufeng Liu, and Yingwei Peng. Modeling clustered long-term survivors using marginal mixture cure model. *Biometrical Journal*, 60:780–796, 2018a.

Yi Niu, Xiaoguang Wang, and Yingwei Peng. geecure: an R-package for marginal proportional hazards mixture cure models. *Computer Methods and Programs in Biomedicine*, 161:115–124, 2018b.

David Oakes. Direct calculation of the information matrix via the EM algorithm. *Journal of the Royal Statistical Society, Series B*, 61:479–482, 1999.

Megan Othus, Yi Li, and Ram C. Tiwari. A class of semiparametric mixture cure survival models with dependent censoring. *Journal of the American Statistical Association*, 104:1241–1250, 2009.

Megan Othus, Bart Barlogie, Michael L. LeBlanc, and John J. Crowley. Cure models as a useful statistical tool for analyzing survival. *Clinical Cancer Research*, 18(14):3731–3736, 2012.

Donald M. Parkin. The evolution of the population-based cancer registry. *Nature Reviews Cancer*, 6(8):603, 2006.

Y. Peng, J. M. G. Taylor, and B. Yu. A marginal regression model for multivariate failure time data with a surviving fraction. *Lifetime Data Analysis*, 13:351–369, 2007a.

Yingwei Peng. Estimating baseline distribution in proportional hazards cure models. *Computational Statistics & Data Analysis*, 42:187–201, 2003a.

Yingwei Peng. Fitting semiparametric cure models. *Computational Statistics & Data Analysis*, 41(3-4):481–490, 2003b.

Yingwei Peng and Keith B. G. Dear. A nonparametric mixture model for cure rate estimation. *Biometrics*, 56:237–243, 2000.

Yingwei Peng and Jeremy M. G. Taylor. Mixture cure model with random effects for the analysis of a multi-centre tonsil cancer study. *Statistics in Medicine*, 30:211–223, 2011.

Yingwei Peng and Jeremy M. G. Taylor. Cure models. In John Klein, Hans van Houwelingen, Joseph G. Ibrahim, and Thomas H. Scheike, editors, *Handbook of Survival Analysis*, Handbooks of Modern Statistical Methods series, chapter 6, pages 113–134. Chapman & Hall, Boca Raton, FL, USA, 2014.

Yingwei Peng and Jeremy M. G. Taylor. Residual-based model diagnosis methods for mixture cure models. *Biometrics*, 73:495–505, 2017.

Yingwei Peng and Jianfeng Xu. An extended cure model and model selection. *Lifetime Data Analysis*, 18:215–233, 2012.

Yingwei Peng and Jiajia Zhang. Estimation method of the semiparametric mixture cure gamma frailty model. *Statistics in Medicine*, 27:5177–5194, 2008a.

Yingwei Peng and Jiajia Zhang. Identifiability of mixture cure frailty model. *Statistics & Probability Letters*, 78:2604–2608, 2008b.

Yingwei Peng, Keith B. G. Dear, and J. W. Denham. A generalized F mixture model for cure rate estimation. *Statistics in Medicine*, 17:813–830, 1998.

Yingwei Peng, Keith B. G. Dear, and K. C. Carriere. Testing for the presence of cured patients: a simulation study. *Statistics in Medicine*, 20:1783–1796, 2001.

Yingwei Peng, Jeremy M. G. Taylor, and Binbing Yu. A marginal regression model for multivariate failure time data with a surviving fraction. *Lifetime Data Analysis*, 13:351–369, 2007b.

José C. Pinheiro, Chuanhai Liu, and Ying Nian Wu. Efficient algorithms for robust estimation in linear mixed-effects models using the multivariate t distribution. *Journal of Computational and Graphical Statistics*, 10(2): 249–276, 2001.

John Platt. Sequential minimal optimization: a fast algorithm for training support vector machines. 1998. URL `https://www.microsoft.com/en-us/research/wp-content/uploads/2016/02/tr-98-14.pdf`.

John Platt et al. Probabilistic outputs for support vector machines and comparisons to regularized likelihood methods. *Advances in large margin classifiers*, 10(3):61–74, 1999.

William H. Press, Saul A. Teukolsky, William T. Vetterling, and Brian P. Flannery. *Numerical Recipes in C: the Art of Scientific Computing*. Cambridge University Press, New York, 1992.

Dionne L. Price and Amita K. Manatunga. Modelling survival data with a cured fraction using frailty models. *Statistics in Medicine*, 20:1515–1527, 2001.

Matthew A. Psioda and Joseph G. Ibrahim. Bayesian design of a survival trial with a cured fraction using historical data. *Statistics in Medicine*, 37(26): 3814–3831, 2018.

Peihua Qiu and Jun Sheng. A two-stage procedure for comparing hazard rate functions. *Journal of the Royal Statistical Society: Series B (Statistical Methodology)*, 70(1):191–208, 2008.

Zhenguo Qiu, Peter X.-K. Song, and Ming Tan. Simplex mixed-effects models for longitudinal proportional data. *Scandinavian Journal of Statistics*, 35: 577–596, 2008.

R Core Team. *R: A Language and Environment for Statistical Computing*. R Foundation for Statistical Computing, Vienna, Austria, 2013. URL http://www.R-project.org/.

Mitra Rahimzadeh, Ebrahim Hajizadeh, and Farzad Eskandari. Non-mixture cure correlated frailty models in Bayesian approach. *Journal of Applied Statistics*, 38(8):1651–1663, 2010.

C. R. Rao. Score test: Historical review and recent developments. In N. Balakrishnan, N. Kannan, and H. N. Nagaraja, editors, *Advances in Ranking and Selection, Multiple Comparisons, and Reliability - Methodology and Applications*, Statistics for Industry and Technology, chapter 1, pages 3–20. Birkhäuser, Boston, USA, 2005.

Samuli Ripatti and Juni Palmgren. Estimation of multivariate frailty models using penalized partial likelihood. *Biometrics*, 56:1016–1022, 2000.

Y. Ritov. Estimation in a linear regression model with censored data. *Annals of Statistics*, 18:303–328, 1990.

Dimitris Rizopoulos. *Joint models for longitudinal and time-to-event data: With applications in R*. Chapman and Hall/CRC, 2012.

Virginie Rondeau, Emmanuel Schaffner, Fabien Corbière, Juan R. Gonzalez, and Simone Mathoulin-Pélissier. Cure frailty models for survival data: Application to recurrences for breast cancer and to hospital readmissions for colorectal cancer. *Statistical Methods in Medical Research*, 22(3):243–260, 2013.

Ori Rosen, Wenxin Jiang, and Martin A. Tanner. Mixtures of marginal models. *Biometrika*, 87:391–404, 2000.

SAS Institute Inc. *SAS/STAT® 9.3 User's Guide*. SAS Institute Inc., Cary, NC, USA, 2011.

Robin Schaffar, Bernard Rachet, Aurélien Belot, and Laura Woods. Cause-specific or relative survival setting to estimate population-based net survival from cancer? An empirical evaluation using women diagnosed with breast cancer in geneva between 1981 and 1991 and followed for 20 years after diagnosis. *Cancer Epidemiology*, 39(3):465–472, 2015.

Robin Schaffar, Bernard Rachet, Auralien Belot, and Laura M. Woods. Estimation of net survival for cancer patients: Relative survival setting more robust to some assumption violations than cause-specific setting, a sensitivity analysis on empirical data. *European Journal of Cancer*, 72:78–83, 2017.

Peter Schmidt and Ann Dryden Witte. Predicting criminal recidivism using 'split population' survival time models. *Journal of Econometrics*, 40(1): 141–159, 1989.

David Schoenfeld. The asymptotic properties of nonparametric tests for comparing survival distributions. *Biometrika*, 68(1):316–319, 1981.

Sylvie Scolas, Anouar El Ghouch, Catherine Legrand, and Abderrahim Oulhaj. Variable selection in a flexible parametric mixture cure model with interval-censored data. *Statistics in Medicine*, 35:1210–1225, 2016.

S. G. Self and K. Y. Liang. Asymptotic properties of maximum likelihood estimators and likelihood ratio tests under nonstandard conditions. *Journal of the American Statistical Association*, 82(398):605–610, 1987.

Karri Seppa, Timo Hakulinen, Hyon-Jung Kim, and Esa Laara. Cure fraction model with random effects for regional variation in cancer survival. *Statistics in Medicine*, 29(27):2781–2793, 2010.

Hua Shen and Richard J. Cook. A dynamic mover–stayer model for recurrent event processes subject to resolution. *Lifetime data analysis*, 20(3):404–423, 2014.

Jun Sheng, Peihua Qiu, and Charles J. Geyer. *TSHRC: Two Stage Hazard Rate Comparison*, 2017. URL `https://CRAN.R-project.org/package=TSHRC`. R package version 0.1-5.

Rebecca L. Siegel, Kimberly D. Miller, and Ahmedin Jemal. Cancer statistics, 2018. *CA: A Cancer Journal for Clinicians*, 68(1):7–30, 2018.

Jeffrey S. Simonoff. *Smoothing methods in statistics.* Springer Science & Business Media, 2012.

Tony Sit, Mengling Liu, Michael Shnaidman, and Zhiliang Ying. Design and analysis of clinical trials in the presence of delayed treatment effect. *Statistics in Medicine*, 35(11):1774–1779, 2016.

Steven Snapinn, Mon-Gy Chen, Qi Jiang, and Tony Koutsoukos. Assessment of futility in clinical trials. *Pharmaceutical Statistics*, 5(4):273–281, 2006.

Hui Song, Yingwei Peng, and Dongsheng Tu. A new approach for joint modeling of longitudinal measurements and survival times with a cure fraction. *Canadian Journal of Statistics*, 40:207–224, 2012.

Hui Song, Yingwei Peng, and Dongsheng Tu. Joint modeling of longitudinal proportional measurements and survival time with a cure fraction. *Science China - Mathematics*, 59(12):2427–2442, 2016a.

Hui Song, Yingwei Peng, and Dongsheng Tu. Recent development in the joint modeling of longitudinal quality of life measurements and survival data from cancer clinical trials. In Ding-Geng (Din) Chen, Jiahua Chen, Xuewen Lu, Grace Yi, and Hao Yu, editors, *Advanced Statistical Methods in Big-Data Sciences*, ICSA Book Series, chapter 8, pages 153–168. Springer, New York, NY, USA, 2016b.

P. X. K. Song and M. Tan. Marginal models for longitudinal continuous proportional data. *Biometrics*, 56:496–502, 2000.

Peter X. K. Song. *Correlated Data Analysis: Modeling, Analytics, and Applications*. Springer, New York, 2007.

Devon Spika, Finian Bannon, Audrey Bonaventure, Laura M. Woods, Rhea Harewood, Helena Carreira, Michel P. Coleman, and Claudia Allemani. Life tables for global surveillance of cancer survival (the concord programme): data sources and methods. *BMC Cancer*, 17(1):159, 2017.

R. Sposto, D. Stablein, and S. Carter-Campbell. A partially grouped logrank test. *Statistics in Medicine*, 16(6):695–704, 1997.

Sibylle Sturtz, Uwe Ligges, and Andrew E. Gelman. R2WinBUGS: a package for running WinBUGS from R. *Journal of Statistical Software*, 12:1–16, 2005.

Chien-Lin Su and Feng-Chang Lin. Analysis of clustered failure time data with cure fraction using copula. *Statistics in Medicine*, 38:3961–3973, 2019.

Zheng Su and Ming Zhu. Is it time for the weighted log-rank test to play a more important role in confirmatory trials? *Contemporary Clinical Trials Communications*, 10:A1, 2018.

Ryan Sun. *reconstructKM: Reconstruct individual-level data from KM plots published in academic journals*, 2019. R package version 0.1.0.

J. P. Sy and J. M. G. Taylor. Standard errors for the Cox proportional hazards cure model. *Mathematical and Computer Modelling*, 33:1237–1251, 2001.

Judy P. Sy and Jeremy M. G. Taylor. Estimation in a Cox proportional hazards cure model. *Biometrics*, 56:227–236, 2000.

R. Szydlo, J. M. Goldman, J. P. Klein, R. P. Gale, R. C. Ash, F. H. Bach, B. A. Bradley, J. T. Casper, N. Flomenberg, J. L. Gajewski, E. Gluckman, P. J. Henslee-Downey, J. M. Hows, N. Jacobsen, H. J. Kolb, B. Lowenberg, T. Masaoka, P. A. Rowlings, P. M. Sondel, D. W. van Bekkum, J. J. van Rood, M. R. Vowels, M. J. Zhang, and M. M. Horowitz. Results of allogeneic bone marrow transplants for leukemia using donors other than HLA-identical siblings. *Journal of Clinical Oncology*, 15(5):1767–1777, 1997.

Martin A. Tanner and Wing Hung Wong. The calculation of posterior distributions by data augmentation. *Journal of the American statistical Association*, 82(398):528–540, 1987.

Richard Tawiah, Geoffrey J. McLachlan, and Shu Kay Ng. Mixture cure models with time-varying and multilevel frailties for recurrent event data. *Statistical Methods in Medical Research*, 2019. In press.

J. M. G. Taylor. Semi-parametric estimation in failure time mixture models. *Biometrics*, 51:899–907, 1995.

Jeremy M. G. Taylor and Ning Liu. Statistical issues involved with extending standard models. In Vijay Nair, editor, *Advances in Statistical Modeling and Inference: Essays in Honor of Kjell a Doksum*, Series in Biostatistics, chapter 15, pages 299–311. World Scientific Publishing Company, 2007.

Terry M. Therneau and Patricia M. Grambsch. *Modeling Survival Data: Extending the Cox Model.* Springer, New York, 2000.

Andrew Thomas, Bob O'Hara, Uwe Ligges, and Sibylle Sturtz. Making BUGS open. *R News*, 6(1):12–17, 2006.

Laine Thomas and Eric M. Reyes. Tutorial: survival estimation for Cox regression models with time-varying coefficients using SAS and R. *Journal of Statistical Software*, 61(c1):1–23, 2014.

R. Tibshirani. Regression shrinkage and selection via the LASSO. *Journal of the Royal Statistical Society, Series B*, 58:267–288, 1996.

Edward N. C. Tong, Christophe Mues, and Lyn C. Thomas. Mixture cure models in credit scoring: If and when borrowers default. *European Journal of Operational Research*, 218(1):132–139, 2012.

Anastasios A. Tsiatis and Marie Davidian. Joint modelling of longitudinal and time-to-event data: an overview. *Statistica Sinica*, 14:809–834, 2004.

A. Tsodikov. Estimation of survival based on proportional hazards when cure is a possibility. *Mathematical and Computer Modelling*, 33:1227–1236, 2001.

A. Tsodikov. Semi-parametric models of long- and short-term survival: an application to the analysis of breast cancer survival in Utah by age and stage. *Statistics in Medicine*, 20:895–920, 2002.

A. Tsodikov. Semiparametric models: a generalized self-consistency approach. *Journal of the Royal Statistical Society, Series B*, 65:759–774, 2003.

A. D. Tsodikov, J. G. Ibrahim, and A. Y. Yakovlev. Estimating cure rates from survival data: an alternative to two-component mixture models. *Journal of the American Statistical Association*, 98(464):1063–1078, 2003.

Alexander Tsodikov. Asymptotic efficiency of a proportional hazards model with cure. *Statistics & Probability Letters*, 39:237–244, 1998a.

Alexander Tsodikov. A proportional hazards model taking account of long-term survivors. *Biometrics*, 54:1508–1516, 1998b.

Alexander Tsodikov, M. Loeffler, and A. Yakovlev. A cure model with time-changing risk factor: an application to the analysis of secondary leukemia. *Statistics in Medicine*, 17:27–40, 1998.

S. L. Tucker and J. M. G. Taylor. Improved models of tumour cure. *International Journal of Radiation Biology*, 70:539–553, 1996.

Geert Verbeke and Geert Molenberghs. *Linear Mixed Models for Longitudinal Data.* Springer Science & Business Media, 2009.

H. T. V. Vu, R. A. Maller, and X. Zhou. Asymptotic properties of a class of mixture models for failure data: the interior and boundary cases. *Annals of the Institute of Statistical Mathematics*, 50:627–653, 1998.

Xiaomin Wan, Liubao Peng, and Yuanjian Li. A review and comparison of methods for recreating individual patient data from published Kaplan-Meier survival curves for economic evaluations: a simulation study. *PLOS One*, 10(3):e0121353, 2015.

Lu Wang, Pang Du, and Hua Liang. Two-component mixture cure rate model with spline estimated nonparametric components. *Biometrics*, 68:726-735, 2012a.

Songfeng Wang, Jiajia Zhang, and Wenbin Lu. Sample size calculation for the proportional hazards cure model. *Statistics in Medicine*, 31(29):3959–3971, 2012b.

G. S. Watson. Smooth regression analysis. *Sankhya: The Indian Journal of Statistics, Series A*, 26:359–372, 1964.

A. Wienke, S. Ripatti, J. Palmgren, and A. Yashin. A bivariate survival model with compound Poisson frailty. *Statistics in Medicine*, 29(2):275–283, 2010.

Andreas Wienke, Paul Lichtenstein, and Anatoli I. Yashin. A bivariate frailty model with a cure fraction for modeling familial correlation in disease. *Biometrics*, 59:1178–1183, 2003.

E. Paul Wileyto, Yimei Li, Jinbo Chen, and Daniel F. Heitjan. Assessing the fit of parametric cure models. *Biostatistics*, 14:340–350, 2013.

Jedd D. Wolchok, Vanna Chiarion-Sileni, Rene Gonzalez, Piotr Rutkowski, Jean-Jacques Grob, C. Lance Cowey, Christopher D. Lao, John Wagstaff, Dirk Schadendorf, Pier F. Ferrucci, et al. Overall survival with combined nivolumab and ipilimumab in advanced melanoma. *New England Journal of Medicine*, 377(14):1345–1356, 2017.

R.F. Woolson. Rank tests and a one-sample log rank test for comparing observed survival data to a standard population. *Biometrics*, 37:687–696, 1981.

Jianrong Wu. *Statistical Methods for Survival Trial Design: With Applications to Cancer Clinical Trials Using R*. CRC Press, 2018.

Yu Wu, Yong Lin, Shou-En Lu, Chin-Shang Li, and Weichung Joe Shih. Extension of a Cox proportional hazards cure model when cure information is partially known. *Biostatistics*, 15(3):540–554, 2014.

Yuanshan Wu and Guosheng Yin. Cure rate quantile regression for censored data with a survival fraction. *Journal of the American Statistical Association*, 108:1517–1531, 2013.

Yuanshan Wu and Guosheng Yin. Multiple imputation for cure rate quantile regression with censored data. *Biometrics*, 73(1):94–103, 2017a.

Yuanshan Wu and Guosheng Yin. Cure rate quantile regression accommodating both finite and infinite survival times. *Canadian Journal of Statistics*, 45(1):29–43, 2017b.

Michael S. Wulfsohn and Anastasios A. Tsiatis. A joint model for survival and longitudinal data measured with error. *Biometrics*, 53:330–339, 1997.

Xiaoping Xiong and Jianrong Wu. A novel sample size formula for the weighted log-rank test under the proportional hazards cure model. *Pharmaceutical Statistics*, 16(1):87–94, 2017.

Jianfeng Xu and Yingwei Peng. Nonparametric cure rate estimation with covariates. *Canadian Journal of Statistics*, 42:1–17, 2014.

Linzhi Xu and Jiajia Zhang. Multiple imputation method for the semiparametric accelerated failure time mixture cure model. *Computational Statistics & Data Analysis*, 54(7):1808–1816, 2010.

Zhenzhen Xu, Boguang Zhen, Yongsoek Park, and Bin Zhu. Designing therapeutic cancer vaccine trials with delayed treatment effect. *Statistics in Medicine*, 36(4):592–605, 2017.

A. Y. Yakovlev, B. Asselain, V. J. Bardou, A. Fourquet, T. Hoang, A. Rochefediere, and A. D. Tsodikov. A simple stochastic model of tumor recurrence and its application to data on premenopausal breast cancer. In B. Asselain, C. Boniface, C. Duby, C. Lopez, J. P. Masson, and J. Tranchefort, editors, *Biometrie et Analyse de Dormees Spatio-Temporelles*, volume 12, pages 66–82. Société Francaise de Biométrie, ENSA Renned, France. C, 1994a.

A. Y. Yakovlev, A. D. Tsodikov, and B. Asselain. *Stochastic Models of Tumor Latency and Their Biostatistical Applications*, volume 1 of *Mathematical Biology and Medicine*. World Scientific, Singapore, 1996.

Andrej Yu Yakovlev, Alan B. Cantor, and Jonathan J. Shuster. Letters to the editor: parametric versus non-parametric methods for estimating cure rates based on censored survival data. *Statistics in Medicine*, 13(9):983–986, 1994b.

K. Yamaguchi. Accelerated failure-time regression models with a regression model of surviving fraction: an application to the analysis of 'permanent employment' in Japan. *Journal of the American Statistical Association*, 87 (418):284–292, 1992.

Kazuo Yamaguchi. Accelerated failure-time Mover-Stayer regression models for the analysis of last-episode data. *Sociological Methodology*, 33(1):81–110, 2003.

Song Yang and Ross Prentice. Semiparametric analysis of short-term and long-term hazard ratios with two-sample survival data. *Biometrika*, 92(1): 1–17, 2005.

Song Yang and Ross Prentice. Improved logrank-type tests for survival data using adaptive weights. *Biometrics*, 66(1):30–38, 2009.

Kelvin K. W. Yau and Angus S. K. Ng. Long-term survivor mixture model with random effects: application to a multi-centre clinical trial of carcinoma. *Statistics in Medicine*, 20(11):1591–1607, 2001.

W. Ye, X. H. Lin, and J. M. G. Taylor. A penalized likelihood approach to joint modeling of longitudinal measurements and time-to-event data. *Statistics and Interface*, 1:33–45, 2008.

Yildiz E. Yilmaz, Jerald F. Lawless, Irene L. Andrulis, and Shelley B. Bull. Insights from mixture cure modeling of molecular markers for prognosis in breast cancer. *Journal of Clinical Oncology*, 31:2047–2054, 2013.

Guosheng Yin. Bayesian cure rate frailty models with application to a root canal therapy study. *Biometrics*, 61:552–558, 2005.

Guosheng Yin. Bayesian transformation cure frailty models with multivariate failure time data. *Statistics in Medicine*, 27:5929–5940, 2008.

Guosheng Yin and Joseph G. Ibrahim. Cure rate models: a unified approach. *The Canadian Journal of Statistics*, 33:559–570, 2005a.

Guosheng Yin and Joseph G. Ibrahim. A general class of Bayesian survival models with zero and nonzero cure fractions. *Biometrics*, 61:403–412, 2005b.

G.-S. Ying, D.F. Heitjan, and T.-T. Chen. Nonparametric prediction of event times in randomized clinical trials. *Clinical Trials*, 1(4):352–361, 2004.

Gui-shuang Ying and Daniel F. Heitjan. Weibull prediction of event times in clinical trials. *Pharmaceutical Statistics*, 7(2):107–120, 2008.

Gui-shuang Ying, Qiang Zhang, Yu Lan, Yimei Li, and Daniel F. Heitjan. Cure modeling in real-time prediction: How much does it help? *Contemporary Clinical Trials*, 59:30–37, 2017.

Binbing Yu. A frailty mixture cure model with application to hospital readmission cata. *Biometrical Journal: Journal of Mathematical Methods in Biosciences*, 50(3):386–394, 2008.

Binbing Yu. A minimum version of log-rank test for testing the existence of cancer cure using relative survival data. *Biometrical Journal*, 54(1):45–60, 2012.

Binbing Yu and Yingwei Peng. Mixture cure models for multivariate survival data. *Computational Statistics & Data Analysis*, 52:1524–1532, 2008.

Binbing Yu and Ram C. Tiwari. A Bayesian approach to mixture cure models with spatial frailties for population-based cancer relative survival data. *Canadian Journal of Statistics*, 40(1):40–54, 2012.

Binbing Yu, Ram C. Tiwari, Kathleen A. Cronin, and Eric J. Feuer. Cure fraction estimation from the mixture cure models for grouped survival data. *Statistics in Medicine*, 23(11):1733–1747, 2004a.

Binbing Yu, Ram C. Tiwari, Kathleen A. Cronin, Chris McDonald, and Eric J. Feuer. CANSURV: a windows program for population-based cancer survival analysis. *Computer Methods and Programs in Biomedicine*, 80(3):195–203, 2005.

Menggang Yu, Ngayee J. Law, Jeremy M. G. Taylor, and Howard M. Sandler. Joint longitudinal-survival-cure models and their application to prostate cancer. *Statistica Sinica*, 14:835–862, 2004b.

Menggang Yu, Jeremy M. G. Taylor, and Howard M. Sandler. Individual prediction in prostate cancer studies using a joint longitudinal survival-cure model. *Journal of the American Statistical Association*, 103:178–187, 2008.

Huibin Yue and K. S. Chan. A dynamic frailty model for multivariate survival data. *Biometrics*, 53:785–793, 1997.

Donglin Zeng and Jianwen Cai. Simultaneous modelling of survival and longitudinal data with an application to repeated quality of life measures. *Lifetime Data Analysis*, 11:151–174, 2005.

Donglin Zeng and D. Y. Lin. Efficient estimation for the accelerated failure time model. *Journal of the American Statistical Association*, 102:1387–1396, 2007.

Donglin Zeng, Guosheng Yin, and Joseph G. Ibrahim. Semiparametric transformation models for survival data with a cure fraction. *Journal of the American Statistical Association*, 101:670–684, 2006.

Jiajia Zhang and Yingwei Peng. A new estimation method for the semiparametric accelerated failure time mixture cure model. *Statistics in Medicine*, 26:3157–3171, 2007.

Jiajia Zhang and Yingwei Peng. Accelerated hazards mixture cure model. *Lifetime Data Analysis*, 15:455–467, 2009a.

Jiajia Zhang and Yingwei Peng. Crossing hazard functions in common survival models. *Statistics & Probability Letters*, 79:2124–2130, 2009b.

Jiajia Zhang and Yingwei Peng. Semiparametric estimation methods for the accelerated failure time mixture cure model. *Journal of the Korean Statistical Society*, 41:415–422, 2012.

Jiajia Zhang, Yingwei Peng, and Haifen Li. A new semiparametric estimation method for accelerated hazards mixture cure model. *Computational Statistics & Data Analysis*, 59:95–102, 2013.

Xiaoxi Zhang and Qi Long. Modeling and prediction of subject accrual and event times in clinical trials: a systematic review. *Clinical Trials*, 9(6): 681–688, 2012.

Yilong Zhang and Yongzhao Shao. Concordance measure and discriminatory accuracy in transformation cure models. *Biostatistics*, 19(1):14–26, 2017.

Yun Zhao, Andy H. Lee, Kelvin KW Yau, Valerie Burke, and Geoffrey J. McLachlan. A score test for assessing the cured proportion in the long-term survivor mixture model. *Statistics in Medicine*, 28(27):3454–3466, 2009.

S. Zhou and R. A. Maller. The likelihood ratio test for the presence of immunes in a censored sample. *Statistics*, 27:181–201, 1995.

Index

Printed in the United States
By Bookmasters